Principles
Equine
Dentistry

David O Klugh

DVM, FAVD/Equine

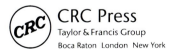

CRC Press
Taylor & Francis Group
Boca Raton London New York

CRC Press is an imprint of the
Taylor & Francis Group, an **informa** business

David O Klugh
DVM, FAVD/Equine

Victor S Cox
DVM, PhD

Jane Quandt
DVM, MS, DACVA

Michael Lowder
DVM, MS

Henry Tremaine
B.Vet Med, M Phil, Cert
ES, Dip ECVS, MRCVS

Randi D Brannan
DVM, FAVD, Dip AVDC

Peter Emily
DDS, Hon

Robert B Wiggs
DVM, Dip AVDC

CRC Press
Taylor & Francis Group
6000 Broken Sound Parkway NW, Suite 300
Boca Raton, FL 33487-2742

© 2010 by Taylor & Francis Group, LLC
CRC Press is an imprint of Taylor & Francis Group, an Informa business

No claim to original U.S. Government works

Printed on acid-free paper
Version Date: 20160224

International Standard Book Number-13: 978-1-84076-114-6 (Hardback)

This book contains information obtained from authentic and highly regarded sources. While all reasonable efforts have been made to publish reliable data and information, neither the author[s] nor the publisher can accept any legal responsibility or liability for any errors or omissions that may be made. The publishers wish to make clear that any views or opinions expressed in this book by individual editors, authors or contributors are personal to them and do not necessarily reflect the views/opinions of the publishers. The information or guidance contained in this book is intended for use by medical, scientific or health-care professionals and is provided strictly as a supplement to the medical or other professional's own judgement, their knowledge of the patient's medical history, relevant manufacturer's instructions and the appropriate best practice guidelines. Because of the rapid advances in medical science, any information or advice on dosages, procedures or diagnoses should be independently verified. The reader is strongly urged to consult the relevant national drug formulary and the drug companies' and device or material manufacturers' printed instructions, and their websites, before administering or utilizing any of the drugs, devices or materials mentioned in this book. This book does not indicate whether a particular treatment is appropriate or suitable for a particular individual. Ultimately it is the sole responsibility of the medical professional to make his or her own professional judgements, so as to advise and treat patients appropriately. The authors and publishers have also attempted to trace the copyright holders of all material reproduced in this publication and apologize to copyright holders if permission to publish in this form has not been obtained. If any copyright material has not been acknowledged please write and let us know so we may rectify in any future reprint.

Visit the Taylor & Francis Web site at
http://www.taylorandfrancis.com

and the CRC Press Web site at
http://www.crcpress.com

CONTENTS

Many have influenced the production of this book. First, I'd like to thank my contributors. I know they have worked long and hard to produce their chapters, and their expertise is much appreciated. To Dr. Randi Brannan, I give my eternal gratitude for her guidance, motivation, her commitment to excellence, her brilliance, and her friendship. To say that without her this would have been impossible is perhaps the greatest understatement in the entire book! To Tony Basil, I want to express my appreciation for sharing a new vision of the world of equine dentistry. To all who have gone before me, especially Drs. Baker, Easley, and Dixon, who served as sounding boards, advisors, and to a significant degree, as trailblazers in the modern world of equine dentistry. There are many others in this category. Names like Becker, Little, Merrilatt, Moriarity, and Jeffrey brought new information to light and left their mark on equine dentistry.

A special thanks to my good friend, Ian Dacre, whose wisdom has been and continues to be gleaned from many late evening discussions of the ideas related in this book prior to its publication. His advice has always been honest. Though we may have disagreed here or there (I think!) he has always kept me focused on accuracy and completeness. Cheers, mate!

Special thanks to Scott Greene, whose energy and innovative mind is well respected and appreciated more than he knows by many in the field of equine dentistry.

Drs. Scott Hansen and Lisa Campbell and the rest of the veterinarians and staff at Columbia Equine Hospital, I thank you for your support. Without it I would have fewer cases from which to learn.

Thanks to all the veterinarians who have referred cases. They have added significantly to the body of knowledge related in these pages.

Last, and certainly importantly, I'd like to thank Beth. Though our paths have diverged, I must express my heartfelt appreciation for your patience and support. To our children, Kacy and Dean, thank you and I love you both more than you know.

David O Klugh

ABBREVIATIONS

AMP	adenosine monophosphate	IM	intramuscularly
bis-GMA	bis-phenol-A glycidyl methacrylate	IV	intravenously
BMP	bone morphogenetic protein	kVp	kilovolt peak
COPD	chronic obstructive pulmonary disease	mAs	milliampere-seconds
		MRI	magnetic resonance imaging
CR	computed radiography	MTA	mineral trioxide aggregate
CRI	constant rate infusion	NMDA	n-methyl-D-asparatate
CT	computed tomography	NSAID	nonsteroidal anti-inflammatory drug
DR	digital radiography	NVPE	nonvital pulp exposure
ECG	electrocardiograph	PaO$_2$	oxygen partial pressure
EDTA	ethylenediaminetetracetic acid	PCO	pulp canal obliteration
FFD	film focal distance	PCV	packed cell volume
FGF	fibroblast growth factor	PDL	periodontal ligament
GABA	gamma-aminobutyric acid	PG	prostaglandin
GCF	gingival crevicular fluid	POC	point of occlusal contact
GI	gastrointestinal	TEGDMA	triethylene glycol dimethacrylate
GIC	glass ionomer cement	TP	total protein
HEMA	hydroxyethyl methacrylate	UDMA	urethane dimethacrylate

When horses functioned as the primary means of draft and transportation, equine dentistry was a very important part of veterinary medicine. This is evidenced by books dedicated to the subject, for example Merillat's book, Veterinary Surgery, Volume 1: *Animal Dentistry and Diseases of the Mouth* published in 1906. Much early literature was based on observation, categorization, and comparison. Examples include dental aging papers that date back to Girard in 1834, Simonds in 1854, and the most famous of all, Galvayne in 1886. Comparative pathology was done brilliantly by Colyer in 1936.

The process of observation, categorization, and comparison might be thought of as classification and is a method common in all branches of science, medicine, veterinary medicine, and dentistry. The next stage is in-depth analysis of physiological and pathological processes and a closer look at anatomy, including histology. The early literature on periodontal disease by Little, Colyer, and Voss falls into this category. Even Aristotle made observations of periodontal disease in equines well before his time!

After the introduction of motorized vehicles, equine dentistry took a back seat to food animal disease. Veterinarians were dealing with infectious diseases that affected food animal production such as hog cholera and foot and mouth disease. Horses were affected by some of these same diseases. However, the growing world population needed to be fed, and veterinarians focused principally on that problem.

At this time veterinarians such as Becker made advanced innovations in instrumentation as well as beginning the next stage of scientific advancement, that is, the application to the equine patient of concepts developed in dentistry of other species. Becker's motorized instruments are still envied by equine dental practitioners today. The many dental impressions he took were examples of application of human dental principles and materials to the equine patient.

After World War II, many parts of the world, especially the US, engaged in economic progress and a financial boom occurred. The result was acquisition of disposable income and equine medicine regained its importance. Evidence of this fact is the formation of the American Association of Equine Practitioners in 1954. People had money to spend on performing horses, and equestrian vocations were either born anew, or expanded significantly.

Equine veterinarians were busy keeping these performers sound and able to do their jobs. While areas of lameness, reproduction, and surgery were rapidly developing, dentistry remained less important, and advancement stagnated. As time went on, a handful of individuals recognized the need for dental care in performing horses and proceeded to fill that niche. Jeffrey, Moriarity, and others who were not veterinarians revived and advanced equine dentistry, with an eye towards bitting comfort.

The stages of advancement overlapped. The second stage of in-depth investigation continued in the 1970s as Baker presented his landmark works. Continuing to current times and knowledge, Dixon and his group, including Kilic and Dacre, made significant contributions with descriptions of dental histology and comparison of normal teeth to diseased teeth. This trend continues in this group today with du Toit's current efforts. They have exponentially advanced knowledge of tooth structure and function.

Continuing to advance the third step in scientific advancement, which we will call cross-species application of dental principles, Dr. Peter Emily pioneered application of human dental principles to all veterinary patients, including the horse. Easley and others have continued the process especially in the area of endodontics, where Easley and Emily collaborated on many surgical endodontic cases.

This book identifies principles found in the world of general dentistry and applies them to the equine species. Since the vast majority of knowledge is based on, and especially the body of literature is comprised of principles of brachydont (human and small animal) dentistry, those principles need to be learned and evaluated in relation to the hypsodont (equine) patient. Their study leads to an understanding of equine dentistry that in many cases fits equine problems, their pathogenesis, evaluation, diagnosis, treatment, and prognosis quite well. When a system, for example, of evaluating the stages of periodontal disease has been well established in brachydont dentistry, it seems to the editor that such an application should be measured in the equine species and its fitness determined. There is no reason to ignore such a system just because it has never before been used in the equine patient. Such a system actually works very well and provides three major benefits: it provides a vocabulary with which equine dental practitioners can communicate with those in the brachydont world; it nullifies the need to 'start from scratch' in staging equine periodontal disease; and it provides a baseline for understanding the disease process itself.

There are many situations where brachydont principles cross species lines. Some are not intuitively obvious, others are. Additionally, many principles that one would assume to cross from brachydont to hypsodont, in fact, do not do so. It is the purpose of this book to identify dental principles, measure them in clinical equine cases, and evaluate the results.

Ideas and principles held dear today become fodder for late night chuckles tomorrow. Other concepts disregarded today become facts of tomorrow. As with all other fields, dentistry continues to evolve. It is hoped that the reader will consider with an open mind the principles of dentistry related to equine patients as discussed in these pages, and continue the process of bringing the larger world of dentistry into that of the equine patient.

EVOLUTION OF THE HYPSODONT TOOTH

David O Klugh   Chapter 1

Equine teeth are described as hypsodont, which is defined as a long-crowned, continuously erupting tooth.[1] The reserve crown is held within the alveolar bone. Equine teeth are further described as *radicular hypsodont*. These teeth have true roots that elongate over the life of the tooth and apices that eventually close. Once the crown is formed within the alveolus, further extension of the tooth's overall length is confined to growth of the root.

By contrast, the teeth of dogs, cats, and man are *brachydont*. These teeth are short-crowned teeth that erupt to occlusal level and stop. Major differences exist between brachydont and hypsodont teeth in the arrangement of the enamel, dentin, and cementum. In brachydont teeth these dental tissues are arranged in layers, with the occlusal crown completely covered by enamel. The root is covered by cementum. The inner part of the tooth is composed of dentin surrounding the pulp (**1**).

The occlusal surface of the hypsodont tooth is composed of the same structures, enamel, dentin, and cementum. Their arrangement is more 'scroll-like' and not in layers. The enamel is arranged in folds, with the dentin contained in the internal parts of the folds adjacent to the pulp and the cementum on the outer surface of the tooth near the alveolar bone. The exceptions are the incisors and the upper cheek teeth. These teeth have an infolding of the peripheral enamel known as the *infundibulum*. This structure is filled variably with cementum. The incisors have one infundibulum each, while the upper cheek teeth have two such infoldings (**2**).

The fossil record of the development of the hypsodont tooth represents adaptation of the needs of the animal to the local environment. Over the millennia, the horse adapted to changes in feeds available, beginning as a foraging animal and gradually changing to the modern grazing creature. The overall form of the animal changed from a small foraging *Hyracotherium* living among forests and consuming leaves and other succulent plants, to the grassland inhabitant. The later animal had longer

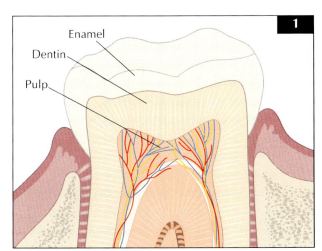

1 A sagittal section of a brachydont tooth shows pulp, dentin, and enamel.

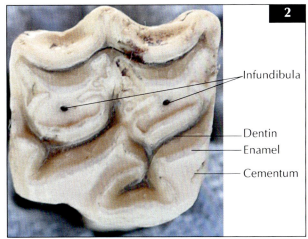

2 The occlusal surface of the hypsodont maxillary cheek teeth shows enamel, dentin, cementum, and two infundibula.

facial structure with eyes set far behind the nose for the purpose of visualizing predators and maintaining herd contact while grazing. The changes in tooth structure mirror the changes in feeding needs that occurred with the transition from forest to grassland environment.

Representation of the development process of *Equus caballus* as a straight line evolutionary process is fallacious. Multiple species of prehistoric horse-like fossils have been found in the same rock strata, indicating co-existence.[2] Many species variations co-existed, with variations in number of toes, ribs, and with differing conformation of teeth. It is instructive to understand the extreme length of time involved in creating a timeline of the fossil record seen in *Table 1*.

This discussion will be limited to the changes that have occurred over millennia in the form and function of teeth of the horse.[3] The earliest fossil records are those of *Eohippus*, also known as *Hyracotherium*, who inhabited much of North America in the Eocene epoch. This 25–50 cm tall (at the shoulder) forest dweller consumed succulent leaves, fruits, vines, and twigs, making it a foraging browser (see figure **3**). Its teeth were short-crowned, or brachydont (**4**). The dental formula contained three incisors, one canine, four premolars, and three molars.

Orohippus, about the same size as *Hyracotherium*, also lived in the Eocene epoch. The major difference was the change in the conformation of the last premolar to be similar in shape to the molars seen in figure **5**. This change is thought to be an adaptation to consumption of some grasses in addition to the browsing diet.

Also in the Eocene epoch, though fossils are generally found in the middle part of this time period, *Epihippus* (**6**) developed molarization of the last two premolars. *Epihippus* was still brachydont, but now had five grinding teeth.

Approximately 40 million years ago, in the late Eocene period, *Mesohippus* appeared on the scene. This animal was about 60 cm tall at the shoulder. The last three premolars were molarized, though *Mesohippus* remained brachydont (**7**). The first premolar remained functional.

Parahippus fossils have been found to date to 23 million years ago, placing it in the Miocene period. Significant dental changes include the presence of a second set of crests or cusps on the lingual or palatal side of the teeth. These crests or cusps merged to form a single crescent or ridge. Still brachydont, these teeth seen in figure **8** were somewhat longer than previously dated fossils.

A major change in dental conformation is seen in the fossil record of *Merychippus*, whose teeth (seen in figure **9**) became the first true hypsodont, with long crowns and cementum surrounding the entire tooth.

Table 1 The enormous length of time included in the fossil record

Prehistoric timeline

Recent 10,000 years ago to present	
Pleistocene	2.5 million years ago (mya) to 10,000 years ago
Pliocene	5.3 mya to 2.5 mya
Miocene	24 mya to 5.3 mya
Oligocene	34 mya to 24 mya
Eocene	54 mya to 34 mya

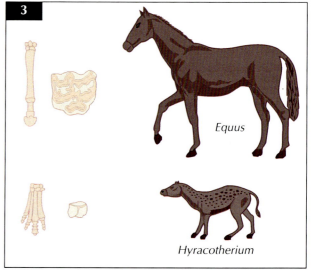

3 Comparison of size of *Hyracotherium* to modern day *Equus caballus*.

These fossils date to the mid-Miocene period. The size of *Merychippus* increased to about that of a small pony. The facial length increased, and their legs lengthened to provide for fast escape from predators.

The first *Equus* fossils (**10**) have been found to date back to about 4 million years ago, in the Pleistocene epoch. They were about the size of ponies, with six molarized cheek teeth and one remnant of a premolar, known later as the wolf tooth.

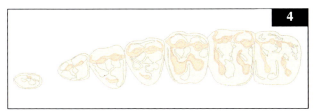

4 The actual size of maxillary cheek teeth, showing short-crowned or brachydont form. Premolars are simpler, having a single palatal cusp, and smaller than molars. (From Matthew and Chubb.[3])

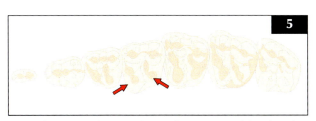

5 *Orohippus* is known for molarization of the fourth premolar. Note the paired cusps on the fourth premolar (arrows). These teeth remain brachydont. (From Matthew and Chubb. (actual size).[3])

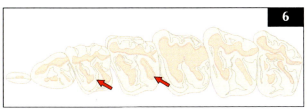

6 *Epihippus* developed molarization, or paired cusps of the palatal occlusal surface of the last two premolars (arrows). ((From Matthew and Chubb. (actual size).[3])

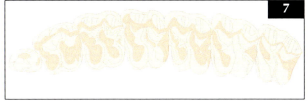

7 *Mesohippus* became slightly larger and finished the process of molarization of the last three premolars. (From Matthew and Chubb. (actual size).[3])

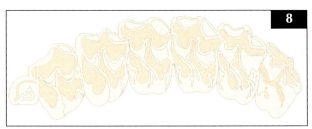

8 *Parahippus* is significant for the increased size of cusps on the occlusal surface that merge into crests. (From Matthew and Chubb. (actual size).[3])

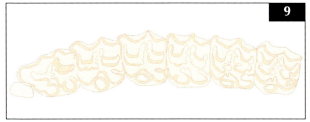

9 *Merychippus* is the first hypsodont in the evolutionary line of horses. (From Matthew and Chubb. (actual size).[3])

10 *Equus* dentition from late Pleistocene shows actual size of premolars only. (From Matthew and Chubb. (actual size).[3])

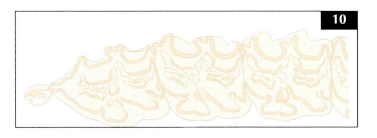

These grazing animals were one-toed grazers from which we have the modern horses, donkeys, asses, zebras, and the onager, a wild ass in Asia and northern Africa.

In summary, it must be kept in mind that horse evolution is not a straight line process. Multiple species co-existed and many species developed suddenly, with no obvious predecessor. Fossils of the Miocene period have the greatest diversity, with numerous species co-existing. Modern *Equus* species fossils are found first in the Pleistocene epoch.

Significant changes from *Hyracotherium* occurred with the first molarization of premolars of *Orohippus*; molarization into six similarly conformed cheek teeth in *Mesohippus*; and development of hypsodont form in *Merychippus*.

REFERENCES

1. Wiggs RB, Lobprise HB. Dental and oral radiology. In: Wiggs RB, Lobprise HB (eds) *Veterinary Dentistry: Principles and Practice*. Philadelphia: Lippincott-Raven, 1997; p. 57.
2. Simpson GG. *Horses: The Story of the Horse Family in the Modern World and Through Sixty Million Years of History*. New York: Anchor Doubleday and the American Museum of Natural History, 1961; pp. 105–116.
3. Matthew WD, Chubb SH. *Evolution of the Horse*, 4th edition. New York: American Museum of Natural History, 1921; pp. 14–23.

DENTAL EXAMINATION

David O Klugh — Chapter 2

The attending veterinarian has primary responsibility for the patient as a whole. Efficient, thorough examination of the patient's general condition, history, and dental anatomy elicits information that may apply to resolution of the presenting problem or may be important in medical management of the patient. It may apply to choice of sedative or other medications. The information gathered may be so significant as to preclude delivery of dental care until other issues are resolved. Specific problems should be prioritized and treatment staged if necessary. Sleuthing problem details and making treatment decisions are, chief responsibilities of the primary care veterinarian.

At the same time, it is important to be efficient in the performance of diagnostic and treatment procedures. Time management is an important part of veterinary practice. Techniques should be developed and practiced that rapidly elicit critical information. Efficient examination procedures also have the benefit of maximizing sedative time for the performance of dental procedures. Efficient yet thorough technique also maximizes safety for all involved, including the patient.

HISTORY AND PRESENTATION

The attending veterinarian usually knows the presenting problem prior to, or shortly after, initial patient contact. Further historical data should be gathered prior to examination. The following is a list of points to elicit in a patient history and the relevance of these points to dental problems:

- **Presenting problem:** the reason for presentation may be routine or may be for a specific concern.
- **Relevant information about the onset, severity, and duration of the problem:** a sudden onset of a problem in a young horse might suggest a retained deciduous tooth, while in an older horse it might suggest periodontal disease or a loose tooth.

- **Other medical problems:** these may impact on patient care or may require resolution prior to delivery of dental care.
- **Other bitting, chewing, or behavioral problems:** these may provide information that gives insight to the origins of the presenting problem. Early recognition of a problem may lead to earlier, less drastic intervention.
- **Previous dental care:** knowledge of previous problems may assist in efficient delivery of services in the current instance, since specific instrumentation can be prepared prior to sedation.
- **Patient's purpose:** breeding, pleasure, performance, or retired. In performance horses, bitting comfort is of critical importance. Every effort should be made to ensure patient comfort during and after the procedure.
- **Diet:** specific changes may be required.
- **Amount of time on pasture:** pasture time may require adjustment. This is very important in correlation with severity of malocclusion present.
- **Turnout time:** greater or less than 6 months out of each year. Also related to severity of malocclusion.

PRELIMINARY PHYSICAL EXAMINATION

When first observing the patient, the general disposition and willingness of the patient to accept strangers and nonroutine procedures is determined. Safety should be kept in the front of the mind of the attending veterinarian at all times, since the veterinarian's liability for injury includes all parties in close proximity. Potential safety concerns are noted and methods instituted for prevention of injury. In some instances it may be appropriate for the owner to handle the patient, while in others a well trained veterinary assistant is best suited. Once the veterinarian has a sense for the safety of the patient, its surroundings, and handlers, the physical examination can continue.

The following are examples of examination parameters noted and entered in medical records:

- **Body condition score:** using the Henneke System of 1 through 9[1] (see *Table 2*).
- **Disposition:** quiet, alert, anxious, fearful.
- **Attitude:** bright and alert, depressed.
- **Appetite:** normal, depressed.
- **Mucous membranes:** moist, dry.
- **Mucous membrane color:** pink, pale.
- **Capillary refill time:** 1–2 s, <1 s, >2 s.
- **Hydration status:** normal, dehydrated.
- **Stool:** normal, loose, dry.
- **Hair coat:** good, fair, poor.
- **Chest auscultation:** clear, dry, moist, wheezes.
- **Respiratory rate.**
- **Heart rate.**
- **Temperature.**
- **Heart rhythm.**
- **Point of occlusal contact:** ½, ⅔, ¾, ⅞ (see Chapter 6 for more discussion of mastication biomechanics).
- **Bars:** normal, exostosis.
- **Lingual mucosa:** normal, laceration.
- **Buccal mucosa:** normal, callused, laceration.

EXAMINATION INSTRUMENTATION

After the patient is sedated, it is evaluated for dental problems. In order to do this, certain instrumentation and equipment are needed to provide the veterinarian with a safe opportunity to perform a thorough yet efficient dental examination. Many devices exist for support of the head, including various head stands. The author's preference is a padded head ring which allows support of the mandible while maintaining flexion of the poll. This device, shown in

Table 2 Henneke body condition scoring chart

1 – Poor:	Emaciated. Prominent spinous processes, ribs, tailhead, and hooks and pins. Noticeable bone structure on withers, shoulders, and neck. No fatty tissues can be palpated.
2 – Very thin:	Emaciated. Slight fat covering over base of spinous processes. Transverse processes of lumbar vertebrae feel rounded. Prominent spinous processes, ribs, tailhead, and hooks and pins. Withers, shoulders, and neck structures faintly discernible.
3 – Thin:	Fat built up about halfway on spinous processes, transverse processes cannot be felt. Slight fat cover over ribs. Spinous processes and ribs easily discernible. Tailhead prominent, but individual vertebrae cannot be visually identified. Hook bones appear rounded, but easily discernible. Pin bones not distinguishable. Withers, shoulders, and neck accentuated.
4 – Moderately thin:	Negative crease along back. Faint outline of ribs discernible. Tailhead prominence depends on conformation, fat can be felt around it. Hook bones not discernible. Withers, shoulders, and neck not obviously thin.
5 – Moderate:	Back is level. Ribs cannot be visually distinguished, but can be easily felt. Fat around tailhead beginning to feel spongy. Withers appear rounded over spinous processes. Shoulders and neck blend smoothly into body.
6 – Moderate to fleshy:	May have slight crease down back. Fat over ribs feels spongy. Fat around tailhead feels soft. Fat beginning to be deposited along the sides of the withers, behind the shoulders, and along the sides of the neck.
7 – Fleshy:	May have crease down back. Individual ribs can be felt, but noticeable filling between ribs with fat. Fat around tailhead is soft. Fat deposits along withers, behind shoulders and along the neck.
8 – Fat:	Crease down back. Difficult to palpate ribs. Fat around tailhead very soft. Area along withers filled with fat. Area behind shoulder filled in flush. Noticeable thickening of neck. Fat deposited along inner buttocks.
9 – Extremely fat:	Obvious crease down back. Patchy fat appearing over ribs. Bulging fat around tailhead, along withers, behind shoulders, and along neck. Fat along inner buttocks may rub together. Flank filled in flush.

figure **11**, is supported by an overhead rope and can be raised and lowered easily. Ropes attached directly to the speculum do not allow the freedom of poll flexion desired for patient comfort.

A full mouth speculum is necessary to provide unfettered access to the entire mouth. Many designs and models exist. One should try several models in order to determine which is most effective for the user.

Stocks provide safety for the patient, the holder, and the veterinarian, and are encouraged whenever possible. An example is shown in figure **12**. They also prevent the patient from moving forward or backward during the procedure. When using stocks, the patient must be aware of its environment to the rear so that rearward-directed kicks may be prevented.

A bright headlight, as seen in figure **13** is necessary for illumination of the entire oral cavity. Many brands and models exist. Some have cooling fans. Battery powered and AC powered models exist. Lights which attach magnetically to the bite plate of the speculum are also available (**14**).

11 The horse's head is supported by a padded, adjustable head ring.

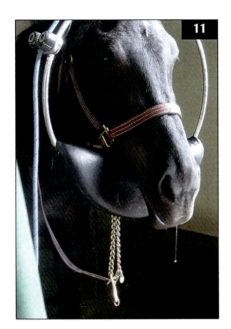

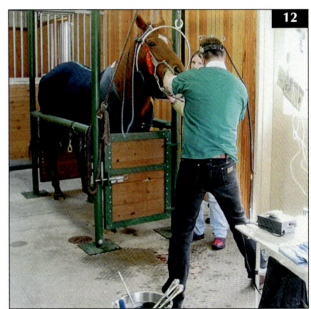

12 Stocks provide a safe working environment.

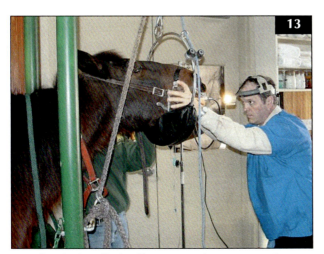

13 A bright headlight illuminates the entire oral cavity.

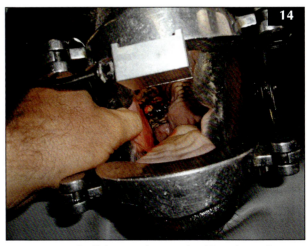

14 A magnetic light attaches to the bite plate of a speculum.

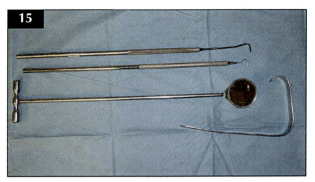

15 Basic examination instrumentation includes a buccal retractor, mirror, explorer, and sickle scaler.

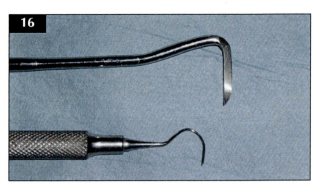

16 The equine sickle scaler (top) has a straight tip that is sharp on three sides and has a sharp pointed tip. The tip of the explorer (bottom) is shaped like a 'shepherd's hook', hence the name 'shepherd's hook explorer'.

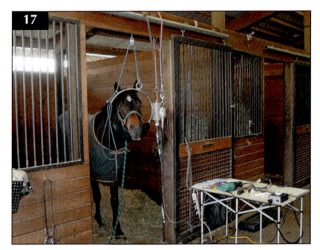

17 A stall-side table is convenient for easy access to instruments.

Basic instrumentation includes a buccal retractor, mirror, explorer, and some instrument, such as a sickle scaler, for removal of feed particles from around and between teeth (15). Figure 16 shows detail of the tips of the explorer and the equine sickle scaler. Molar forceps are also useful in the examination process for quantifying the stage of mobility of loose teeth.

Finally, a table on which instruments can be placed provides easy access to the multitude of instruments necessary for providing complete dental care to the patient (17). Camping style folding or roll-up tables are inexpensive, very portable, and easily replaced.

DENTAL EXAMINATION

After performing the basic physical examination, a specific and detailed evaluation of the head and mouth is carried out. External evaluation includes observation and palpation of the temporomandibular joint (18), the cheek overlying sharp enamel points of the buccal aspect of the maxillary cheek teeth (19), alignment of the incisors and their manner of occlusion, alignment and symmetry of the head and arcades, and any lumps, enlargements, or depressions in the region of the teeth. Nasal passages are evaluated for discharge and any abnormal odors are noted. In most cases, the owner will present the patient for abnormalities found on external examination. Any abnormalities are charted, the most common of which are found by pain elicited on palpation or movement.

Prior to introduction of the speculum, a functional examination is performed. The head is placed in the padded ring or other support device and the buccal retractor is used to examine the arcades for the determination of the point of occlusal contact (POC). This is done by retracting the cheek and centering the mandible (20–22).

The mandible is then moved palatally to determine the point on the occlusal surface of the maxillary arcade where the lateral margin of the mandibular arcade initially comes into contact. This point is noted on both sides. The importance of this evaluation is that this point represents the endpoint of the power stroke of mastication. The POC is discussed further in Chapter 6.

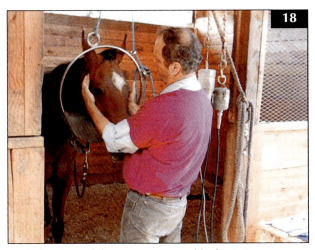

18 Palpation of the temporomandibular joint.

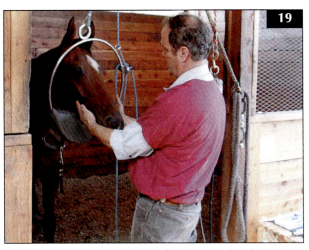

19 Palpation of sharp enamel points under the cheeks.

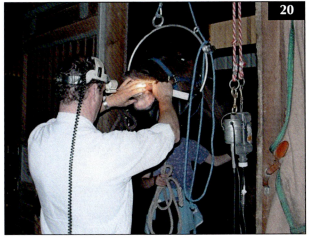

20 The cheek is retracted to demonstrate the point of occlusal contact (POC).

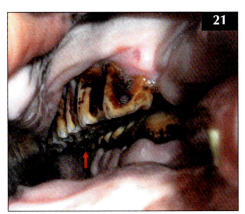

21 The POC is demonstrated (arrow). All teeth contact at the same time. This measurement is repeated after occlusal equilibration.

22 The mandible is moved palatally to demonstrate even interdental space, and parallel occlusal surfaces. This measurement is repeated after occlusal equilibration. In this example the amount of overlong tooth can also be estimated. Arrows indicate slightly overlong 408 and 109 (steps).

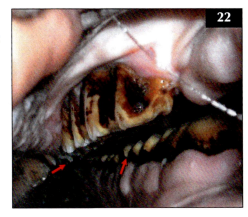

This measurement is easily recognized and is a reproducible way to measure the function of mastication objectively. A goal of dental care is to reproduce this measurement after the performance of occlusal equilibration procedures.

The importance of the POC is understood when considering mastication physiology. After opening, the mandible moves in three directions. As it closes, it moves in a lateral to medial and caudal to rostral angle across the maxillary arcade. All aspects of the range of motion are important when considering the development of malocclusions and their treatment. If one of these directions is limited by an abnormally long tooth, the patient develops problems that only worsen as time passes, since the horse cannot resolve such an abnormality without outside intervention. When examining the POC, the occlusal surfaces are examined further. Both upper and lower surfaces should be parallel and the space between them should be even from front to back. The two surfaces should meet together. This evaluation process should be repeated after occlusal equilibration is completed so as to ensure normal functional physiology.

Normal horses have occlusion that is centered and even at the incisors. Cheek teeth have an occlusal angle of around 15°. When viewed from the side, the cheek teeth occlude evenly in a straight line that curves upward relative to the degree of curvature of Spee. When viewed with a buccal retractor, the arcades have even, though not flat, occlusion with several sharp enamel points on the buccal side of the upper cheek teeth, and the lingual side of the lower cheek teeth.

The presence and degree of abnormality can be determined initially by evaluation with the buccal retractor. With the cheek retracted and viewing the occlusal surface, the amount of overlong tooth can be estimated. It is critical to determine this abnormality by correct determination of the normal line and angle of occlusion. It is helpful to slide the mandible palatally to open the occlusal space for best evaluation. Once the space is sufficiently open, the occlusal surfaces of both upper and lower arcades can be evaluated for abnormalities and degree of correction required.

DETAILED DENTAL EXAMINATION

Each tooth is then briefly examined using a headlight and mirror for abnormalities. Pulp horns are checked with a dental explorer for potential exposure. Infundibula are examined for decay and, when present, the disease process is staged. Arcades are examined for periodontal disease, abnormally shaped or positioned teeth, fractured teeth, and the full range of potential dental problems. All abnormalities are charted. Figures **23** and **24** demonstrate the examination process.

With repetition, this detailed examination can become very efficient, and recognition of problems very acute. It is a learning process that requires regular, deliberate technique that, with time and diligence, will yield maximum information with minimal effort.

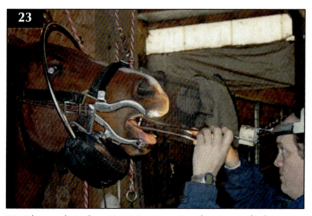

23 The sedated patient is examined using a light source, speculum, and hand instruments.

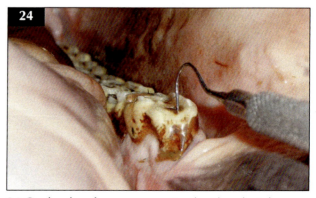

24 Occlusal surfaces are examined with a dental explorer for the presence of necrotic dentin which may correspond to a nonvital pulp exposure. The explorer is drawn across the surface of the tooth. If it 'catches' or penetrates the surface slightly, the dentin is necrotic.

CHARTING

Accurate charting is integral to good medical record keeping. Problem progress can be monitored and adjustments made to treatments as needed.

Many options exist for dental charting. A plethora of handwritten charts exists. Examples of a chart and exam form are given in figures **25–27**.

25 Sample form for charting.

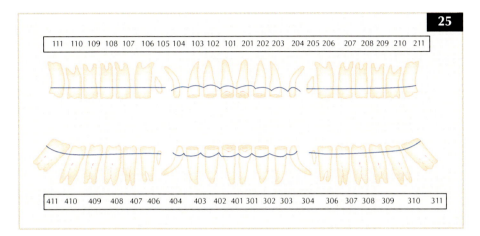

25

|111 110 109 108 107 106 105 104 103 102 101 201 202 203 204 205 206 207 208 209 210 211|

|411 410 409 408 407 406 404 403 402 401 301 302 303 304 306 307 308 309 310 311|

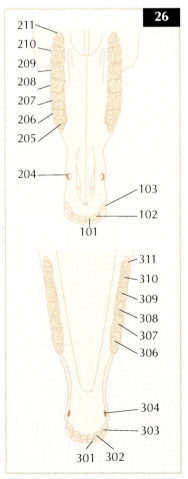

211
210
209
208
207
206
205
204
103
102
101
311
310
309
308
307
306
304
303
301 302

26

26 Sample form for charting.

27

Veterinary Clinic Name
Medical History and General Examination Form

Barn _____   Date _____
Owner _____   Patient_____
Address _____   Breed_____ DOB_____
_____   Sex___ Color___ Wt_____
City_____ State____ Zip _____   Insurance: Medical/Life_____
Phone (D)_____ (N) _____
Email_____
History: Patient's purpose: _____   Diet:_____
Pasture:____ hrs/day _____   mos/yr
Presenting problem: Routine follow-up Last done: _____
      Wt. Loss Dropping feed Abnormal chewing Quidding
      Head tossing Resisting R/L Head tilt Colic Swelling
      Feed packing Foul odor Behavioral Soaking feed Eating slowly
Previous medical problems:_____
Physical Examination:
Attitude:_____ Disposition:____ HR____ RR____ Temp ____
App: ____ MM: Moist/dry Color_____ CRT_____ Hyd ____
Stool +/– N/A _____
Body condition____ Hair coat____ Manure: fine/med/coarse
Soft tissue: left/right; abrasion/laceration/swelling/normal:
L/R : A/L/S/N
Lips: L/R : A/L/S/N   Tongue: L/R : A/L/S/N
Palate: L/R: A/L/S/N   Gingiva: L/R : A/L/S N
Bars: L/R/A/L/S/N
Occlusal table angle: normal/steep/flat/
sheared: N/S/F/Sh
    Left Side: N/S/F/Sh   Right Side: N/S/F/Sh
Palpation response: +/– @ _____
Point of occlusal contact:

       Before   After

27 Sample examination form.

Computerized charting is also available. Documentation of dental problems can also be done with digital or other photography. Radiographs can be reproduced as digital images. Digital or computerized radiographs can be included in the chart and can be made available to the client.

Use of the modified Triadan system of dental nomenclature as discussed in Chapter 3 is the currently accepted method of tooth identification.

EQUINE DENTAL TERMS ABBREVIATIONS

The following terms and abbreviations are currently in use and accepted by the American College of Veterinary Dentistry and the Academy of Veterinary Dentistry.[2] In order for these terms and abbreviations to gain approval by the Academy of Veterinary Dentistry and the American College of Veterinary Dentistry, they must first be approved by an agency referred to as SNOMED, an acronym for **S**ystemized **No**menclature for **Med**icine. This organization is traditionally used for approval of nomenclature in all medical fields. The approval by this agency for veterinary dental terminology gives authority to any list of terms and abbreviations used by the AVD and AVDC. More information about this agency is available at www.snomed.org.

Each figure shows a particular condition which is defined and lists the accepted abbreviation for dental charting.

Diagnostic problems and their codes
Incisors

Figures **28–34** illustrate problems in incisor teeth. The codes for these are given in the figure legends.

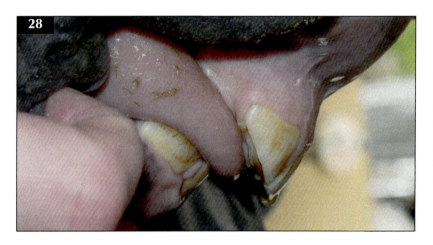

28 Overbite, brachygnathism, mandibular brachygnathism (code MAL2): extension of upper teeth vertically beyond lower teeth.[3] Defined by the term *distoclusion*, where some or all of the mandibular teeth are distal in relationship to their maxillary counterparts. A class II malocclusion.

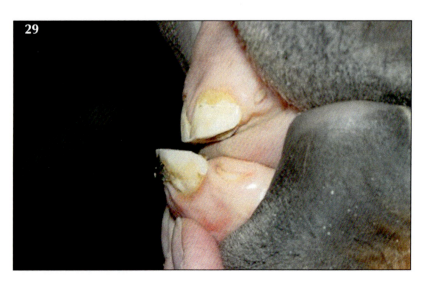

29 Underbite, prognathism, mandibular prognathism (code MAL3): defined by the term *mesioclusion*[3], where some or all of the mandibular teeth are mesial in their relationship to their maxillary counterparts. A class III malocclusion.

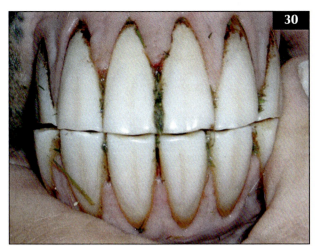

30 Ventral curvature (code CV): the upper central incisors are protuberant beyond the level of the upper intermediate and corner incisors.

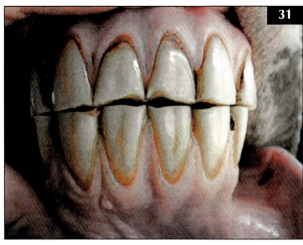

31 Dorsal curvature (code CD): the lower central incisors are protuberant beyond the level of the lower intermediate and corner incisors.

32 Diagonal (code DGL): the lower incisors are longer on either the left side or right side. Mandibular incisors are longer on arcade number 3 or 4. Arcade 400 is longer in this figure (code DGL/4).

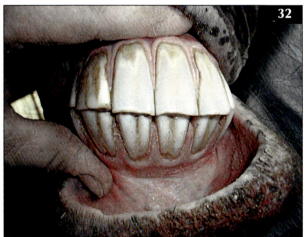

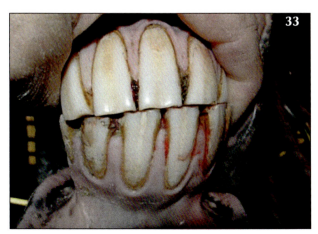

33 Diagonal: arcade 300 is longer (code DGL/3).

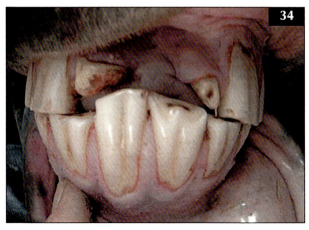

34 Overlong (code TO): refers to a protuberant tooth (or teeth) not conforming to usual patterns. The term used is for 'tooth overgrowth'.

Cheek teeth

Problems in cheek teeth are shown in figures **35–48**, with the codes in the legends.

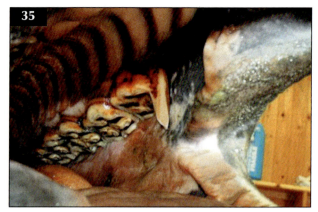

35 Hook (code HK): a protuberant crown longer than it is wide.[4]

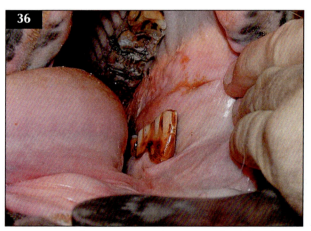

36 Ramp (code RMP): protuberant tooth wider than it is long.[4]

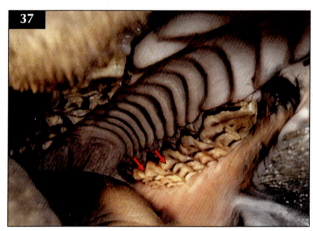

37 Wave (code WV): there is more than one tooth with excess crown in a single arcade (arrows).[4]

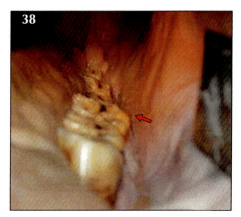

38 Waves (arrow) involve both the upper and lower arcades. Charting should designate all teeth concerned on both arcades.

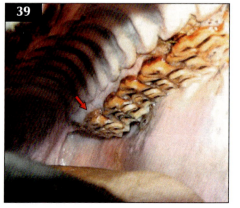

39 Step (code STP): there is one tooth only with excess crown (arrow).[4]

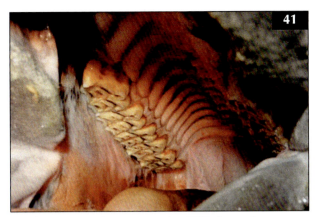

40 Excessive transverse ridges (code ETR): there are ridges in excess of 3 mm in height.[4]

41 Sharp enamel points (codes PTS): buccal cusps on uppers and lingual cusps on lowers are sharpened from wear.

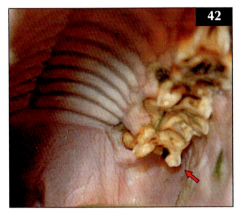

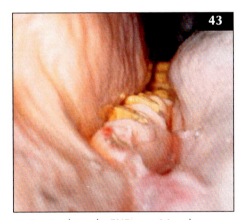

42 Cupped (code CUPD): the crown is worn past the infundibulum (uppers only) (arrow). The tooth still has the crown above the gingival margin.

43 Expired (code EXP): attrition has occurred to gingival level with thin crown connecting all roots.

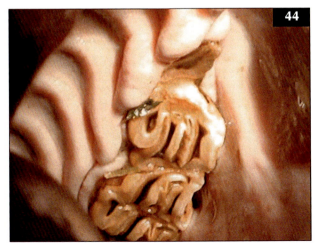

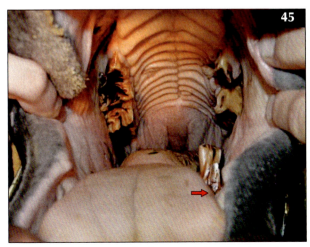

44 Expired/retained tooth root (code EXP/RTR): attrition has occurred to gingival level with no crown present connecting root fragments.

45 Missing/absent (code 0, arrow): in charting, the tooth is circled.

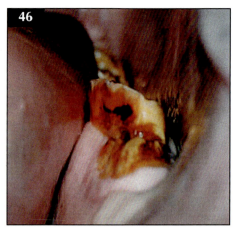

46 Retained deciduous (code RD): caps.

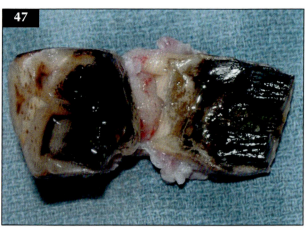

47 Fracture (code FX). A sagittal fracture (code FX/SAG) below the gum line through the infundibulum is shown.

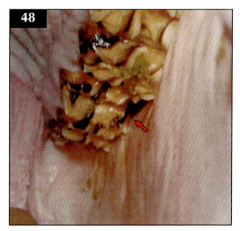

48 Wedge fracture (code FX/WDG): outside infundibulum, usually through pulp horns (arrow).

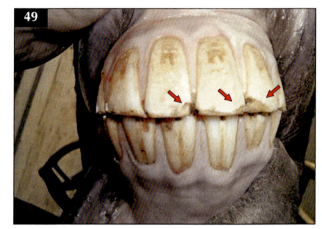

49 Chip fracture (code FX/CHP): occlusal margin only (arrows). The tooth is not fractured down to gingiva.

Fractures are coded according to type of fracture and location. The code for a frature is FX. Fractures may be sagittal (FX/SAG) (**47**), wedge (FX/WDG) (**48**), or chip (FX/CHP) (**49**). Codes are also given for region:

- **Interproximal region:** Mesial or distal (code: IP/M or D).
- **Buccal** (code B).
- **Palatal** (code P).
- **Lingual** (code L).

Example: Fractured 109 on palatal margin not extending to gingiva: 109 FX/CHP/P. This fracture is possibly reduced with normal odontoplasty.

Example: Wedge fracture of 209 on distal interproximal surface extending to gingival margin: 209 FX/WDG/IP. This fracture will not be reduced completely with routine odontoplasty, and may be restored, with any periodontal disease treated as well.

Wolf teeth

Figures **50–52** illustrate problems in the wolf teeth. The codes for these are given in the figure legends.

50 'Blind' (code TU): the accurate term is 'unerupted'. The tooth is not completely erupted, and is partly or fully covered by bone or soft tissue. The term used is 'tooth unerupted' (arrow).

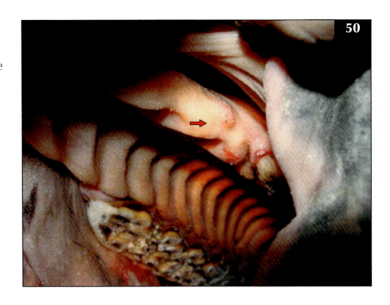

51 Fragment/root fragment: commonly seen as a remnant of a deciduous tooth root. The figure shows a retained root tip (code RRT): a portion of root or tip is retained (arrow).

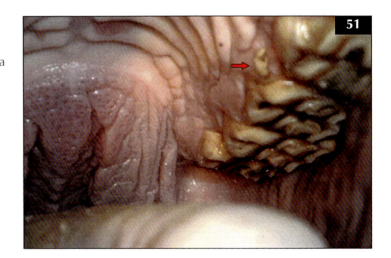

52 Retained tooth root (code RTR): the entire root is retained (arrow).

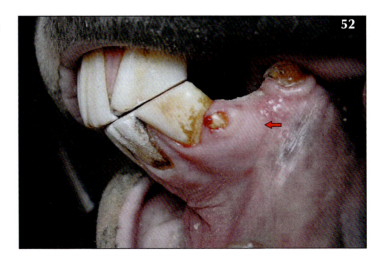

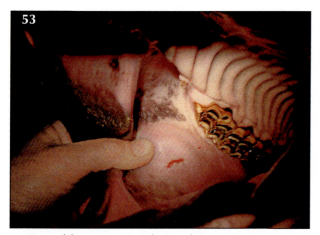

53 Buccal laceration (code LAC/B).

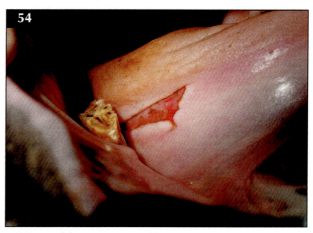

54 Lingual laceration (code LAC/L).

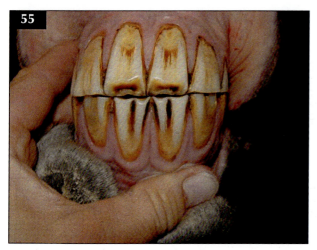

55 Abrasion (code AB): a tooth suffering wear as a result of trauma from a foreign material such as a bit, cribbing, or when grazing very short pasture and abrading the teeth on dirt and sod. This can occur on any tooth.

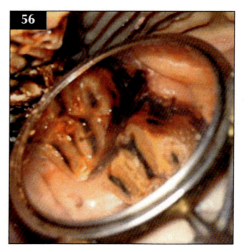

56 Periodontal disease (code PD).

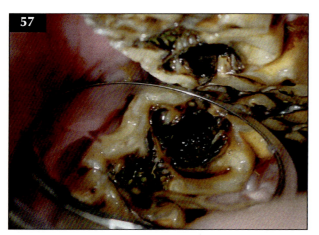

57 Infundibular cavity (code INF/CA): decay of the infundibulum of maxillary cheek teeth.

Soft tissue and other problems

Figures **53–56** show soft tissues problems. Periodontal disease (code PD) is classified as stage 1–4 (see Chapter 16 for complete description). A periodontal pocket is coded as PP. An infundibular cavity is illustrated in figure **57** (see Chapter 15 for complete discussion). Caries (code CA) describes decay present in any location on a tooth.

Procedures

The codes for dental procedures are as follows:
- **Odontoplasty (code OD):** reduction of excessive crown of occlusal surface.
- **Float (code FLT):** reduction of lingual and buccal enamel points.

- **Bit seat (code BS):** rounding of mesial margins of second premolars.
- **Intraoral extractions:**
  - Extraction, simple (code X).
  - Extraction, sectioned (code XS).
  - Surgical extraction (code XSS).
- **Cap extraction or retained deciduous extraction (code 506X, 606X, and so on)**.
- **Wolf tooth extraction (code 105X, and so on)**.
- **Incisor reduction (code I/OD):** term used is 'incisor odontoplasty'.

AGE-SPECIFIC PROBLEMS

BIRTH TO 18 MONTHS

Newborn foals should be examined as soon after birth as possible for congenital defects in bite alignment and head formation. Eruption sequence of deciduous teeth is rarely abnormal, though when present can result in significant malalignments. Sharp enamel points can affect mastication and nursing. When young horses suffer eating or apparent appetite disorders, oral examination is indicated.

AGE 18–60 MONTHS

The young performance horse learning how to handle a bit is losing 24 teeth and gaining 36–44 adult teeth over this period of time. The dramatic change in occlusion, and the discomfort of deciduous exfoliation and adult tooth eruption create an environment that is not necessarily conducive to successful training. Close monitoring of young horses at this time is helpful in assisting proper training. Many bitting problems are corrected by close observation of deciduous exfoliation. It is also important in maintaining proper adult tooth alignment.

Asymmetrical deciduous shedding of premolars can be a significant contributing factor to the development of adult malocclusions. Figure **58** shows asynchronous exfoliation of deciduous 8s that is a major factor in the development of wave malocclusion. Upper 8s are shed long after lowers, resulting in eruption of lower 8s beyond the normal level of occlusion.

AGE 5–12 YEARS

At 5 years of age, all adult teeth should be in full normal function. These horses are frequently at their peak of athletic performance. It is the goal of most

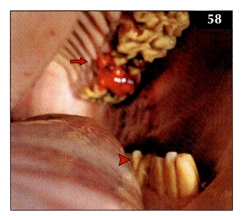

58 The arrowhead indicates the level of the lower 8 above the occlusal plane of the 7. The arrow indicates the level of the upper 8 immediately after extraction of the deciduous tooth. This disparity in occlusal level resulting from asynchronous exfoliation is a major contributing factor in the development of waves.

owners that their horse performs at the highest level for the longest time possible. Maintenance of good dentition is an important part of overall healthcare. Since longevity and comfort are both of primary concern at this time in the horse's life, it is imperative that the attending veterinarian understand dental physiology and the development of malocclusions. Many dental problems are prevented by correction of abnormal forces of mastication. This is the primary focus of dental care at this time of the horse's life. Dental comfort in mastication and bitting is almost as important.

Most patients are best cared for on an annual basis. More frequent dental care may be necessary in some cases. One must be extremely careful in delivering routine occlusal equilibration on a semi-annual basis. One of the goals of regular dental care is to equate the rate of eruption and the rate of attrition of all teeth. In doing so, the rate of attrition slows down and the teeth last longer. As the rate of attrition slows, so does the rate of eruption. Increased frequency of occlusal equilibration can negate this benefit by removal of excessive dental tissue. Great care must be taken in the balanced adult mouth that excess tooth is not removed and the life of the tooth shortened.

AGE 13–19 YEARS

The teenage horse has problems similar to those of the young adult. Additionally, it is in this age range that age-related tooth breakdown problems can begin to occur. Periodontal disease affects many older horses. If regular occlusal equilibration is correctly performed, periodontal disease is less frequent and less severe. When present it can be reversed in most cases. Infundibular disease is also more frequent in this age range. Yearly examination allows the attending veterinarian to intervene early in this problem and prevent complications such as tooth fracture.

AGE 20 YEARS AND OLDER

Geriatric horses typically have teeth that are erupting near the end of their reserve crown. They are prone to periodontal disease, fracture, decay, and other complications. Teeth undergo excessive wear in many cases. Many malocclusions develop that cannot be completely corrected. At this time of life most dental procedures are 'salvage' type procedures, designed to relieve pain and minimize damage to the arcade.

The focus of dental care in the geriatric patient is pain relief, and not correction of abnormal forces. If attempts are made to address the presence of abnormal forces aggressively by excess reduction of occlusal crown, there is high risk of post-treatment pain associated with dentinal exposure, temporo-mandibular joint inflammation, mastication muscle irritation, or irritation of a tooth with short roots and reserve crown. In geriatric patients the development of post-treatment complications can be life threatening.

It is important to address geriatrics carefully. The attending veterinarian should carefully consider the condition and status of the entire animal. A full and complete medical history and examination should be performed in every case and at every appointment for an individual.

Staging of dental procedures in geriatrics is an effective method for minimizing risk exposure. In doing so, the worst problem is addressed first and the patient is allowed to recover. For instance, diseased teeth may be extracted on one arcade prior to occlusal equilibration on a following appointment. As many episodes of dental care as necessary are scheduled until the treatment is finished. It is important to maintain normal occlusal balance during these treatments. Other medical problems may require resolution prior to dental care.

SUMMARY

Dental examination is the basis for treatment planning. Safety is a primary concern. Efficient, thorough examination is facilitated with a full range of instrumentation and repeated practice. Charting assists in treatment planning, prognosis, follow-up, and accurate adjustments to treatment. Common terminology facilitates communication among dental professionals.

REFERENCES

1. Henneke DR, Potte GD, Kreider JL, Yeates BF. Relationship between condition score, physical measurements and body fat percentage in mares. *Equine Veterinary Journal* 1983: **15**(4); 1–2.
2. Klugh DO, Brannan, RD. Terminology and abbreviations for equine charting. *Conference Proceedings 15th Annual Veterinary Dental Forum* 2001; pp. 188–192.
3. Wiggs RB, Lobprise HB. *Veterinary Dentistry: Principles and Practice.* Philadelphia: Lippincott-Raven, 1997; pp. 628–676.
4. Greene S. Personal communication.

ANATOMICAL CHARACTERISTICS OF EQUINE DENTITION

David O Klugh   Chapter 3

TRIADAN SYSTEM OF IDENTIFICATION

Historically, equine tooth anatomy has been referred to descriptively. For instance an incisor was called a central or intermediate incisor and a cheek tooth was called a second premolar or first molar. In 1991, Dr. Michael Floyd[1] introduced the Triadan system of dental nomenclature to veterinary dentistry. In such a system arcades are given a first number and teeth are given an additional number. In a description of the location of a tooth, 208 for instance, the number '2' or '200' refers to the arcade in which the tooth resides, and the '8' refers to the tooth itself.

Arcades are numbered beginning with number 1 at the horse's upper right. The sequence is continued in a clockwise direction when observing the horse from the front. The upper left is number 2, lower left is number 3, and lower right is number 4. This sequence is illustrated in figure **59**.

Teeth are numbered 1 through 11 on each arcade beginning with the central incisor as tooth number 1 and continuing distally in each arcade to the last molar which is numbered 11. This numbering system is demonstrated in figure **60**.

In the Triadan system teeth such as the wolf tooth and canines are numbered whether they are present or not, so that in a patient that has neither a wolf tooth nor a canine, the first cheek tooth is always number 6, the first molar is always number 9, and the last molar is always number 11.

Deciduous teeth are enumerated separately from the permanent teeth. Arcade number 1 is referred to as arcade 5 when referring to deciduous teeth, with arcade 2 becoming number 6, arcade 3 known as number 7, and arcade 4 referred to as

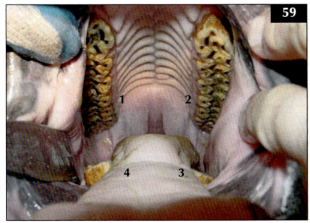

59 Arcades are numbered 1 to 4 beginning with the upper right arcade and continuing clockwise around the mouth.

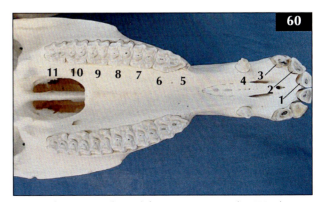

60 Teeth are numbered from 1 to 11 in the Triadan system.

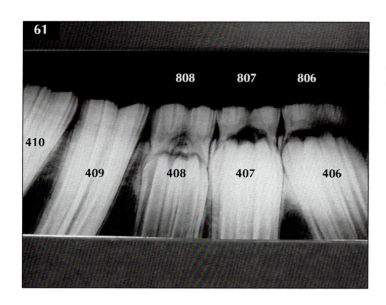

61 The Triadan system incorporates separate numbering for deciduous teeth, with the arcades numbered 5, 6, 7, and 8, starting with the upper right arcade and continuing in a clockwise direction. The arcade in the radiograph is the lower right.

number 8. In such a system the upper left second premolar would be 206 for a permanent tooth and 606 for the comparable dediduous tooth. The deciduous premolars are identified with their counterparts in figure **61**.

When identifying a tooth using the Triadan system both the arcade number and the tooth number are used. The arcade designation is used first and the tooth number is second. Since there are up to 11 teeth the designation for individual teeth requires the use of two digits. For this reason, arcade designations are often referred to as 100, 200, 300, and 400.

In identifying specific teeth a three-digit number is employed. In teeth enumerated with a single digit, a '0' is added so that a logical sequence is created. 101, 102, and 103 would be the right upper first through third incisors.

The Triadan system makes tooth identification much easier and faster while facilitating communication between the practitioners of dentistry on any species.

DENTAL TERMINOLOGY

Specific terminology is used in describing relationships of position and tooth surfaces within the arcades.[2] These terms are demonstrated in figure **62**. The following definitions apply:
- **Labial:** surface toward lips of canine and incisors.
- **Buccal:** surface toward the cheeks of premolars and molars.

- **Facial:** the labial and buccal surfaces are known collectively as the facial surfaces.
- **Lingual:** towards the tongue. This term is sometimes used interchangeably with 'palatal' to describe that surface of the upper teeth related to the palate.
- **Occlusal:** surface in contact with opposite arcade.
- **Proximal:** surface contacting next tooth in sequence in the same arcade.
- **Interproximal space:** between two proximal teeth.
- **Distal:** proximal tooth surface or space positioned or facing away from the median line.
- **Mesial:** proximal tooth surface or space positioned or facing toward the median line.
- **Apical:** direction toward the root tip and/or away from the occlusal surface.
- **Coronal:** direction toward the occlusal surface.
- **Apex:** root tip.
- **Apical foramen:** opening in the apex where vessels and nerves enter the pulp.

Equine teeth have a distinct root separate from a continuously erupting long crown that is worn down over time. These teeth are therefore known as *radicular hypsodont*.

The crown is divided into clinical and reserve crown. The clinical crown is that portion of the crown above the gingiva and lying within the oral cavity. The reserve crown lies below the gingiva. It can be further divided into gingival crown and alveolar crown.[3] Gingival crown is below the gingiva and above the alveolar bone. Alveolar crown is surrounded by alveolar bone.

Since the entire tooth is surrounded by cementum, equine teeth have no cementoenamel junction. There is no 'neck' or constriction in equine permanent teeth. The crown is that portion of the tooth that contains enamel. Beyond the termination of the enamel lies the root, which is composed of peripheral cementum surrounding dentin and enclosing the pulp. The pulp cavity is the entire space within both the crown and the root that contains the nutritive and sensory organ known as the pulp (**63**).

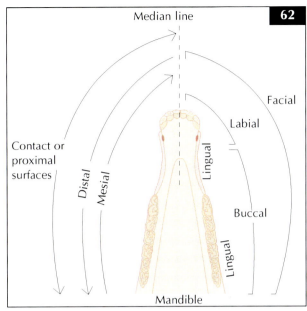

62 Directional terms are indicated.

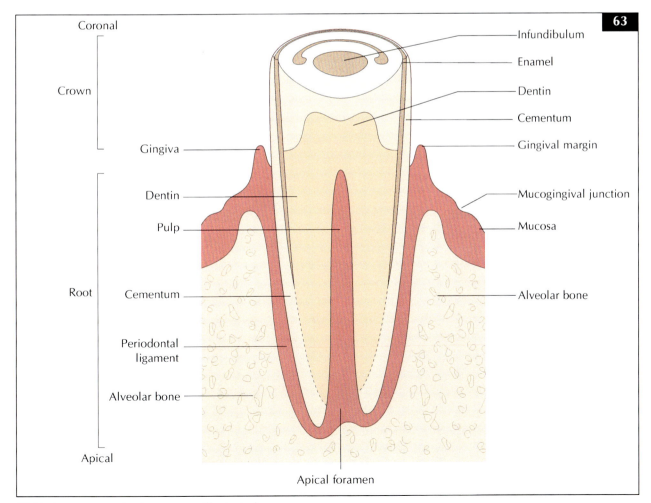

63 Various anatomical terms are illustrated.

ANATOMY OF DECIDUOUS EQUINE TEETH

There are up to 28 deciduous equine teeth. The dental formula for equine deciduous teeth is:

Di 3/3 Dc 1/1 Dp 3/3.

The central deciduous incisors (Triadan 1s) erupt within the first week of life if they are not present at birth. The intermediate incisors (2s) erupt by 6 weeks of age, and the corner incisors (3s) erupt around 6–9 months of age.

Deciduous incisors are smaller than their permanent counterparts. The labial surface of the occlusal crown is more triangular. There are numerous longitudinal lines or ridges on the labial surface. The infundibulum is wide and shallow. The occlusal surface is wide mesiodistally and narrow labiolingually. Deciduous incisors have a distinct 'neck' where the crown terminates and the root begins. Figure **64** shows some of these features.

The presence of deciduous canine teeth has been debated. The radiograph in figure **65** demonstrates their presence. There can be up to four deciduous canine teeth. They are small spicules that lie within the gingiva and are lost during the eruption process of the deciduous 3s. There are three deciduous premolars in each arcade. In the Triadan system they are numbered 6, 7, and 8. These numbers correspond to the second, third, and fourth premolars.

The occlusal surface area of the crown of deciduous premolars is approximately as large as that of permanents. In most cases they are present at birth, though many erupt within the first week of life. The erupting deciduous tooth may have very sharp enamel points. These sharp points can be a cause of dysmastication in young foals. Therefore, it is prudent for the clinician to examine teeth when presented with a foal that is not eating well.

The crown of deciduous premolars is shorter than that of the permanents, being 3–4 cm in length. These teeth have a distinctive 'neck' where the crown terminates and the root originates.

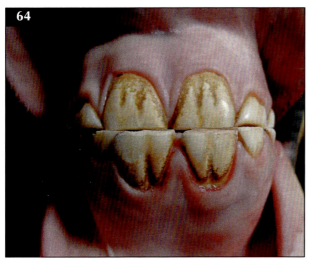

64 The permanent 1s are wide compared to the smaller, more triangular deciduous 2s.

ANATOMY OF PERMANENT EQUINE TEETH

There can be up to 44 permanent teeth in equines. The formula for permanent teeth is:

I 3/3 C 1/1 P 4/4 M 3/3.

There are three permanent incisors in each of the four arcades. Incisors are embedded in the mandible and premaxilla or incisive bone. The permanent incisors are longer and wider than deciduous incisors. The upper incisors are wider than the lowers. They curve longitudinally and taper toward the apex. Their average length when initially in wear is about 7 cm.[4] In some cases incisors can be as long as 8 cm.

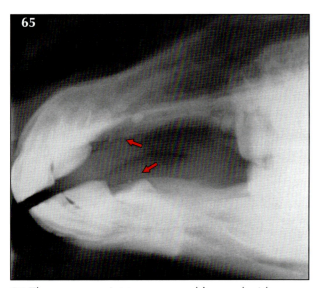

65 The arrows point to upper and lower deciduous canine teeth.

The view from the occlusal surface of the curvature of the arch made by incisors begins as a semicircle in young horses, as seen in figure **66**. As aging occurs, the semicircle becomes more linear (**67**).

In profile, the angle made by the labial borders of the upper and lower incisors begins as nearly a straight line (**68**). As the horse ages, this angle becomes more acute (**69**).

The angle of occlusion of the incisors should not change with age. It should not parallel that of the cheek teeth when viewed from the side. A line drawn over the incisor angle of occlusion should continue directly across the eye or ear of the horse, shown in figure **70**.

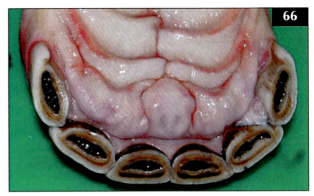

66 The incisor arch begins as a semicircle in the young adult.

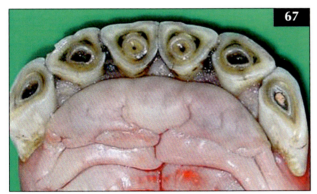

67 The incisor arch becomes more linear in the aged horse.

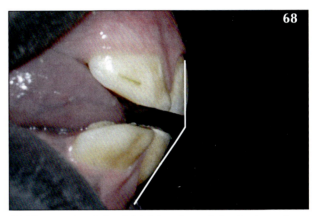

68 The angle of the labial borders of the incisors is nearly straight in the young horse.

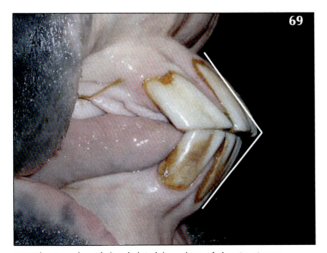

69 The angle of the labial border of the incisors becomes more acute in the aging patient.

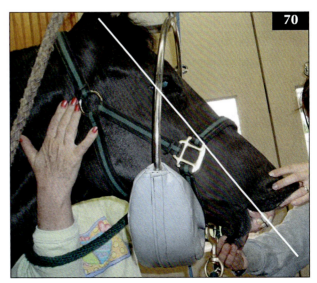

70 The angle of occlusion of the incisors is in a direct line with the eye or ear.

The occlusal surface of the incisors changes with age. In young adults it is oval (**71**). The long diameter is in a mesial-to-distal direction. With age, the occlusal surface becomes round or trapezoid shaped (**72**). By the early teens, the occlusal surface is triangular in shape (**73**). In the twenties and thirties it becomes oval again, as in figure **74**, but with the long diameter of the oval in a labial-to-lingual direction.

The longitudinal *Galvayne's groove* on the labial surface of the upper third incisor (103 and 203) has been used in aging horses. Traditionally, it is said to appear at the gingival margin at 10 years of age. At about 15 years of age, the groove's margin is at the midpoint of the occlusal crown. By 20 years, it reaches the occlusal border. By 25 the apical margin of the groove is at the crown's midpoint, and by 30 the groove disappears. This groove is inconsistent in its appearance. Figure **75a,b** shows the inconsistency in a 20-year-old patient, with the groove less than half way down on the 103 and not yet reaching the occlusal border on the 203.

The infundibulum of incisors is wide in a mesiodistal direction. It is compressed labiolingually into an oval that is larger than that of a deciduous tooth. It is deeper on upper incisors in general, but its depth on all teeth is variable.

The infundibulum is a cone-shaped ring of enamel extending apically from the occlusal surface. It is filled to a variable degree with cementum, and is referred to by the common name of the 'cup'. The disappearance of the cup has long been used in aging horses. Typically, disappearance from the lower 1s is considered to occur by the age of 6 years; from the 2s by 7 years; and from the 3s by age 8 years. There is much individual variation, however, in the amount of cementum filling the infundibulum, making unreliable the process of aging based on the presence or absence of cups.

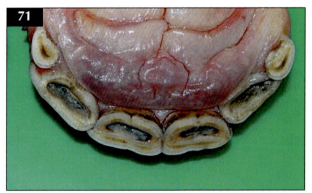

71 The oval-shaped occlusal surface of the young horse has its longer diameter in the mesial-to-distal direction.

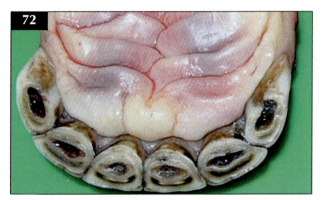

72 The occlusal surface of the adult incisors becomes more round or trapezoid.

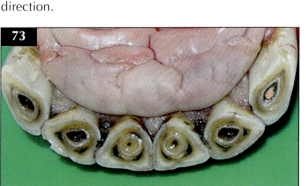

73 The occlusal surface of the teenage horse becomes triangular.

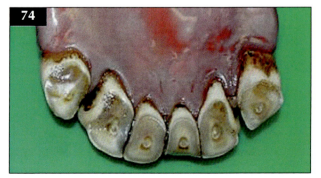

74 The occlusal surface of the 30-year-old horse becomes oval. The long diameter is in the labial-to-lingual direction.

After the cup wears down the remaining infundibulum is filled with cementum. This is commonly called the 'mark'. It is also traditionally used in aging, but is also highly variable, and therefore unreliable.

Between the infundibulum and the labial surface lies the pulp cavity. This space becomes filled with dentin as the tooth erupts and is visible on the occlusal surface as the 'dental star'. When first seen it is wide in a mesiodistal direction, being compressed in its position by the infundibulum (**76**). As eruption and attrition continue, and the infundibulum becomes smaller, the dental star becomes more round and moves to the central part of the occlusal surface (**77**).

In general, the dental star appears on the 1s between 4½ and 5 years of age; on the 2s between 5½ and 6 years of age; and on the 3s between 6½ and 8 years of age.

The dental star is composed of secondary dentin peripherally and tertiary dentin centrally. The secondary dentin of incisors has dentinal tubules with no intratubular dentin and thus takes up pigments from feeds to create the brown stain.

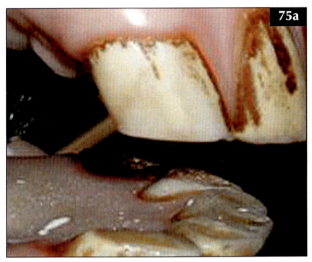 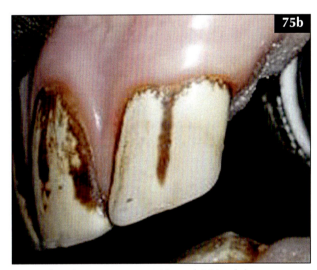

75a,b The location of Galvayne's groove is inconsistent. Pictured is the groove on 103 and 203 of the same patient.

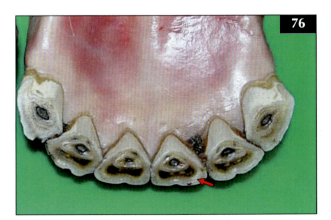 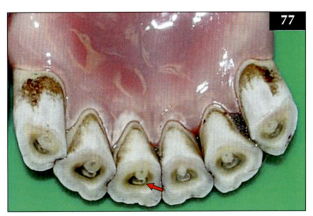

76 The dental star is compressed by the infundibulum and is located between the infundibulum and the labial surface (arrow).

77 In the aging horse the dental star moves to a more central location on the occlusal surface (arrow).

In the center of the dental star is an area of tertiary dentin. Dentinal tubules in this location are small in diameter, fewer in number, and are arranged irregularly.[5] This area does not, therefore, take up any pigments from feeds, and is pale in comparison to the periphery.

The central pale portion of the dental star appears on the 1s between 7 and 8 years of age; on the 2s between 7 and 11 years of age; and on the 3s between 10 and 15 years of age.

The accuracy of determination of age by dental examination declines as the horse ages. Eruption times are reasonably dependable. The rest are estimates. Rather than specifically identifying age of the patient, the clinician should consider identifying a range of years when asked to determine the patient's age.

The root of the tooth is defined as that portion formed apically from the termination of the enamel. It is comprised of dentin and cementum. Root formation adds to the length of the tooth as the crown undergoes attrition, so that the overall length of the tooth may remain at about 70 mm up to the mid to late teenage years. In geriatric years (>20) root formation slows, as does eruption. The result is an ever shortening overall length.

The pulp cavity of adult equine incisors begins as a large cone-shaped space with a large apical foramen, as in figure **78**. The space is filled as odontoblasts lay down dentin. Understanding of the shape of the canal is important in root canal therapy. The occlusal third of the canal is compressed labiolingually by the presence of the infundibulum (**79**). This compression may be so severe as to split the pulp canal into a bipartite or ribbon shape, as evidenced by the shape of the dental star.

Moving in an apical direction past the infundibulum, the maturing canal of the aging horse becomes cylindrical in shape for as much as 2–3 cm (**80**). As the canal reaches the apical crown and proceeds into the root it is compressed laterally. Mandibular incisors (**81**) are more convergent than maxillary incisors (**82**).

The fact that all incisors are apically convergent leads to another anatomical condition related to the canal. The apical part of the canal is compressed laterally into a ribbon or oblong shape (**83**).

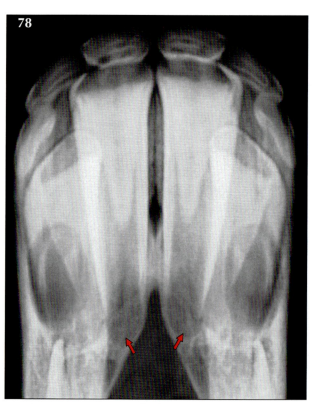

78 The arrows point to the large apical foramina of the pulp canal of pre-erupted 101 and 201.

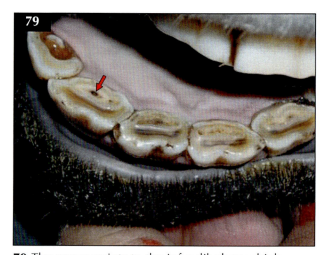

79 The arrow points to the infundibulum which compresses the shape of the pulp in this part of the crown. The dental star in this tooth is compressed into a ribbon shape.

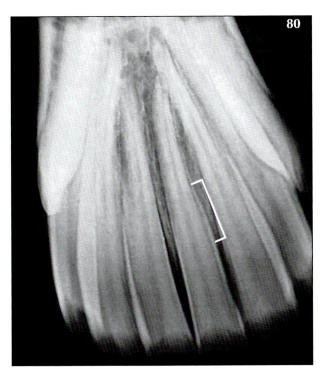

80 A radiograph of an incisor in an 18-year-old patient shows the cylindrical shape of the middle third of the pulp canal (bracket).

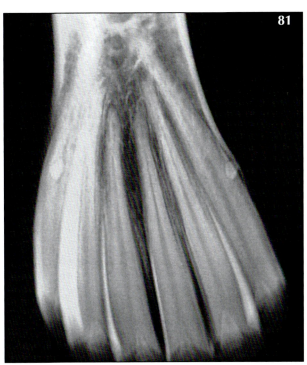

81 The radiograph of the mandibular incisors demonstrates the degree of convergence of the roots.

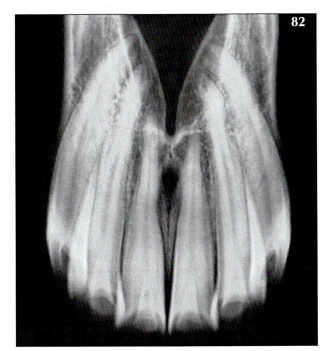

82 The radiograph of the maxillary incisors demonstrates that the roots are less convergent than those of the mandibular arcades.

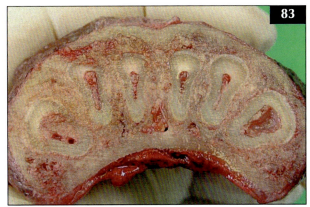

83 The effect of lateral compression of the pulp canal into an oval or oblong shape is shown on these incisors.

In many cases the canal is compressed such that it becomes divergent into two parts. This is demonstrated in figure **84**, where a cut has been made through the mandibular arcades of a cadaver specimen.

Canal divergence is most common in the lower 2s, though it is seen occasionally in all incisors. It may be present within the first 1½ to 2 years of tooth age. In divergent canals, the lingual branch fills with dentin first. During development it may be a blind pouch, receiving circulation from the coronal pulp. In the geriatric horse the lingual canal is filled with dentin, with only the single labial canal present. Divergence is not visible radiographically.

The various shapes of the incisor pulp cavity are not always amenable to instrumentation in root canal therapy. Therefore, chemical debridement and sterilization are critical in thorough treatment of pulp disease.

The position of the apical foramen in geriatric teeth is highly variable. It may be at the apical terminus of the root tip, or it may be positioned as a lateral aperture either mesially or distally (**85**, **86**). These foramina may be in addition to or instead of a foramen at the true apex.

Each incisor has a single root composed of dentin surrounding the pulp and a peripheral layer of cementum. The roots of hypsodont teeth elongate during adulthood by apical extension of peripheral cementum and central dentin. The peripheral cementum is of a 'cellular' nature. This means that cementoblasts are surrounded by the cementum they produce. These cells become cementocytes. The mineralized cementum incorporates fibers of the periodontal ligament (PDL). These fibers are *Sharpey's fibers* which attach the tooth to the PDL.

Odontoblasts of the pulp produce secondary dentin as the length of the root increases. The root canal is both extended in length and narrowed in diameter. As root length increases, the diameter of the apical foramen decreases. In equine incisors there may be two or three apical foramina positioned variably at the root tip.

In geriatric teeth with termination of the pulp via a lateral foramen, the entire root tip located apically to the foramen is composed of cellular cementum. This tissue can easily be fractured during extraction. Postoperative radiographs assist in determination of the presence of a retained root tip.

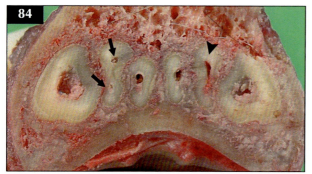

84 This specimen shows the effects of lateral compression of the pulp canal. The arrowhead indicates the ribbon shape of the canal in 302. The arrows show the divergent canal in 402.

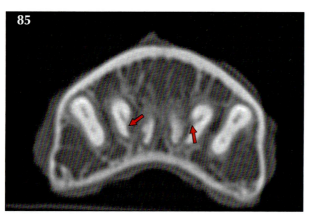

85 The arrows indicate the mesially located apical foramina of the lower 2s captured on computed tomography.

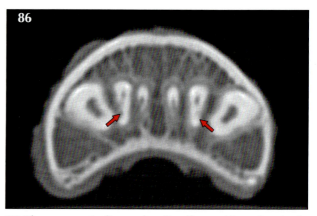

86 The arrows indicate the distally positioned apical foramina of the lower 2s captured on computed tomography.

In geriatric teeth, the overall length of the tooth shortens as the rate of eruption, though slowed, remains faster than the rate of root formation. In some cases root tip resorption contributes to overall reduction in tooth length.

Canine teeth are absent or rudimentary in most mares, as in figure **87**. Canines in mares are reported to have an incidence of 28%.[6] Occasionally, mares have normal canine teeth.

The normal canine tooth in geldings is curved distally (**88**), with a crown that is somewhat compressed laterally at its occlusal margin. There is a small sharp ridge mesially and distally that extends several millimeters apically from the occlusal border.

The pulp in the young horse in figure **88** is very large and relatively close to the occlusal margin. It can easily be exposed by excessive reduction in a newly erupted tooth. Eruption of canines occurs very slowly.[7]

The first premolar, or wolf tooth, is number 05 in the Triadan system. It is most commonly present in the maxillary arcades (**89**), though rarely mandibular wolf teeth do occur (**90**). The incidence of wolf teeth is reported to be 24.4% in mares and 14.9% in geldings and stallions.[8] Other studies show a variation in incidence from 13%[9] to 31.9%.[10]

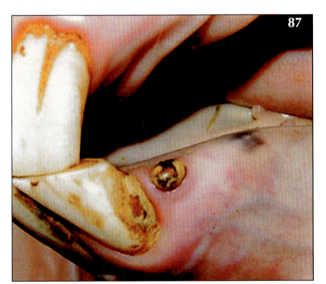

87 A small canine tooth of a mare is shown after removal of calculus. Mild gingivitis is common in such cases.

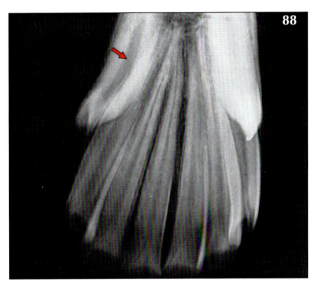

88 The arrow points to the large pulp of a newly erupted canine tooth in a 5-year-old gelding.

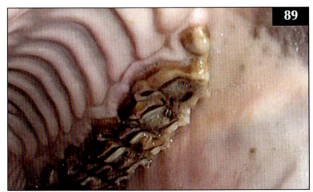

89 This yearling patient has a normally positioned wolf tooth.

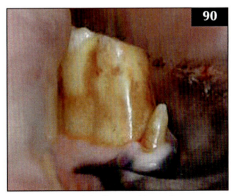

90 Rare mandibular wolf tooth.

The position of the wolf tooth in the maxillary arcade is variable. It may be immediately adjacent mesial to the 6 as in figure **89**; it may be positioned palatally (**91**); or it may be several millimeters mesial to the 6 (**92**).

The wolf tooth erupts at between 9 and 12 months of age. The length of the tooth varies from 1–2.5 cm. The root may be straight, curved, or spiral shaped. It may be long and slender or short and blunt. The crown may be small and simple or large and molariform. Varieties are seen in figure **93**. In some cases the crown is somewhat molariform with longitudinal ridges of folding enamel creating cusps on the occlusal surface (**94**).

When positioned palatally to the 6, the crown of the wolf tooth may suffer attrition from mastication forces, as the mandibular arcade moves in its lateral to medial motion (**95**).

The six cheek teeth in each arcade are premolars 2, 3, and 4, and molars 1, 2, and 3 (**96**). These

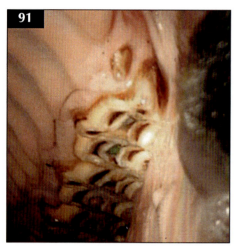

91 A palatally displaced wolf tooth is very common.

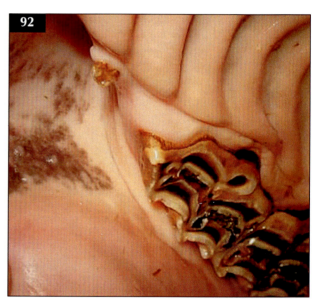

92 The wolf tooth may be displaced several millimeters mesially.

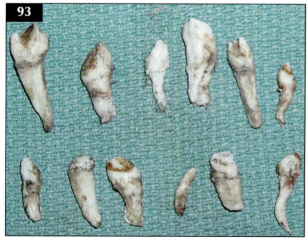

93 Several wolf teeth with different shaped roots and crowns.

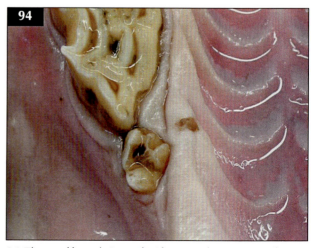

94 The wolf tooth is molariform with cusps on the occlusal surface.

correspond to teeth numbered 6 through 11 in the Triadan system.

The cheek teeth are large quadrilaterals, nearly rectangular in cross-section except the 6 and 11 which are approximately triangular (**97**).

The maxillary cheek teeth are wider in the buccolingual direction than the mandibulars. This is due to the presence of two deep infundibula in each of the upper cheek teeth. The comparison is demonstrated in figures **98** and **99**. Maxillary cheek teeth are about 2.5–3 cm wide. Mandibular cheek teeth are about 1.5–2 cm wide.

The infundibula are somewhat crescent-shaped infoldings of enamel seen on the occlusal surface.

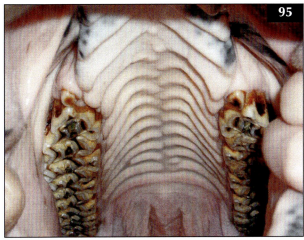

95 These wolf teeth in a 13-year-old patient have suffered attrition from mastication.

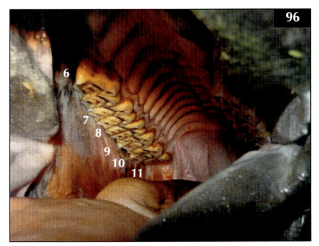

96 The cheek teeth are numbered 6 to 11 in the Triadan system.

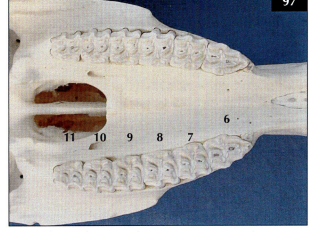

97 Teeth number 6 and 11 are more triangular in shape than those in the rest of the arcade.

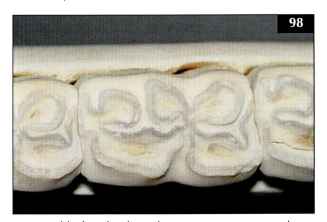

98 Mandibular cheek teeth are narrow compared to maxillary cheek teeth.

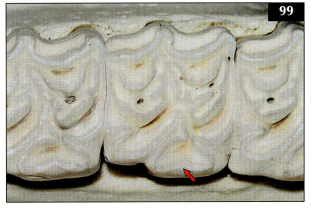

99 The presence of two infundibula makes maxillary cheek teeth wider than mandibulars. The arrow points to the palatal ridge of upper cheek teeth.

They are deep infoldings that extend apically for most of the length of the crown. Cementum fills these 'enamel lakes'[11] to a varying degree. The depth of the infundibulum is shown in figure **100**.

The process of cemental filling of the infundibulum begins on the occlusal surface and proceeds apically.[12] This cementum is supplied by an artery from the occlusal surface via the embryological dental sac. The two infundibular arteries are connected. The distal infundibulum fills with cementum first. This is due to the distal-to-mesial direction of blood flow and tissue development. When these teeth erupt, the blood supply is disrupted and cementogenesis terminates. The infundibular cement becomes a nonviable tissue. The disruption of blood supply may occur prior to complete filling of the infundibulum, resulting in infundibular cemental hypoplasia. This condition plays a role in the development of infundibular cavities.

The upper cheek teeth have two prominent ridges mesially and one less prominent ridge distally on their buccal surfaces separated by two deep grooves, except the 6s which may have three or four ridges and grooves. As these teeth undergo attrition, the enamel ridges become sharp enamel points that may lacerate the cheek. Buccal lacerations are seen in figure **101**.

The palatal aspect of upper cheek teeth has a single longitudinal ridge (see **99**). This ridge is located slightly mesial to the center in all maxillary cheek teeth and can serve to assist the clinician in identifying which direction is mesial when viewing the occlusal surface. This ridge is less prominent and more rounded than those on the buccal surface. Because of its rounded form and location on the palatal aspect of the tooth, it rarely becomes sharp as a result of attrition from mastication.

Mandibular premolars and molars have enamel infoldings as seen in figure **102**. One infolding or groove is present buccally. This groove separates two rounded ridges well covered by cementum. Lingually there are two deep and one shallow infolding. While these grooves are well covered by cementum, mastication forces frequently expose the enamel ridges and attrition results in development of sharp enamel points.

When observing a single mandibular cheek tooth, determination of its general spatial position can be made by noting occlusal surface angulation and position of sharp enamel cusps. The mandibular teeth are always angled with the lingual aspect taller than the buccal side. The two deep longitudinal grooves separate the lingual surface into mesial and distal parts. On the mesial part a shallow longitudinal

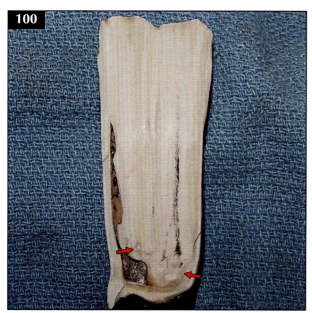

100 The arrows point to the apical termination of the infundibula. The mesial infundibulum on the right is incompletely filled with cementum.

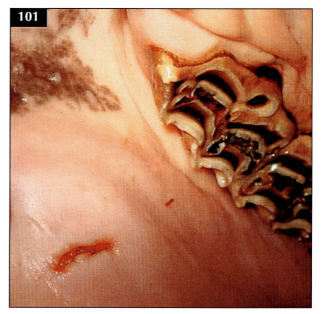

101 The buccal laceration was caused by the sharp enamel points on the buccal aspect of the maxillary teeth.

groove splits the mesial fold. This separation of the mesial folds is uniform on all mandibular cheek teeth, and denotes the mesiolingual corner of the tooth by the presence of two cusps with the appearance of 'mouse ears' (**102**).

Enamel points develop from worn cusps or ridges on the occlusal surface of the erupting tooth. These ridges form after the newly erupted tooth enters occlusion and begins to suffer attrition. The erupting tooth has four to five protrusions called 'styles', which resemble an 'egg carton' (**103**).

The newly erupted cheek tooth and its enamel protrusions or styles undergo attrition. As the worn tooth erupts the longitudinal enamel ridges and cusps become evident as the infoldings continue apically. These ridges become the sharp enamel points that may lacerate the buccal mucosa.

The development of sharp enamel points is particularly evident on the distal aspects of both upper and lower arcades (**104, 105**). This is a primary reason for performance of annual dental care in all patients. These points can be very uncomfortable

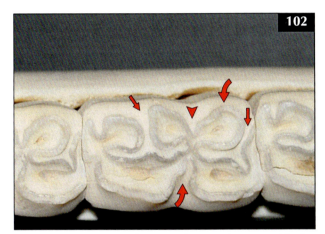

102 The pattern of infolding of enamel in mandibular cheek teeth is demonstrated. Lingual aspect of mandibular cheek tooth with 2 deep (small arrows) and 1 shallow (arrowhead) enamel infoldings. This groove lies between the two 'mouse ears' which denote the mesiolingual corner of the tooth (curved arrows). The buccal aspect of mandibular cheek teeth has a single deep infolding of enamel.

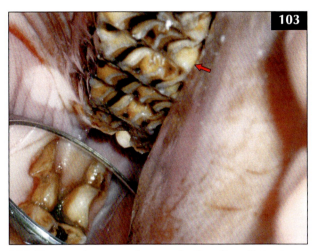

103 The newly erupted premolar has five distinct 'styles' (arrow) resembling an egg carton. These 'styles' become sharp enamel points as the tooth erupts and undergoes attrition. The condition of the infundibula in this tooth are not to be confused with those of the aging patient.

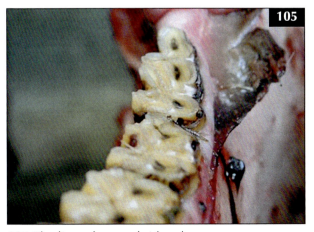

105 The lingual enamel ridges become more prominent distally in the mandibular arcade of this cadaver specimen.

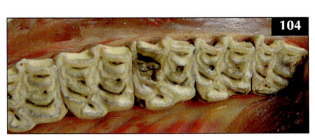

104 The buccal ridges are more prominent on the distal arcade (to the right in the picture).

during mastication and bitting. They may even cause lacerations to the adjacent mucosa. They do not have to cause lacerations to be painful. Sharp points may cause only indentations and not lacerations on the mucosa. The pressure causing these indentations may be uncomfortable. This is evidenced by the improvement in bitting response or mastication comfort and efficiency after routine dental care.

Enamel points may cause hyperkeratosis or callus formation on the buccal mucosa over long exposure (**106**). These calluses are not normal, they are an adaptive response to pathology. Removal of the underlying cause, the sharp enamel points, relieves the hyperkeratotic response and returns the mucosa to normal.

Infundibular foldings are also present on the surface of the new tooth. The condition of the newly erupted infundibulum is not to be confused with the infundibular hypoplasia of an aging patient.

Permanent upper and lower premolars and molars are up to 8 cm long. Merrillat[13] made the measurements shown in *Table 3*.

The mandibular premolars and molars are somewhat longer and may be up to 90 mm in length.

The 6s are usually 0.5–1 cm broader in a mesial-to-distal distance. All 6s are angled distally. The 7s, 8s, and 9s are approximately vertical or have a slight mesial angulation. The 10s and 11s have a significant mesial inclination. This arrangement is seen in figure **107**.

Forces of eruption and mesial drift keep these teeth in close contact with minimal interproximal space. In this way a single masticating battery is created and maintained. The 6 serves as the base or 'retaining wall' for the forces that compress the dental battery. Its broad mesiodistal width and distal angulation 'retain' the forces of eruption of the mesially inclined distal teeth and the force of mesial drift of all teeth.

Not only are the teeth angulated in their position, maxillary cheek teeth are curved slightly in a buccolingual direction when viewed in a facial plane. Maxillary and mandibular premolars are generally straight when viewed laterally. The 8 may have a slight distal curvature. All molars are curved distally, with the degree of curvature increasing distally in the arcade (**107**).

Table 3 Tooth length as measured by Merrillat[13]

Tooth number	Length (mm)
6	48
7	55
8	73
9	68
10	65
11	60

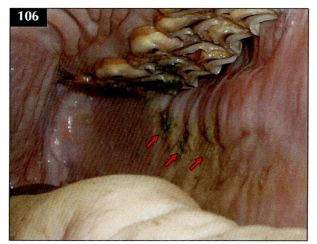

106 Hyperkeratosis of the buccal mucosa occurs from chronic irritation of sharp enamel points (arrows). This condition returns to normal when sharp points are removed.

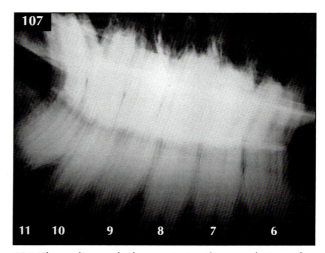

107 The radiograph demonstrates the angulation of the cheek teeth. The teeth are identified by the Triadan system.

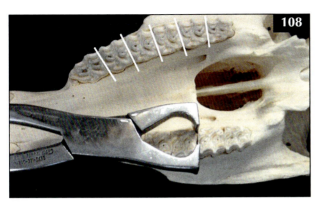

108 The laterally divergent pattern of interproximal spaces on the maxillary arcade is important in placement of molar spreaders.

The interproximal spaces of the upper arcade form a laterally divergent or 'fan-shaped' pattern when viewed from the occlusal surface (**108**). This is important in placement of molar spreader forceps during the extraction process. Mandibular teeth have variably angulated interproximal spaces (**109**), though this variation is regular from horse to horse.

The maxillary arcades are 23% wider than the mandibular arcades.[14] This disparity is termed anisognathism. When the mouth is closed and the incisors are aligned, the maxillary arcades laterally overlap the mandibulars (**110**).

The width between the arcades was measured by Merrillat[13] (*Table 4*). In this study the arcades were measured at about 18–20 cm in length.

When centered and aligned, the equine bite is a closed, level bite anteriorly (incisors) and open posteriorly (cheek teeth).[15] This is opposed to the scissor bite of dogs and cats and the closed bite of man, where posteriors occlude directly and anteriors close in a scissors fashion, with the uppers closing labially to the lowers.

The occlusal angle of cheek teeth has been measured at approximately 10°.[16] This method compared the occlusal surface with the longitudinal axis of mandibular teeth. Cheek teeth are angled buccally, with the apices of the left side angled toward those of the right and the occlusal surfaces angled apart (**111**).

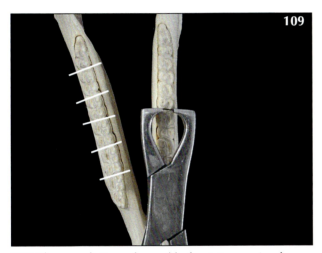

109 The angulation of mandibular interproximal spaces varies within the arcade.

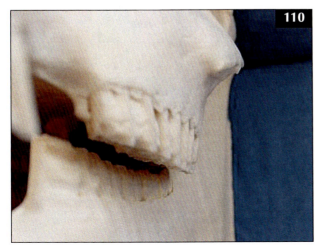

110 The maxillary arcade laterally overlaps the mandibular arcade.

Table 4 Distances between various points on the arcades as determined by Merrillat[13]	
Maxillary arcade	
Teeth number	**Distance between teeth**
6s	57 mm
9s	75 mm
11s	83 mm
Mandibular arcade	
Teeth number	**Distance between teeth**
6s	50 mm
9s	60 mm
11s	75 mm

The result of this angulation is to make the occlusal angle appear to be somewhat steeper, and may explain previous reports suggesting a 15–25° occlusal angle.

The frequently reported observation that distal cheek teeth have a flatter occlusal angle than those located more mesially is not shown in Carmalt's paper in a statistically significant fashion. However, the explanation is in measurement of the angle related to the long axis of the tooth and not to the mandible. In figure **111**, the flatter angle distally in the arcade as related to the mandible is demonstrated. The reason is the more vertical distal cheek teeth versus the slightly more laterally inclined mesial cheek teeth as they lie within the mandible. Thus the occlusal angle

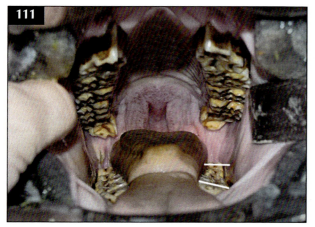

111 The occlusal angle is demonstrated. When measuring the angle as related to the mandible, the occlusal angle becomes flatter distally in the arcade.

may be measured at 10° when referring to the angle of the tooth itself, and 15–25° when observing clinically.

The maxillary arcades form a slightly curved row with the convexity oriented buccally. The degree of curvature varies greatly on an individual, breed, and age basis. Short-headed horses have greater curvature. In general the curvature decreases with age. The curvature of the maxillary arcades is seen in figure **108**. In many individuals the curvature is such that the buccal cusps of upper 10s and 11s are difficult to address unless the clinician has instruments specifically designed for access to this area (**112**, **113**).

The mandibular arcades are straighter or even slightly 'S' curved in some cases (**114**, **115**). This becomes important in addressing the lingual enamel points of the lower 10s. It is important to change the angulation of a file such that it can contact these surfaces. The handle of the file must be moved lingually to contact the lingual surface of the lower 10s. Figure **116** shows failure to contact the lingual 10, while figure **117** shows the slight angulation necessary to reduce these sharp points.

When viewed from the side the occlusal line of the last two and rarely the last three cheek teeth curves dorsally (**118**). This line follows the curvature of the mandible as it continues to the anterior border of the ramus and the curvature of the maxilla as it terminates caudally in the tubercle housing the last molar. This curvature on both arcades is termed the curvature of Spee.[17] Some have mistakenly termed the curvature on the maxillary arcade as the curvature of Wilson;

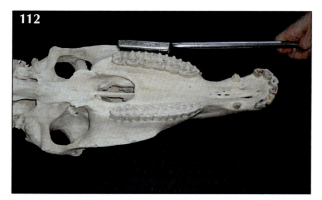

112 A straight file will not reach the buccal cusps of the upper 11s.

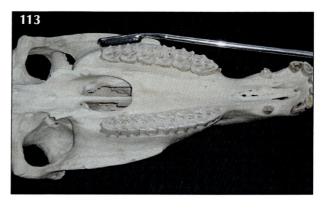

113 A closed angle file reaches the buccal cusps of the upper 10s and 11s.

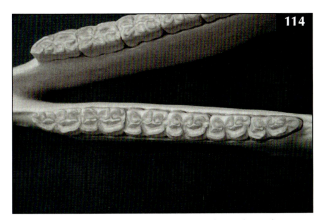

114 The mandibular arcade is straighter than the maxillary arcade.

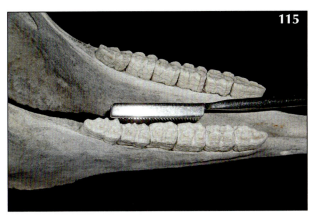

115 Some mandibular arcades have a slight 'S' curve with the lower 10 positioned buccally relative to the other aligned teeth in the arcade.

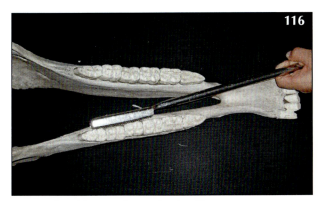

116 In the 'S' curved arcade the file cannot contact the lingual points of the lower 10s if held straight.

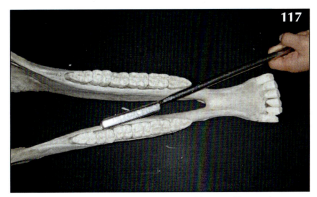

117 When the 10s are positioned buccally in the 'S' curved arcade, the handle of the file is moved lingually in order to contact the lingual enamel points.

118 The curvature of Spee is the term for the dorsal curvature of both upper and lower arcades at their distal termination.

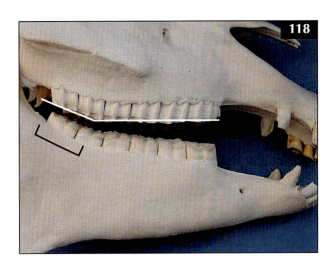

however, this term applies to the angulation of the maxillary molars in the frontal plane in man.[17] It would relate to the occlusal angle in the horse.

The internal space of the tooth occupied by pulp tissue is the *pulp cavity*. The newly erupted cheek tooth has a very large pulp cavity. During the aging process, the pulp cavity is separated into various anatomical parts by further elongation of the tooth and deposition of secondary dentin within the pulp cavity.

The following terms apply to the anatomical divisions of the pulp cavity and are demonstrated in figure **119**:
- **Root canal:** the space in the root occupied by the pulp.
- **Pulp chamber:** the pulp space in the apical part, or base, of the crown from which extend the other parts of the pulp cavity.
- **Pulp horns:** the pulpal extensions into the coronal structure.

Kirkland *et al.*[18] observed various changes in the pulp cavity associated with age. Within 2 years after eruption, roots are formed (**120**).

Four to five years after eruption, the tooth matures by addition of secondary dentin to separate the pulp chamber into mesial and distal parts. In maxillary cheek teeth the presence of the infundibulum does not hasten buccolingual separation of the pulp chamber. The tooth in figure **121** is from an 18-year-old patient whose pulp chamber opens to pulp horns palatally and buccally from the pulp chamber. Teeth at least 7 years of age have completely separated mesial and distal pulp chambers.

Each cheek tooth has at least five pulp horns. Dacre[19] describes a system of numbering pulp horns on the occlusal surface. The general approach to numbering begins by observing the side of the tooth with the sharp enamel points. On maxillary teeth this would be the buccal side and on mandibular teeth this is the lingual side. Once the long side is noted, the most mesial pulp horn on the long side of the tooth is number one. The pulp horns are the brown stained spots on the occlusal surface. On maxillary teeth pulp horn number two is the next distal horn. Horn three is the mesiopalatal brown spot, four is distopalatal, and five is the midpalatal horn. The sequence is followed as one might read a book. The mandibular horns are similarly numbered. The lingual side of the mandibular tooth has three horns numbered one through three from mesial to distal.

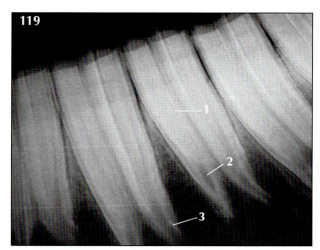

119 The divisions of the pulp cavity are identified. **1**: Pulp horn; **2**: Pulp chambe;r **3**: Root canal.

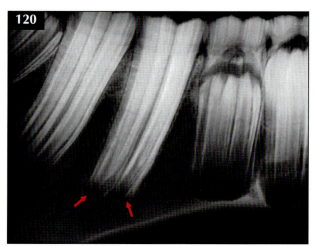

120 The roots of the lower 9 (arrows) are forming in this 3-year-old patient.

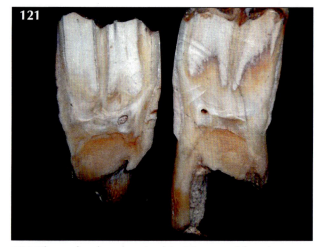

121 The pulp chamber in this 18-year-old patient communicates with pulp horns both palatally and buccally.

The mesiobuccal horn is number four and the distobuccal horn is number five. The normal second premolar has an additional mesial horn numbered six. The numbering system holds that when referring to 'pulp horn six', it is understood to always refer to the mesial pulp horn of the second premolar. The third molar also has additional pulp horns, though the number six is skipped in this sequence. The additional horns are numbered beginning with the number seven, so that seven and eight (when present) are the most distal two horns. Third molars may have up to 11 pulp horns. Figure **122** demonstrates the numbering system for mandibular teeth and figure **123** shows the maxillary system.

The clinical importance of understanding the aging process as it relates to the pulp cavity is in treatment of endodontic disease. In teeth at least 7 years of age, endodontic disease affecting one tooth root can usually be addressed by treatment of only the affected root and pulp chamber. In teeth less than 7 years of age, endodontic disease of one root will spread to involve the entire pulp. Thus in these younger teeth, the entire pulp must be debrided and the cavity treated.

Adult maxillary teeth have three or four roots. Two roots form buccally and one palatally, as seen in figure **124**. The palatal root may split into two roots, a mesial and a distal root, making four in total. Mandibular teeth have two roots, a mesial and a distal root (**125**). The exception is the lower 11 which may have three roots. Mandibular roots are longer than maxillary roots.

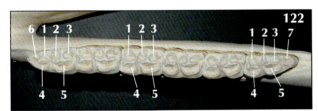

122 The pulp horn numbering system for mandibular cheek teeth is demonstrated.

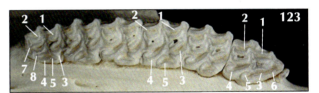

123 The pulp horn numbering system for maxillary cheek teeth is demonstrated.

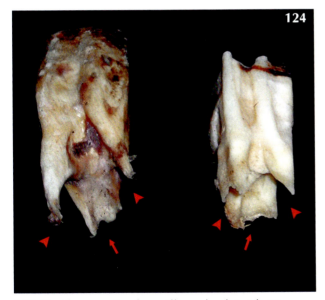

124 The three roots of maxillary cheek teeth are shown. Both teeth have their single palatal root down (arrows) and the two buccal roots up (arrowheads).

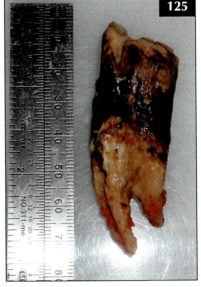

125 The two roots of mandibular cheek teeth are shown.

The lower cheek teeth reside within the mandible, while the upper cheek teeth reside within the maxilla. In young horses the reserve crowns of some of the cheek teeth occupy significant space within the sinuses. In the young adult horse the 6s and 7s do not occupy space within the sinus. The distal 8s and all of the 9s are within the rostral maxillary sinus. The 10s and 11s are within the caudal maxillary sinus. These positons may vary with individuals.

As the head and sinuses lengthen with age and the teeth erupt, less volume of tooth resides within the sinuses. The teeth also undergo mesial drift and therefore their position within the sinuses changes with age. In 1895 Goodall[20] demonstrated these changes by noting the change in position related to the orbit. In the 180-day fetus, this position is located between the last two premolars. At birth it is posterior to the last premolar. At 2 years it is posterior to the second molar, and at 19 years it is posterior to the third molar. Radiographic examination of each patient determines its exact anatomical relationship.

SUMMARY

Detailed understanding and knowledge of dental anatomy are critical in understanding how teeth function; how pathology develops; and correction methods. It also provides a three-dimensional picture in the mind of the operator when performing corrections or surgical treatments. Lack of in-depth anatomical knowledge and relationships of dental structures can result in either failure of treatment or even in further damage. Good patient management requires good anatomical understanding.

REFERENCES

1. Floyd MR. The modified Triadan system: nomenclature for veterinary dentistry. *Journal of Veterinary Dentistry* 1991: **8**(4); 18–19.
2. Wiggs RB, Lobprise HB. *Veterinary Dentistry: Principles and Practice*. Philadelphia: Lippincott-Raven, 1997; pp. 69–70.
3. Mitchell SR, Kempson SA, Dixon PM. Structure of peripheral cementum of normal equine cheek teeth. *Journal of Veterinary Dentistry* 2003: **20**(4); 199–208.
4. St. Clair LE. Teeth. In: Getty R (ed) *Sisson and Grossman's: The Anatomy of the Domestic Animals*, 5th edition, Volume 1. Philadelphia: WB Saunders, 1975; p. 460.
5. Muylle S. Aging. In: Baker GJ, Easley KJ (eds) *Equine Dentistry*, 2nd edition. London: Elsevier Limited, 2005; pp. 55–68.
6. Eisenmenger E, Zetner K. *Veterinary Dentistry*. Philadelphia: Lea and Febiger, 1985; pp. 55–57.
7. St. Clair LE. Teeth. In: Getty R (ed) *Sisson and Grossman's: The Anatomy of the Domestic Animals*, 5th edition, Volume 1. Philadelphia: WB Saunders, 1975; p 465.
8. Colyer JF. Variations and diseases of teeth of horses. *Transactions of the Odontological Society of Great Britain* 1906: **38**; 47–74.
9. Baker GJ. *A Study of Dental Disease in the Horse*. PhD thesis, Glasgow University, 1979; pp. 3–96.
10. Wafa NSY. *A Study of Dental Disease in the Horse*. MVM thesis, University College Dublin, 1974; pp. 1–203.
11. Baker GJ. Some aspects of equine dental decay *Equine Veterinary Journal* 1974: **6**(3); 127–130.
12. Baker GJ. Infundibular embryology, morphology, pathology, and clinical signs in horses. *Conference Proceedings 14th Annual Veterinary Dental Forum* 2000; pp. 296–300.
13. Merrillat LA. *Veterinary Surgery*, Volume 1. Chicago: Alexander Eger, 1906; pp. 32–34.
14. Taylor AC. *An Investigation of Mandibular Width and Related Dental Disorders in the Equine Oral Cavity*. PhD thesis, Coventry University 2001.
15. Wiggs RB. Unpublished manuscript.
16. Carmalt JL. Observations of the cheek tooth occlusal angle in the horse. *Journal of Veterinary Dentistry* 2004: **21**(2); 70–75.
17. Jablonsky S. *Jablonsky's Dictionary of Dentistry*. Florida: Kreiger Pub Co, 1992; p. 221.
18. Kirkland KD, Baker GJ, Marretta SM, *et al*. Effects of aging on the endodontic system, reserve crown, and roots of equine mandibular cheek teeth. *American Journal of Veterinary Research* 1996: **57**(1); 31–38.
19. Dacre I. *A Pathological Study of Equine Dental Disorders*. PhD thesis, The University of Edinburgh, 2003.
20. Goodall TB. The teeth of the horse and illusions to equine dentistry. *Journal of Comparative Pathology and Therapeutics* 1895: **8**; 126–140.

EMBRYOLOGY

David O Klugh   Chapter 4

The embryological development of the tooth is an orderly process of successive steps. Each individual tooth develops as a distinct unit. The process of embryological tooth maturation is similar for all teeth. Interaction between embryological oral epithelial cells and underlying ectomesenchymal cells produces specific stages of development, including bud, cap, and bell stages. Cells undergo proliferation during early stages and subsequently differentiate into progenitors of dentin, enamel, pulp, cementum, and periodontal structures in the later stages of development.

Crown structures, including cusp formation, begin early as thickenings of the internal enamel epithelium during the bell stage. Mineralization of the crown begins at the occlusal surface and proceeds apically. Root formation begins after the crown is fully formed. Periodontal structures develop concomitant with crown lengthening.

INITIAL DEVELOPMENT

During embryogenesis, neural crest cells proliferate and condense to form the dental lamina. Odontogenesis is initiated by chemical signals originating from the epithelium of the dental lamina. The genetically controlled production of signaling molecules such as bone morphogenetic proteins (BMP-2 and BMP-4) initiates precise location and timing of odontogenesis. As tooth formation occurs, epithelium and ectomesenchymal cells proliferate. Both cell types are from neural crest, and therefore ectodermal origin.

Tooth development begins with an ingrowth of epithelial cells of the dental lamina into ectomesenchyme. Studies show that the mitotic index of the epithelial cells is slightly lower than that of the ectomesenchyme, suggesting that part of the process of 'ingrowth' is actually upgrowth of ectomesenchyme.[1]

Tooth development requires both epithelial cells and ectomesenchymal cells. *Initiation* is the process by which development begins via a complex molecular interaction between these two cell types. The timing of the signals to begin the initiation phase is very specific. Multiple molecular interactions are expressed by genetic codes, indicating a predetermined stepwise process.

BUD STAGE

After initiation of odontogenesis, epithelial cells proliferate into the underlying ectomesenchyme, where cells become crowded adjacent to the epithelial bud (**126**).

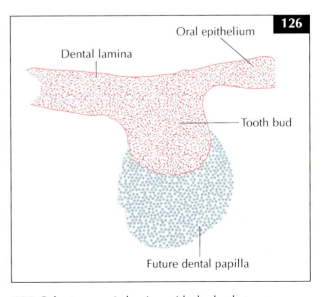

126 Odontogenesis begins with the bud stage.

CAP STAGE

The primary feature of the cap stage is *proliferation* of the epithelial bud accompanied by increased cellular density of adjacent ectomesenchyme. This process is classically referred to as *condensation*. The combined structure of the epithelium and condensed ectomesenchyme is called the *dental organ* or *enamel organ*.

The condensed ectomesenchyme is now referred to as the *dental papilla*. It gives rise to the dentin and pulp of the mature tooth. Another layer of condensed ectomesenchyme cells surrounds the dental organ. This layer is called the *dental follicle*, and gives rise to the supporting tissues of the tooth (cementum, PDL, and alveolar bone) (**127**).

BELL STAGE

Further tooth development is characterized by *differentiation*. The tooth germ proliferates and the collection of related cell types transforms into cells of different morphology and function (**128**). Formation of the *stellate reticulum* occurs as cells in the center of

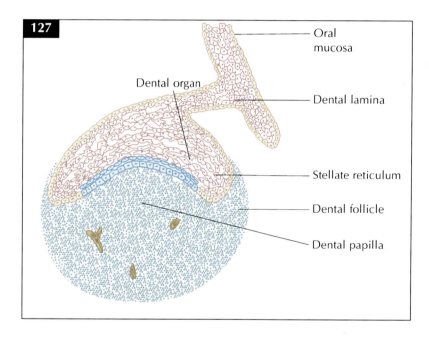

Oral mucosa

Dental organ

Dental lamina

Stellate reticulum

Dental follicle

Dental papilla

127 Cap stage: The dental organ, dental follicle, and dental papilla together constitute the *tooth germ*.

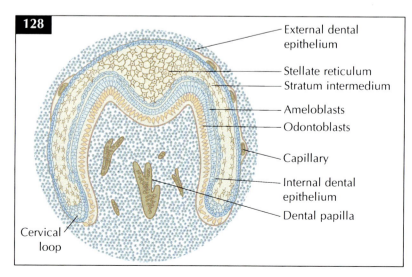

External dental epithelium

Stellate reticulum
Stratum intermedium

Ameloblasts
Odontoblasts

Capillary

Internal dental epithelium

Dental papilla

Cervical loop

128 Tooth development at the bell stage.

the dental organ produce glycosaminoglycans into the extracellular space. As water is attracted by these hydrophilic molecules the space between them increases. Cells maintain desmosomal contact and thus become star-shaped. These cells are destined to become part of the epithelial attachment of the tooth which coalesces with oral epithelium during eruption to form the gingival attachment apparatus.

At the periphery of the dental organ, cells differentiate into cuboidal form to become the *external dental epithelium*. The cells adjacent to the dental papilla form two histologically separate layers. The layer next to the papilla is the *internal dental epithelium*. Between this layer and the stellate reticulum lies the *stratum intermedium*. Together these layers are responsible for formation of enamel.

The junction of the internal dental epithelium and the external dental epithelium is the *cervical loop*. This structure gives rise to the root.

CUSP FORMATION

During the late bud stage of tooth development, a new signaling center develops near the center of the tooth germ. These nondividing cells form a transient population called the *enamel knot*, which serves to regulate the transition from bud to cap stage.[2] As odontogenesis progresses through the cap and bell stages, the primary enamel knot is involved in signaling cervical loop cell proliferation via chemical messengers. When its duties are completed it undergoes apoptosis and disappears almost entirely except for a portion which forms the secondary enamel knot.

It has been suggested that cap stage dental ectomesenchyme regulates primary knot formation, which determines location and morphology of the crown base and location of secondary enamel knots.[2] Secondary enamel knots determine the position and shape of enamel cusps (**129**).

Cellular regulation is carried out by antagonistic interactions of cusp activator messenger molecules such as fibroblast growth factors (FGFs) and cusp inhibitory messenger molecules such as BMPs. These chemical messengers are part of the transforming growth factor-beta family of cytokines.

Cusp formation is another example of the complex interaction between epithelium and mesenchyme. The signaling molecules are transcribed at specific times from genetic codes. The timing of the expression of

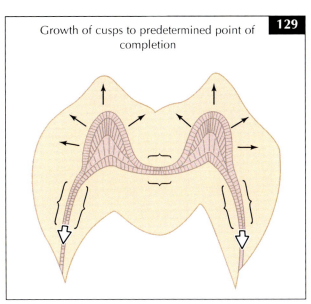

Growth of cusps to predetermined point of completion

129

129 Location of enamel knots determines cusp position and shape.

these genes is a function of genes known as *homeobox genes*, a large group of genes that code the transcription factors responsible for regulating the expression of downstream target genes.[3] These genes code signals that turn on (upregulate) the transcription of other specific genes that produce molecules signaling cells to undergo morphogenesis or discontinue function.

The complex interaction between epithelial and mesenchymal cells is required for tooth generation. Prior to the bud stage the potential to induce tooth morphogenesis resides in the epithelium. At this stage of development only local epithelium is capable of inducing underlying ectomesenchyme differentiation into dental papilla. Additionally, the epithelium of the dental lamina can only specify tooth development in mesenchyme of neural crest origin. After the bud stage, the induction capability of the epithelium shifts to the ectomesenchyme.[3]

CROWN STAGE

DENTINOGENESIS

Formation of dentin (dentinogenesis) precedes formation of enamel (amelogenesis) and signals the beginning of the crown stage of odontogenesis. Cells of the internal dental epithelium located at the tips of the future cusps cease proliferation and undergo morphogenesis into tall columnar cells. Adjacent dental papillary cells differentiate into odontoblasts, the dentin-forming cells. The process of differentiation of the papillary cells is a function of molecular messengers from the internal dental epithelium. If epithelial cells are not present, dentin will not form.[1]

Progressive maturation of internal dental epithelium down the cusp slopes continues tooth development. Production of an organic matrix of collagen, dentin, and ground substance by odontoblasts begins the process of dentinogenesis (**130**). As the matrix is produced, the odontoblasts move toward the center of the dental papilla, leaving behind an extension of cytoplasm around which more matrix is produced. This extension is the odontoblastic process which lies inside the developing dentinal tubule.

AMELOGENESIS

Amelogenesis is the development of enamel (**131**). It starts after a few millimeters of dentin are formed. Ameloblasts develop as the internal dental epithelium cells transform into tall columnar cells. As ameloblasts

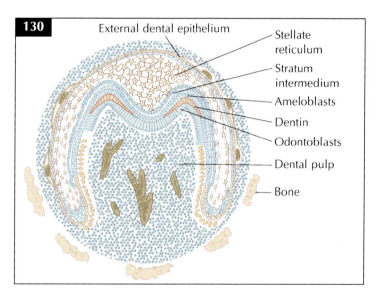

130 Diagram of dentinogenesis.

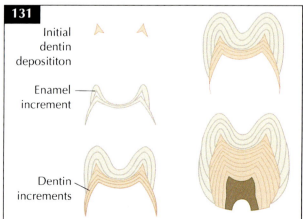

131 The pattern of amelogenesis involves incremental formation of dentin and enamel.

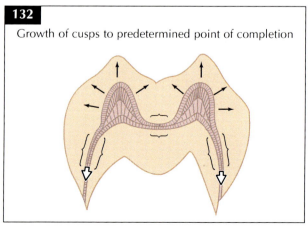

132 Enamel and dentin formation begins at the tips of the cusps.

begin secretion of enamel matrix, overlying cells of the stratum intermedium differentiate into cells assisting in enamel production. Enamel production begins at the occlusal surface.

CROWN MATURATION

The shape of the crown is determined by the internal dental epithelium. In multicusped teeth, such as equine cheek teeth, enamel production begins at the cusp tips and proceeds peripherally as in figure **132**.

As previously described, dentin production by odontobalsts cannot begin without the presence of internal dental epithelium cells. Epithelial cells undergo morphological and functional changes that precede differentiation of papillary cells into odontoblasts. After dentin formation begins, internal dental epithelium cells transform into ameloblasts and produce enamel. This transformation cannot happen without the presence of some already formed dentin. This is an example of reciprocal induction. This process is demonstrated in figure **133**.

133 Reciprocal induction is demonstrated by transformation of internal dental epithelium cells into ameloblasts by the presence of dentin created by odontoblasts. (1) The internal dental epithelium is separated from the dental papilla by the acellular zone. (2) Dental epithelial cells transform and odontoblasts develop from the dental papilla. The cell-free zone has disappeared. (3) Odontoblasts form dentin and retreat towards the pulp. (4) The internal dental epithelium cells have become ameloblasts and form enamel.

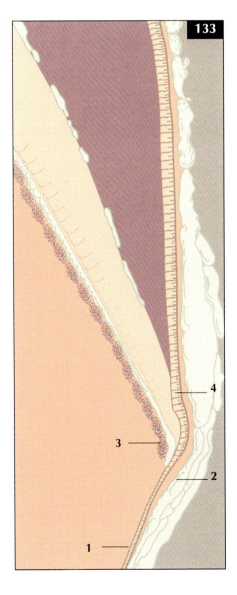

Mineralization of equine teeth begins at the cusp tips and proceeds apically, following the pattern of enamel and dentin formation as in figure **134**. Tooth mineralization begins shortly after enamel deposition and continues after eruption. In cheek teeth, mineralization continues 6–12 months after eruption.[4] Total time of mineralization ranges from 1.5–2.8 years.

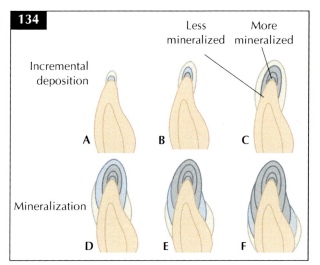

134 Mineralization begins at the occlusal surface and proceeds apically, following the pattern of enamel formation.

ROOT FORMATION

Cell proliferation at the base of the enamel organ continues as the crown develops. The *cervical loop* (junction of the internal and external dental epithelium) becomes *Hertwig's epithelial root sheath*. This structure determines root growth, shape, length, and form. Root formation begins after crown formation is completed. The root begins at the point where enamel formation terminates. Cells of the internal dental epithelium induce more papillary cells to differentiate into odontoblasts of the root. Cells of the outer root sheath differentiate into cementoblasts. These cells produce root cementum. Root elongation occurs as cells of the root sheath proliferate similarly to those that formed the crown.

Multiple roots are formed when a furcation zone develops. This is a process of separation of a single root into two or more roots. Cells of the root sheath in two or more foci grow more rapidly than the rest of the root sheath. These cells grow toward the center of the tooth as a 'tongue' extending centrally in the pulp. Coalescence of these extensions results in the formation of two or three roots (**135**).

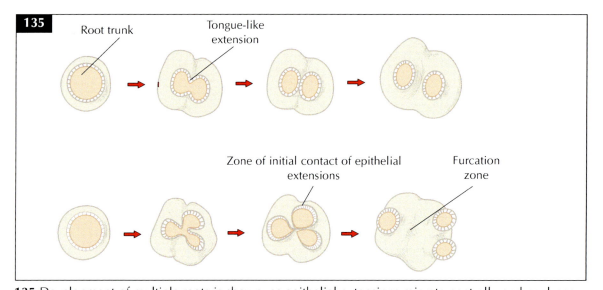

135 Development of multiple roots is shown, as epithelial extensions migrate centrally and coalesce.

SUPPORTING STRUCTURES

The dental follicle is the fibrocellular layer surrounding the dental papilla and dental organ (**136**). Some of these cells migrate peripherally to form alveolar bone. As the root sheath fragments, ectomesenchymal cells of the dental follicle migrate through these spaces and contact dentin. This contact induces them to transform into cementoblasts. Other cells form collagen bundles and produce the PDL. Collagen fiber bundles are imbedded in the cementum on the tooth and in alveolar bone at their other attachment.

SUMMARY

Tooth development requires the interaction of two cell types, epithelium and ectomesenchyme. Both are derived from neural ectoderm. Specific timing of cell morphogenesis, initiation, and termination of function is closely directed by genetic codes transcribing specifically acting molecular messengers. Development through bud, cap, and bell stages involves proliferation and differentiation of soft tissue cells. Dentinogenesis and amelogenesis begin the development of hard tissues. Crown development with cusp formation follows. Cusp form, size, and location are controlled by internal dental epithelium which determines the location of enamel knots. Enamel knots form at the tips of the cusps, and crown maturation extends peripherally and apically from that location. Tooth mineralization continues after eruption for up to 12 months and follows the same occlusal-to-apical pattern of tooth development. Root formation begins after crown formation terminates. Form, length, size, and number of roots are functions of Hertwig's epithelial root sheath. Supporting structures develop concomitant with crown formation from the embryological dental follicle cells. Odontogenesis is summarized in figure **137**.

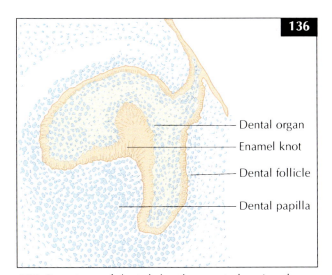

136 Cap stage of dental development showing the dental follicle surrounding the dental organ and dental papilla.

— Dental organ
— Enamel knot
— Dental follicle
— Dental papilla

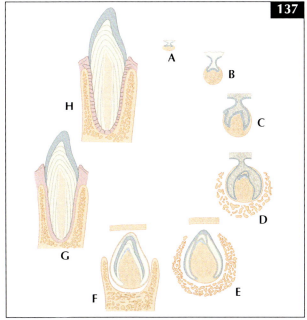

137 Summary of stages of odontogenesis. **A.** Bud; **B.** Cap; **C.** Bell; **D.** and **E.** Dentinogenesis and amelogenesis; **F.** Crown formation; **G.** Root formation and eruption; **H.** Function.

REFERENCES

1. Ten Cate AR. Development of the tooth and its supporting structures. In: Ten Cate, AR (ed) *Oral Histology: Development, Structure, and Function*, 5th edition. St. Louis: Mosby, 1998.
2. Wang X. *Molecular Mechanisms Underlying Morphogenesis and Cell Differentiation*. PhD thesis, University of Helsinki, 2004.
3. Cobourne M. The genetic control of early odontogenesis. *British Journal of Orthodontics* 1999: **26**(1); 21–28.
4. Hoppe KA, Stover SM, Pascoe JR, Amundson R. Tooth enamel biomineralization in extant horses: implications for isotopic microsampling. *Palaeogeography, Palaeoclimatology, Palaeoecology* 2004: **206**; 355–365.

MUSCLES OF MASTICATION

Victor S Cox and David O Klugh   Chapter 5

Mastication is a complex process involving both chewing and manipulation of a food bolus. Tongue and cheek muscles are responsible for movement of the bolus while the muscles of the mandible produce chewing movements. Six muscles move the mandible. All except the sternocepahlicus muscle originate from the skull. These muscles and their main relationship to the mandible are:

- Masseter muscle (lateral).
- Temporalis muscle (dorsal).
- Medial pterygoid muscle (medial).
- Lateral pterygoid muscle (medial).
- Digastricus muscle (medial).
- Occipitomandibularis part (caudal).
- Sternocephalicus muscle (caudal).

All muscles can act individually or to varying degrees in concert with others to create the diverse mandibular motion and forces of mastication. Several authors have described the anatomical features of the muscles of mastication.[1–7]

The masseter muscle is the largest of the six. It is a fan-shaped muscle that originates from the facial crest and zygomatic arch and inserts on the lateral surface of the mandibular body and ramus (**138**).

The action of the masseter muscle is to close the mouth. Contraction also pulls the mandible somewhat rostrally because the muscle fibers originate rostral to their insertion. Likewise, the origin is lateral to the insertion so that when contracted unilaterally the massester muscle pulls the mandible laterally toward the contracting side. The masseter muscle is supplied by the facial, transverse facial, and masseteric arteries. The mandibular nerve supplies the masseter, temporalis, pterygoid, and digastric muscles.

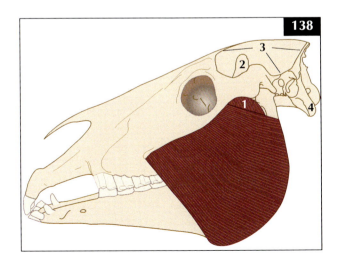

138 The rostral pull of the masseter muscle on the mandible is indicated by the fiber direction of the major part which is superficial. The deep part of the masseter (1) originates from the zygomatic arch. The coronoid process (2) and temporal fossa (3) are attachment sites of the temporalis muscle. The digastricus muscle originates from the paracondylar process (4). (From Cox[3], used by permission.)

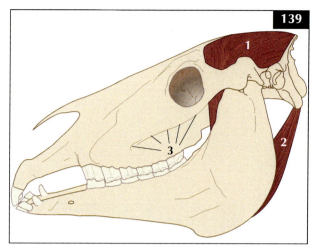

139 The temporalis muscle (1) lies deep to the zygomatic arch and closes the mouth. The occipitomandibularis muscle (2) is shown originating from the paracondylar process. The facial crest (3) is the origin of the masseter muscle. (From Cox[3], used by permission.)

The temporalis muscle originates from the temporal fossa (**138**) and the medial aspect of the zygomatic arch. It inserts on the coronoid process of the mandible and the cranial aspect of the mandibular ramus as shown in figure **139**. Its action is to close the mouth. It is supplied by the superficial, deep temporal, and caudal meningeal arteries.

The pterygoid muscles occupy approximately the same place on the medial side of the mandible as does the masseter muscle on the lateral side. The medial pterygoid muscle is large and has vertically directed fibers while the lateral ptergoid muscle is smaller and has horizontal fibers (**140**).

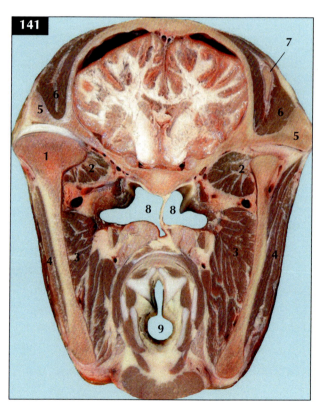

141 Transverse section through the temporomandibular joint (left). 1 = mandibular condyle; 2 = lateral pterygoid muscle; 3 = medial pterygoid muscle; 4 = masseter muscle; 5 = zygomatic arch; 6 = temporalis muscle; 7 = coronoid process of mandible; 8 = guttural pouch; 9 = laryngeal lumen. The articular disc is between 1 and 5 on the left. The right side is more rostral; the skin was removed before cryosectioning. (From Cox[3], used by permission.)

140 Midline view of a bisected skull. The medial pterygoid muscle has a main part (1) and a smaller deep part (2). The lateral pterygoid muscle (3) is dorsal to most of the medial muscle but both are medial to the mandible. Also seen are the digastricus muscle caudal (4), rostral (5), and occipitomandibular (6) parts. (From Cox[3], used by permission.)

The medial pterygoid muscle originates from the crest formed by the pterygoid process of the basisphenoid and palatine bones. It fans out and inserts on the concave medial surface of the ramus of the mandible and continues to the medial lip of the ventral border of the mandible. Unilateral contraction moves the mandible somewhat sidewards while bilateral contraction raises the mandible. The medial pterygoid muscle is supplied by the maxillary and mandibular arteries.

The lateral pterygoid muscle (**140**) lies between the mandibular condyle and the guttural pouch where it is best observed in a cross-section of the head at the level of the temporomandibular joint (**141**). It originates on the lateral surface of the pterygoid process of the basisphenoid bone. It inserts on the medial surface of the neck and rostral border of the mandibular condyle (**141**) and also the articular disc. Contracting bilaterally, these muscles cause protrusion or rostal movement of the mandible. Unilateral contraction causes the attached mandibular condyle to move medially (sidewards movement of the mandible as a whole).

The digastricus muscle (**140**) is a complex muscle made up of rostral and caudal bellies connected by an intermediate tendon. These three segments of the muscle could be referred to as the digastricus proper. In addition, the occitipitomandibularis portion of the muscle and the caudal belly of the digastricus proper have a common origin from the paracondylar process of the occipital bone. This process is so named because it lies adjacent to the occipital condyle. The occipitomandibularis part inserts on the caudal border of the mandible but the digastricus proper inserts on the medial surface of the ventral border of the mandible. The intermediate tendon penetrates the tendon of insertion of the stylohyoideus muscle near the rostral belly.[4] The digastricus muscle is the main muscle for opening the mouth. When the mouth is held closed by other muscles, bilateral contraction of the digastricus proper causes upward movement of the tongue and larynx due to the connection with the stylohyoideus muscle tendon of insertion. This is the first step in deglutition. While the caudal parts of the digastricus muscle are innervated by the mandibular nerve, the rostral belly is supplied by the facial nerve. Arterial supply is from the external carotid and lingual arteries.

The sternocephalicus muscle (**142**) is a long muscle extending along the ventral neck from the sternum to the caudal border of the mandibular ramus. The tendon of insertion is thinly covered by the parotid salivary gland but is easily palpated when made tense by elevation and extension of the head. Such palpation is key to locating Viborg's triangle for which the sternocephalicus muscle forms the dorsal/caudal border. It assists in flexing and inclining the head in addition to opening the mouth and pulling the mandible in a caudal direction when the head is extended. It is supplied by the carotid artery and the ventral branch of the accessory nerve (cranial nerve XI).

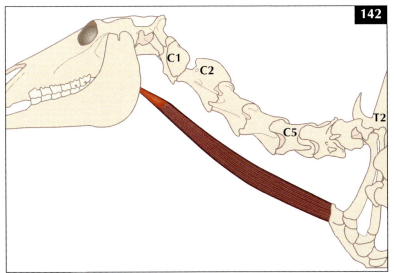

142 The sternocephalicus muscle extends from the sternum to the caudal edge of the ramus of the mandible. (From Cox[3], used by permission.)

Multiple influences cause opening of the mouth. Gravity is assisted by contraction of the digastricus and sternocephalicus muscles. The mandible is pulled caudally by the sternocephalicus and laterally by the contraction of the contralateral medial and lateral pterygoid muscles. The caudal-to-rostral and lateral-to-medial diagonal movement together with the closing movement of the mandible are accomplished by contraction of the masseter and temporalis muscles and the ipsilateral pterygoid muscles. The extent of caudal movement can be measured clinically[8] and is due to tensing the sternocephalicus muscle as the head is raised and extended by the observer.

The mandible can move in many directions. The articulation of the condyle is structured so that the primary motion is hinge-like around a transverse axis. In protrusion and retraction the mandible glides on the articular surface. Transverse movements are accomplished by protrusion of one side and retraction of the opposite side. Subtle movements of mastication can be achieved by unilateral contraction of one muscle group or another.

SUMMARY

The muscles of mastication deliver varying forces to the teeth during mastication in compensation for feed characteristics. Knowledge of the origins, insertions, and actions of both unilateral and bilateral contraction of these muscles, alone and in concert, assists in clarification of the effects of mastication forces on teeth. These forces can result in abnormal attrition of teeth and malocclusions. The practitioner's ability to correct malocclusions is greatly enhanced by understanding the actions of muscles during mastication.

REFERENCES

1. Budras K-D. *Anatomy of the Horse: an Illustrated Text*. Hannover: Schlütersche GmbH, 2003; pp. 34–35.
2. Clayton HM, Flood PF, Rosenstein DS. *Clinical Anatomy of the Horse*. Edinburgh: Mosby, Elsevier, 2005; pp. 12, 23.
3. Cox VS. *Minnesota Ungulate Dissection Guide*, 3rd edition. St. Paul: Self published, 2006.
4. Dyce KM, Sack WO, Wensing CJG. *Textbook of Veterinary Anatomy*, 3rd edition. Philadelphia: WB Saunders, 2002; pp. 495–496.
5. Konig HE, Liebich HG. *Veterinary Anatomy of Domestic Mammals: Textbook and Colour Atlas*. Stuttgart: Schattauer, 2004; pp. 103–106.
6. Nickel R, Schummer A, Seiferle E. *The Anatomy of the Domestic Animals, Volume 1, The Locomotor System*. Berlin: Verlag Paul Parey, 1986; pp. 261–263.
7. Sisson S. Equine myology. In: Getty R (ed) *Sisson and Grossman's: The Anatomy of Domestic Animals*, Volume 1, 5th Edition. Philadelphia: WB Saunders, 1985; pp. 384–386.
8. Carmalt JL, Townsend HGG, Allen AL. A preliminary study to examine the effects of dental floatation on rostro-caudal movement of the equine mandible. *Journal of the American Veterinary Medical Association* 2003: **223**(5); 666–669.

PRINCIPLES OF MASTICATION BIOMECHANICS

David O Klugh   Chapter 6

The malocclusions commonly seen in equine dental practice are a result of the complex interactions of the range of motion of the mandible in mastication and the variety of forces within that range of motion that are delivered to the tooth. Mastication forces and motion cause attrition of teeth from abrasion by feeds. Certain teeth may suffer more attrition than others in the same arcade. Opposing teeth erupt to compensate and maintain dental contact. While some teeth in an arcade suffer attrition, others endure overgrowth. The result is an uneven arcade with a malocclusion. The combination of attrition and overgrowth within the same arcade demonstrates the extent and variation in forces produced in mastication, and sensed and compensated for by adapting teeth and associated structures.

Attrition reflects forces delivered to occluding teeth. It is instructive to understand and observe the physiology and biomechanics of mandibular motion and the responses of teeth to forces of mastication. Deviations from normal attrition rate affect both the future development of a malocclusion and the longevity of the tooth and arcade. Faster attrition results in premature expiration of a tooth. Slower attrition improves tooth longevity. Rates of attrition are difficult to quantify. Eruption reflects attrition. Therefore, measurement of eruption rates is an accurate reflection of the forces delivered to, and attrition suffered by, the tooth.

A review of the anatomical structures involved in mandibular motion is helpful to gain a clear understanding of mastication motion and the effects on teeth and surrounding structures.

ANATOMY OF THE TEMPOROMANDIBULAR JOINT

The temporomandibular joint is the articulation between the temporal bone of the skull and the mandible. The right and left mandibles are connected at the mandibular symphysis, making the movements of both sides connected. The articulation may, therefore, be considered as the 'craniomandibular articulation'.[1]

When viewed laterally the temporal articulation consists of a mandibular fossa, a concave structure, and the articular tubercle, a convex structure[2] seen in figure **143**. Caudal to the mandibular fossa is the

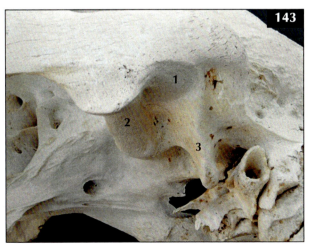

143 Lateral view of the temporal articulation of the temporomandibular joint. The concave mandibular fossa (1), convex articular tubercle (2), and retroarticular process (3) are identified.

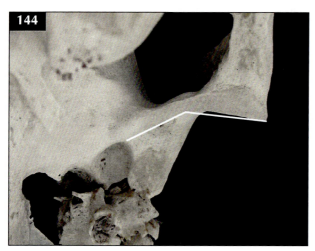

144 Frontal plane of the articular tubercle. The tubercle is concave in this plane.

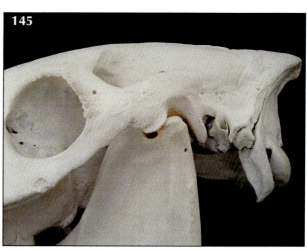

145 The mandible is in a closed position with the mandibular condyle in the mandibular fossa of the temporal bone.

retroarticular process. In a frontal plane the articular tubercle is concave (**144**).

The mandible has an articular condyle which is convex and elongated transversely. The joint surfaces are composed of fibrocartilage instead of hyaline cartilage.[3]

The temporomandibular joint is a diarthrodial or synovial joint[4] with a fibrocartilaginous disk. This disk is molded to fit the surfaces of the articular tubercle of the temporal bone and the condyle of the mandible. The perimeter of the disk is connected to the joint capsule.[5]

The articular disk separates the joint into two compartments, dorsal and ventral. The dorsal compartment is larger. All compartments were connected in a study of six cadavers.[6] Another study of 12 cadavers observed separation of the dorsal and ventral compartments.[7]

FUNCTION OF THE TEMPOROMANDIBULAR JOINT MOTION

The temporomandibular joint is classified as a ginglymoarthrodial joint.[8] It has two types of motion: ginglymoid or hinge motion, and arthrodial or sliding motion.

When the mouth is closed the mandibular condyle rests in the mandibular fossa of the temporal bone (**145**).

When the mouth is open slightly, as in nipping grass, the primary action is ginglymoid (hinge) movement of the ventral compartment[9] of the joint. When wider opening occurs, as in prehending hay or an apple, or when grinding soft feeds, arthrodial (sliding) movement of the dorsal compartment[9] predominates as the mouth is opened and the mandible is protruded. Protrusion (anterior movement) and retrusion (posterior movement) involve sliding of the mandible and articular disk over the articular tubercle and mandibular fossa.[10]

In the horse, passive protrusion and retrusion have been demonstrated by position change of the mandible when the head is raised and lowered.[11] Active protrusion is observed when horses eat grass. The mandible is protruded to maximize incisor contact in nipping of grass stems and leaves (**146**).

NORMAL MASTICATION MOTION

In mastication, mandibular movement involves complex combinations of the above motions. Protrusion or retrusion on one side is compensated for by opposite motion on the contralateral side. Mastication involves both diarthrodial and ginglymoid motion.

Repetitive motions of opening, closing, and sliding of the mandible and mandibular teeth across the maxillary arcades comprise the mastication cycle. In equines the mastication cycle is divided into three

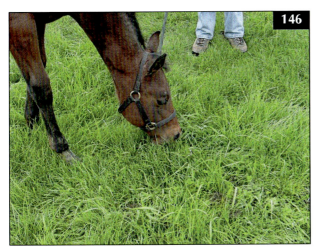

146 Active protrusion of the mandible in grass consumption is demonstrated in this foal with a mild overbite. Note the stretching of the throatlatch accompanying mandibular protrusion.

phases: the opening stroke, the closing stroke, and the power stroke.[12]

The opening stroke involves mandibular depression, lateral movement, and slight retrusion on the side of mastication. The closing stroke involves mandibular elevation and slight medial and rostral movement. When feed becomes compressed between the arcades, the power stroke begins. This stroke involves compression by the mandible, with shearing forces resulting from grinding motion of the mandible moving diagonally across the maxillary arcade in a lateral-to-medial and caudal-to-rostral direction.

The horse first selects feed material with its lips and grasps it with its incisors and tongue. Blades of grass are grasped with the incisors and severed as the horse tips or twists its head. Then the tongue and cheeks work with the first and second cheek teeth to begin the process of feedstuff breakdown by funneling feed into the grinding apparatus. It is helpful to think of the first two cheek teeth as a 'prehensile apparatus' grasping and positioning feed for the mastication battery. Repeated mandibular movement previously described breaks feed materials into smaller pieces as it is moved caudally and finally swallowed. Hardest feeds are crushed in the most distal part of the arcades. Softer feeds are ground by the middle portion of the arcades.

It is important to understand the importance of the caudal-to-rostral direction of mastication and the associated forces delivered to the tooth. As previously described, the arthrodial (sliding) motion of the mandible allows for caudal-to-rostral movement of the mandible. The fibers of the masseter muscle are directed in a disto-lateral and only slightly ventral direction from the facial crest to the ramus of the mandible (see **138**). The angulation as viewed from the side of teeth at the curvature of Spee presents a perfect occlusal surface angle for maximal force distribution in crushing hard feeds during caudal-to-rostral mandibular movement. As these feeds are crushed, the mandible moves palatally, finishing the job of mastication.

The caudal-to-rostral motion is also important in grinding soft feeds in the rostral portion of the arcade. The mandible undergoes more of the caudal-to-rostral motion in masticating soft feeds (see Changes in mastication range of motion, below).

The angulation of the occlusal surface and motion of the mandible in its caudolateral to rostromedial direction are assisted by the tongue, cheeks, and the 18 pairs of palatal ridges to gradually 'auger' feed material caudally.[13] Confirmation of this action is observed in many geriatric horses when reduced occlusion results in quidding, or dropping partly chewed boluses of hay or grass (see **155**). Many of these boluses are in the form of twisted spirals of long stemmed hay or grass as they are discharged from the oral cavity instead of swallowed.

NORMAL OCCLUSION

The normal equine bite is closed anteriorly (incisors in contact) and open posteriorly (premolars and molars not in contact) when the mandible is at rest in centric relationship. The jaws should be of similar length, and the arcades should be exactly the same length. The anisognathic relationship of the premolars and molars should have the lingual cusps of the mandibular teeth positioned immediately below the palatal cusps of the maxillary teeth (see further discussion in Chapter 18: Principles of orthodontics). With the cheek retracted and viewed as described in Chapter 2: Dental examination, the cheek teeth can be further evaluated for normal functional relationship:
1. The occlusal surfaces should be even, though not flat, back to the curvature of Spee.
2. The occlusal surfaces of both arcades should be parallel.

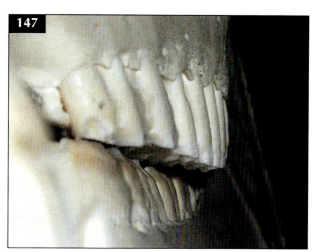

147 Normal occlusion involves contact of all teeth on one side at the same time.

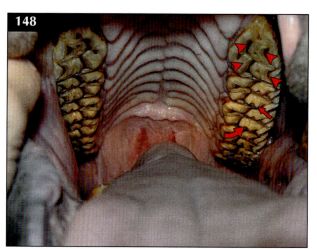

148 The infundibulum is positioned in the middle of the tooth. On either side it is associated with pulp horns, easily identified as brown stained spots on the tooth surface (arrowheads). When the mouth is viewed as in this picture, the pulp horns are aligned distally, facilitating their identification. The borders of the infundibulum are identified as slightly protuberant enamel ridges next to the pulp horns. The buccal border is identified with an arrow, while the palatal ridge is marked with a curved arrow.

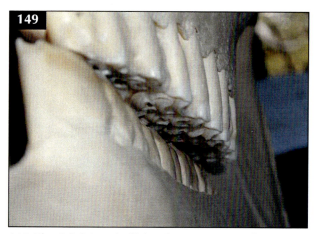

149 The POC is at half the distance across the maxillary occlusal surface in a horse on a pasture diet.

3. The occlusal angle should be about 15°.
4. The mandible is moved laterally, moving the teeth into contact. All teeth should contact at the same time (**147**).
5. The lateral margin of the lower arcade contacts the occlusal surface of the maxillary arcade at the POC. This point is noted.

The POC is best observed on the upper third or fourth premolar when the cheek is retracted and the mouth closed. It represents the end point of the power stroke of the mastication, where incisor contact occurs. As incisor contact occurs, the power stroke terminates and the mandible is returned to the opening stroke and the cycle repeats. In most horses, the POC is half to two-thirds of the distance from medial to lateral on the upper arcade. The half-way point is easily located in most patients as the palatal border of the infundibulum. This anatomical location is demonstrated in figure **148**. In horses on pasture, the POC is commonly at the half-way point, or at the palatal border of the infundibulum (**149**). In horses stabled and fed hay and grain the POC lies near the 'two-thirds point', or at the buccal margin of the infundibulum (**150**). This point is positioned at the lateral border of the infundibulum in most patients. The POC represents a baseline measurement of occlusal contact.

When viewed from the side, there is a normal line of occlusion from the 6 to the 11. This line should be straight from the 6 to the 9 or 10 until the curvature of Spee carries it dorsally. This line is demonstrated in figure **151**.

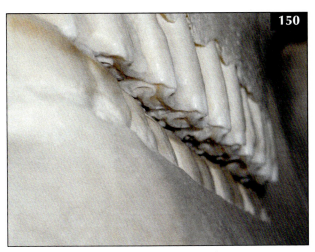

150 The POC at is two-thirds of the distance across the maxillary occlusal surface in a horse on a diet of hay and grain.

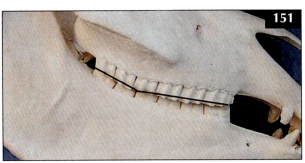

151 The line of occlusion viewed from the side is straight from the 6 to the 9 or 10, from which point it curves dorsally as the curvature of Spee involving the 10s and 11s.

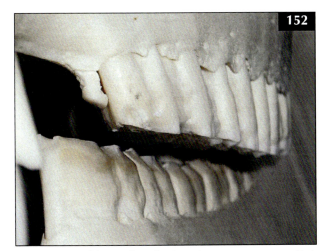

152 A normal line of occlusion demonstrates parallel occlusal surfaces, even interdental space, and normal occlusal angle.

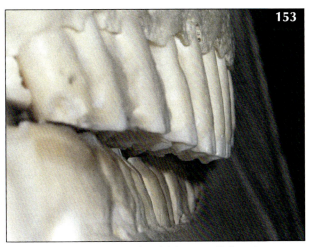

153 Occlusal surfaces should be parallel and meet together.

The line of occlusion can be best observed in the patient with the cheek retracted. The occlusal plane is noted, and any alterations to the normal even line are identified. These overlong teeth are characterized and estimations of the amount of reduction necessary for correction are made. The normal view at rest is seen in figure **152**.

When observing the occlusal line with buccal retractor and head light, the arcades should present parallel occlusal surfaces. When passively moving the mandible laterally, all teeth should contact together (**153**).

EFFECTS ON RATE OF ERUPTION AND ATTRITION

When forces and motion are normal, and occlusion is therefore normal, the rate of eruption of teeth is equal to the rate of attrition in the hypsodont patient. Factors adversely affecting the rate of attrition of the horse's teeth include abnormally high forces delivered to the occlusal surface and abnormal construction of the teeth.

When the tooth is constructed of developmentally abnormal enamel or dentin, or when mineralization of these tissues is reduced, abnormally high rates of attrition may occur.

Abnormal development is random. Excessive attrition of teeth appears to have regular patterns. This suggests that the primary cause of excessive attrition is related more to the forces delivered to the tooth than to its construction.

Physiology of eruption is discussed in Chapter 8: Eruption and shedding of teeth. Responsibility for dental eruption lies with the PDL. As discussed earlier, eruption compensates attrition. However, tooth support structures, including the PDL and alveolar bone, undergo certain adaptations to increased stress. The PDL responds to stresses placed on it during mastication by increasing the size and number of principal fibers when forces are increased. Rates of eruption are higher if stress is beyond a compensatory threshold. Alveolar bone undergoes sclerosis.

The eruption rate of equine teeth is generally thought to be about 2–3 mm per year.[14] In clinical practice rates of eruption vary. In all newly erupting adult teeth the rate is rapid until normal occlusion is reached. As the horse ages, the rate of eruption slows until in a geriatric horse the rate is quite slow.

Rates of eruption vary with other factors such as age, diet, and frequency of occlusal equilibration.[15] Horses on lush pasture for at least 12 hr/day for at least 6 months of the year have slower eruption rates that are more even throughout the arcade. In horses that have at least three occlusal equilibrations performed 1 year apart, rates of eruption are slowed.

The reduction in rate of eruption results from more even force distribution on the arcade; since forces are not focused on one spot on the arcade, the tooth is under less stress during mastication. PDL fiber size and number return to normal and the rate of eruption slows to normal.

CHANGES IN MASTICATION RANGE OF MOTION

The range of motion of the mandible can be affected by numerous conditions induced by traumatic, congenital, idiopathic, and iatrogenic influences. Individual style or habitual variations are probably involved. This concept is demonstrated in the subtle variations observed among horses with the same basic malocclusion pattern. One horse may have a large upper hook, while another's may be small. The forces causing the development of both are similar.

Diet also affects mandibular range of motion. Observations of horses eating lush, moist feeds such as green pasture reveal that their range of motion is larger than that of horses on drier, harder feeds.[16–18] This principle is demonstrated in figure **154** as a summary of research done by Leue in 1941.[17] There is wider lateral excursion with more caudal-to-rostral component in soft feeds since they require less crushing force. These feeds are masticated in a grinding motion.

The concept of the 'vicious cycle' is important in the development of malocclusions. That is to say, all malocclusions left untreated get worse instead of

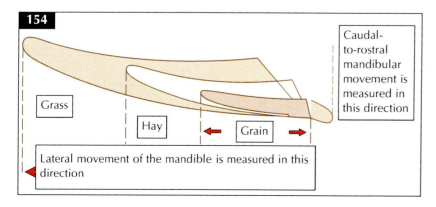

154 Mandibular range of motion varies with hardness of feeds. This diagram demonstrates variation with grains, hay, and grass. (Redrawn from Leue.[17])

better as time progresses. Any alteration in the range of motion of the mandible causes the full, complete, maximum range of motion to be reduced. As range of motion is reduced, uneven attrition results. While eruption continues, a protuberance develops on the arcade. Since there is suboptimal range of motion, this condition never resolves without outside intervention.

DEVELOPMENT OF MALOCCLUSIONS

Forces of mastication delivered to the tooth are sensed by the PDL and alveolar bone. These structures are designed to manage a wide range of forces. Forces of a magnitude within normal range are sensed by these structures and initiate certain adaptive changes in their structure. Forces of a magnitude outside this range result in different adaptive changes.

Sensation of a range of forces is necessary for the entire periodontium to maintain its structural integrity. Forces below normal result in atrophy of the PDL and decreased density of alveolar bone. Forces greater than normal result in significant structural changes.

Forces delivered to the tooth during mastication are both tipping and compressive. Increased magnitude of forces may be light or heavy. Light forces result in structural changes that are significantly different from those resulting from heavy forces.

When light forces are sensed by the PDL, principal fibers increase in size and number, while alveolar bone and trabeculae become more dense. Tooth contact is maintained by the eruptive process as opposing teeth suffer attrition. Eruption rates increase as numbers of fibroblasts escalate with addition of principal fibers. This is a compensation mechanism for excessive attrition, and reflects the forces of mastication at this site on the arcade.

When forces become heavy, and well beyond the threshold of compensation by the periodontium, further pathological changes occur. PDL fibers mineralize, alveolar bone becomes thicker and more dense, and the periodontium becomes sclerosed. Eruption is slowed or arrested if ankylosis occurs.

Differences in range of motion of the mandible during mastication of hard versus soft feeds have been shown. Changes in magnitude of the forces delivered within the range of motion also exist. When mandibular range of motion is reduced, shearing forces are reduced and crushing forces are increased. Additionally, crushing forces are localized on specific segments of the arcade. This phenomenon is demonstrated by the repeatable pattern of wave malocclusion.

In a normal range of motion, as in consumption of green grass pasture, crushing forces are minimized and shearing forces of grinding motion are maximized. Larger range of motion distributes forces over a larger proportion of the arcade.

PHYSIOLOGY OF MALOCCLUSION CORRECTION

What are the specific observable conditions seen during examination of malocclusions? What are the underlying changes in physiology that cause them? What exactly do corrective methods achieve physiologically? These questions lie at the heart of diagnosis of equine dental disorders. Full understanding of their answers leads to correct treatment with resolution of underlying pathology.

The basic observable condition in malocclusions is a disharmony in the rates of attrition and eruption. An overlong tooth has either undergone decreased attrition or increased rate of eruption, or possibly both. A short tooth may be normal, have excessive attrition or decreased eruption, or may have undergone ankylosis of the alveolar bone and PDL.

Exaggerated attrition and eruption result from forces of a magnitude greater than normal that are focused on specific arcade segments. The malocclusion develops further as dental interlock results in a vicious cycle of ever increasing forces that cannot resolve without outside intervention.

Economically and technically feasible procedures and materials do not yet exist for rebuilding the excessively worn tooth to a normal occlusal level. As time passes, materials and techniques will be developed.

An overlong tooth that has undergone a decreased rate of attrition is easily addressed by routine occlusal equilibration.

PDL ankylosis is not uncommon, especially in geriatric patients. In such cases, longstanding malocclusions cannot routinely be returned to normal.

The underlying goal of correction of malocclusions is to return occlusion and mastication range of motion to normal.

This produces mastication forces that result in equal, balanced occlusion. Occlusal equilibration should achieve even arcades and normal occlusion. In so doing, exaggerated rates of eruption are reduced, reduced range of motion is returned to normal and forces are spread more evenly across the arcades.

SUMMARY

Normal occlusion is recognized as even occlusion. The normal alignment of teeth is a straight line from the 6s to the 10s where the line curves dorsally to include the 11s. Individual variations occur, where the dorsal curvature (of Spee) begins at the 9s.

Abnormal physiological events leading to the development of malocclusions include uneven and abnormal rates of attrition and eruption. Increased or decreased forces resulting from reduced range of motion are delivered to specific arcade segments. Changes in mandibular range of motion related to feed types are major factors in the development of abnormal forces. Dental physiology responds to the abnormal forces by creating malocclusions.

Correction of pathological events involves addressing abnormal forces, i.e. return to normal. Equilibration of forces involves correction of anatomical and physiological events. Occlusal equilibration is the process of reduction of the clinical crown in order to facilitate correction of pathological force distribution during mastication.

REFERENCES

1. Dubrul EL. Oral anatomy. In: Sicher H, Dubrul EL (eds) *The Craniomandibular Articulation*, 8th edition. India: AITBS Publishers & Distributor, 1996; pp. 107–131.
2. Hillmann DJ. Skull. In: Getty R (ed) *Sisson and Grossman's: The Anatomy of the Domestic Animals*, 5th edition, Volume 1. Philadelphia: WB Saunders, 1975; pp. 318–348.
3. Moll HD, May KA. A review of conditions of the equine temporomandibular joint. *Proceedings 48th Annual Convention of American Assocation of Equine Practitioners* 2002; pp. 240–243.
4. Baker GJ. Equine temporomandibular joints (TMJ); morphology, function, and clinical disease. *Proceedings 48th Annual Convention of American Assocation of Equine Practitioners* 2002; pp. 442–447.
5. Sisson S. Equine syndesmology. In: Getty R (ed) *Sisson and Grossman's: The Anatomy of the Domestic Animals*, 5th edition, Volume 1. Philadelphia: WB Saunders, 1975; pp. 349–375.
6. Rosenstein DS, Bullock MF, Ocelo PJ, Clayton, HM. Arthrocentesis of the temporomandibular joint in adult horses. *American Journal of Veterinary Research* 2001: **62**; 729–733.
7. Rodriguez MJ, Agut A, Gil F, Latorre R. Anatomy of the temporomandibular joint: a study by gross dissection vascular injection and section. *Equine Veterinary Journal* 2006: **38**(2); 143–147.
8. Jablonsky S. *Jablonsky's Dictionary of Dentistry*. Florida: Kreiger Pub Co., 1992; p. 432.
9. Ramzan PHL. The temporomandibular joint: component of clinical complexity. *Equine Veterinary Journal* 2006: **38**(2); 102–104.
10. Gray H. The Articulations. In: Pick TP, Howden R (eds) *Anatomy, Descriptive and Surgical*. New York: Gramercy Books, 1977; p. 233.
11. Carmalt JL, Townsend HGG, Allen AL. A preliminary study to examine the effects of dental flotation on rostro-caudal movement of the equine mandible. *Journal of the American Veterinary Medical Association* 2003: **223**(5); 666–669.
12. Baker GJ. Dental physiology. In: Baker, GJ and Easley J (eds) *Equine Dentistry*, 2nd edition. London: WB Saunders, 2005; 49–54.
13. Baker GJ. Dental physiology. In: Baker, GJ and Easley J (eds) *Equine Dentistry*, 2nd edition. London: WB Saunders, 2005; pp. 29–34.
14. Baker GJ. Oral examination and diagnosis: management of oral diseases. In: Harvey CE (ed) *Veterinary Dentistry*. Philadelphia: WB Saunders, 1985; pp. 217–228.
15. Klugh DO. Measurement of rates of eruption in equine 2nd premolars. *Conference Proceedings 15th Annual Veterinary Dental Forum* 2001; pp. 178–183.
16. Easley J. Equine dental development and anatomy. *Proceedings 42nd Annual Convention of the American Association of Equine Practitioners* 1996; p. 1.
17. Leue G. *Beizehungen zwischen Zahnanomalien und Verdaungsstorungen biem Pferde unter Heranzeihung von Kaubildern*. Veterinary Medicine thesis, Hanover; pp. 170–174.
18. Bonin SJ. *Three dimensional kinematics of the equine temporomandibular joint*. MS thesis, Michigan State University, 2001.

PRINCIPLES OF OCCLUSAL EQUILIBRATION

David O Klugh   Chapter 7

The basic task of equine dentistry is occlusal equilibration. This term refers to the reduction of tooth overgrowth to a normal occlusal level for the purpose of correcting abnormal forces of mastication, equalizing forces delivered throughout the arcade, and relieving abnormal conditions causing discomfort.

The hypsodont nature of the equine tooth gives it a very dynamic character. It is by definition continuously erupting. This means that the tooth undergoes constant physical and physiological activity. Continuous metabolic and physical activity means high cellular activity and active remodeling of tissue. Hypsodont teeth are therefore primed to readily respond to forces, both normal and abnormal. They do so by altering rates of eruption and by changing attachment character, such as in alveolar sclerosis or thickened and more numerous PDL fibers. The constant dynamics and ability to compensate separates hypsodont teeth from brachydont teeth. Consideration of these dynamics, therefore, separates equine dentistry from dentistry of other species and must be kept in the front of the mind of the equine dental practitioner.

The need for dental care in equine veterinary dentistry is no different from the need for dental care in other species. There are three reasons horses need dental care:

- Relief of immediate causes of pain.
- Proper alignment of teeth and arcades.
- Longevity of all teeth.

All contribute to patient comfort and efficient mastication.

Historically, various clinical signs have been used as indicators for the need for dental care in the equine patient. These include such problems as:

- Foul breath.
- Weight loss.
- Head tossing.
- Dropping feed (quidding) (**155**).
- Bitting problems: stiffness, resisting, refusal to take a lead (**156**).

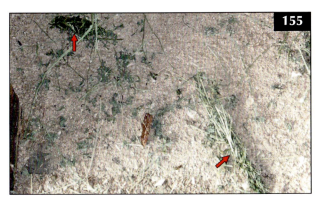

155 Partly chewed boluses, or quids, of hay are lost by the patient (arrows). The hay is twisted during the early part of mastication as the feed enters the mastication 'auger'.

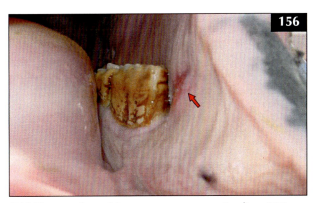

156 Trauma from bit pressure on a protruding 306 (arrow).

- Soaking food before eating.
- Large pieces of undigested food in feces.
- Facial swelling (**157**).
- Feed packing (**158**).
- Colic.
- Eating slowly.
- Chewing abnormalities.

While these signs frequently indicate dental disease, they are usually only present in cases of severe dental disease. Many of these problems are irreversible by the time they are clinically evident. In

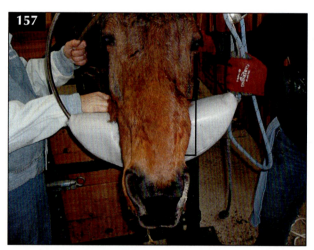

157 The bracket indicates an area of facial swelling.

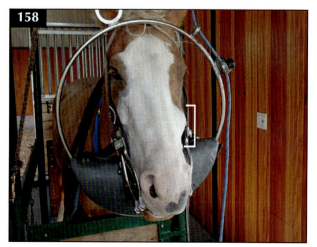

158 This patient exhibits signs referable to feed packing on the buccal aspect of the left maxillary arcade (bracket).

such cases, necessary dental procedures are usually salvage procedures. The ideal approach is early recognition and prevention. This is achieved by regular dental care.

The purpose of occlusal equilibration is correction of abnormal forces, by the correction of uneven arcades and return of the arcades to normal occlusal relationship. This is achieved by reduction of the least amount of crown possible. On initial treatment of a malocclusion, rates of attrition are pathological and rates of eruption are exaggerated. Until these dynamics are completely corrected, rates of eruption and attrition will not be corrected. Malocclusions and the forces that created them will remain in play. Once forces are corrected, the rate of development of malocclusions slows. Thus, the goal to promote longevity of the arcade is achieved.

It should be the goal for every patient to have annual dental care. More frequent occlusal equilibration in a corrected patient can result in excessive crown removal. In early stages of correction of a malocclusion, increased frequency of care is often necessary in order to correct underlying pathophysiology.

There are four factors involved in efficient delivery of dental care:
1. Restraint.
2. Access.
3. Proper equipment.
4. Instruction in the use of the instrumentation.

Patient comfort, health, and welfare are maintained by efficient delivery of service and minimal use of sedatives. In order to address problems effectively anywhere in the mouth, but especially in the molar region, the patient must first be well sedated. Insufficient sedation results in patient motion, which can result in injury to the patient, operator, or handler, and can prolong the time required for job completion.

The use of a dental speculum provides appropriate access to the cheek teeth. Many styles exist (**159–161**). The practitioner should try several models and use the one which is most comfortable. It may be helpful to have multiple models available for use in different procedures.

Specific instrumentation for occlusal equilibration is the decision of each individual practitioner. Instructions for correct use of the instrumentation are best acquired from the manufacturer. The reader is referred to other texts for instructions on specifics of

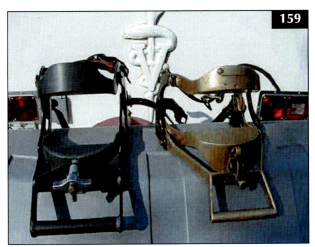

159 Examples of oral speculums: on the left is a Lochner speculum; on the right is a McAllen speculum. (Courtesy of Dr. Mike Lowder.)

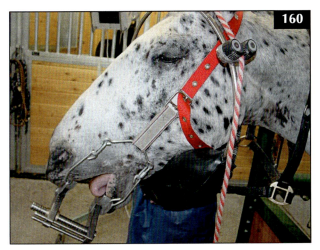

160 A Stubbs speculum is used in this patient.

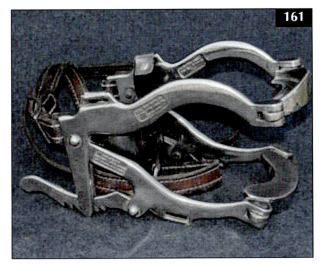

161 A MacPherson speculum.

instrumentation. It is the aim of this chapter to address principles involved in procedures and decisions, and principles that apply to problems that may arise.

The following steps should each be addressed in occlusal equilibration:

1. Odontoplasty, or reduction of overlong occlusal crown.
2. Floating, or reduction of cusps and rounding edges of arcades.
3. Bit seat application.
4. Occlusal angle.
5. Wolf teeth.
6. Canines when present.
7. Deciduous teeth.
8. Incisors.

ODONTOPLASTY

After finishing the examination process, the first step in the procedure is reduction of overlong occlusal crowns. This process is referred to as odontoplasty. The goal of this procedure is to return crown height to normal such that occlusal surfaces of opposing arcades are even and forces are normal. The patient benefits from improved alignment of the arcades and in promotion of longevity of the teeth.

The amount of tooth removed at any one time is determined by a balance between the need to achieve normal occlusal relationships and preservation of viable reserve crown and odontoblastic processes. Research has determined the presence of odontoblastic processes that appear viable within 4 mm of the occlusal surface.[1] Exposure of viable odontoblastic processes may be one of the causes of post-treatment dysmastication; in other species, exposure of odontoblastic processes is painful.[2]

As a general rule, when addressing nongeriatric patients overlong teeth are reduced to the tallest point of the normal teeth in the arcade. All teeth in the arcade are thus even. The results are: all teeth meet evenly during mastication motion; the interdental space is parallel on inspection with a buccal retractor with the speculum removed; and occlusion is maximized. If a tooth is overworn it may be rested and taken out of occlusion by reduction of its occlusal partner. This allows the overworn tooth to erupt to the normal level of the rest of the arcade. This concept is discussed further in Chapter 6: Principles of mastication biomechanics.

An example of appropriate reduction is shown in figures **162** and **163**.

Geriatric patients are treated to remove causes of immediate pain. There is rarely sufficient reserve or occlusal crown to correct abnormal forces. In geriatrics, removal of sharp points and reduction of unopposed crowns is usually sufficient. An example of a geriatric patient with a severe, uncorrectable malocclusion is shown in figure **164**.

Most patients require less than 4 mm of crown reduction. When reduction of more than 4 mm of crown is necessary two options exist. Further reduction to normal occlusal level can be followed by coating the tooth surface with three successive layers of light cured dentinal bonding agent (see Chapter 17: Principles of endodontics). A second option is to stage further crown reduction over two or three sessions. Since the underlying problem is, in part, an excessive rate of eruption, the rapid eruption process will not be corrected until reduction to normal is completed. For example, if a 4 mm overlong crown is erupting at a rate of 4 mm/year and 3 mm of crown is reduced at each appointment, it would require two appointments within 1 year to achieve normal occlusion. If only one appointment is scheduled each year and only 3 mm is reduced at each appointment the patient will never be corrected. Conversely, consider a malocclusion that includes a tooth with 6 mm of overlong crown and an eruption rate of 4 mm/year. If 3 mm of crown reduction is done at each appointment, this patient would require three appointments for complete resolution within 1 year. If only addressed twice in a year, the malocclusion will never be corrected.

Aside from hand instruments, three basic types of motorized instruments are available for odontoplasty. All have benefits and drawbacks.

Reciprocating instruments (figures **165**, **166**) allow for very rapid reduction of crown when used with sharp carbide blades. They can be injurious to tissue in the distal arcade when used incorrectly or when the

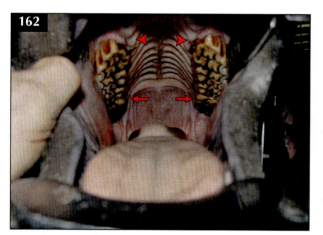

162 The arrowheads indicate the small hooks on the upper 6s. The arrows identify the wave on the upper 9s and 10s.

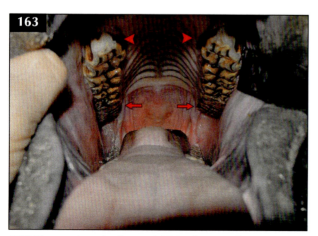

163 The patient in figure **162** is shown after correction of the malocclusion. The hooks are reduced and the mesial edges are rounded. The wave involving the 9s and 10s is reduced. Buccal cusps are rounded.

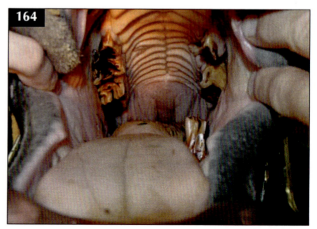

164 Geriatric patients may have malocclusions that cannot be corrected. In such cases, relief of painful conditions should be the priority.

patient is not well sedated and moves its head from side to side. Laceration of buccal or pharyngeal mucosa, gingiva, or palate, or damage to tooth or bone may result. This style of instrument requires careful, prolonged practice for perfection; when mastered, it is extremely efficient.

A second style of instrument is the rotary instrument where the cutting wheel rotates perpendicular to the shaft (**167**). Guarded cutting wheels are diamond, carbide chip, or solid-cut carbide. These instruments are quickly mastered. They are less likely to injure soft tissue, unless it is caught between the guard and the cutting wheel. Odontoplasty is usually somewhat less efficient with this style of instrument than with the reciprocating instrument.

A third style is the rotary instrument with the cutting bur rotating in line with the shaft. These instruments are usually guarded (**168**). Some come with irrigation, vacuum, or light attachments. With minimal practice and sharp diamond chip, carbide chip, or solid-cut carbide burs, they can be quickly mastered. They are quite safe to operate. Overheating of the tooth is prevented in most cases by water irrigation. These instruments allow for very controlled and focused reduction of occlusal crown.

Instrument choice depends on operator experience and comfort. Reciprocating instruments require more skill and practice to master. When mastered, reciprocating instruments are extremely efficient. Rotary equipment is usually safer for the beginner, but not as efficient.

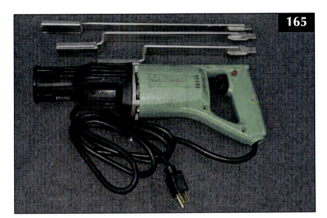

165 The large reciprocating float.

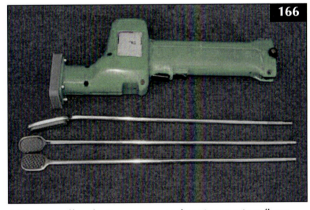

166 A smaller, battery-powered reciprocating float.

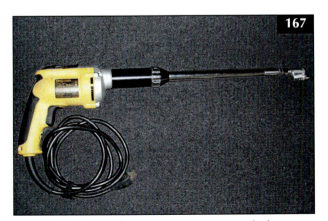

167 An example of a rotary instrument with the cutting wheel rotating perpendicular to the shaft.

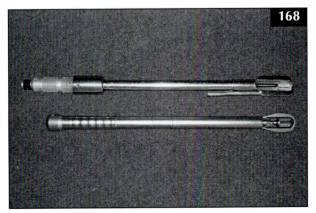

168 Examples are shown of rotary instruments with an in-line rotating cutting bur.

FLOATING

The second step in occlusal equilibration is floating, or reduction of sharp edges and enamel points. The lingual edges of lower cheek teeth and buccal edges of upper cheek teeth are rounded and cusps removed. Figures **169** and **170** show a patient with sharp enamel points that are reduced appropriately. Figure **171** shows a patient with severely excessive reduction of buccal cusps. These cusps are reduced almost to the pulp chambers.

The purpose of floating is to maximize patient comfort in bitting and mastication. In many cases, patients protect soft tissue from injury by sharp enamel points by limiting the range of mandibular motion. Lateral mandibular movement is limited. Buccal muscle tone necessary in positioning the food

bolus between chewing surfaces is reduced. The result is accumulation of a food bolus on the buccal aspect of maxillary teeth. Other patients demonstrate bitting resistance, as response to bit manipulation is delayed or resisted while the patient avoids sharp points.

Care must be taken to avoid damage to gingiva when filing or grinding buccal borders of maxillary teeth. Figure **172** shows the result of gingival trauma. The distance dorsally from the occlusal surface that buccal cusps are reduced depends on frequency of dental care. If edges are rounded 5–7 mm from the occlusal surface on the buccal aspect of maxillary teeth, and if done annually, the reappearance of sharp points will be minimized. If buccal cusps are aggressively removed to the gingival margin, there is potential for damage to gingiva and buccal mucosa and underlying tissue.

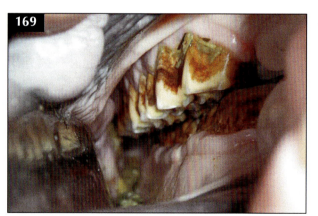

169 Sharp enamel points on the buccal aspect of the right maxillary arcade.

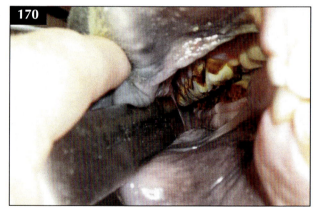

170 After reduction, the enamel cusps are rounded and smooth.

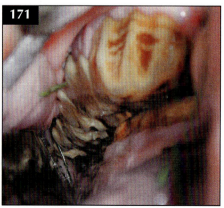

171 Severely excessive reduction of buccal cusps may potentially expose the pulp. This must be avoided.

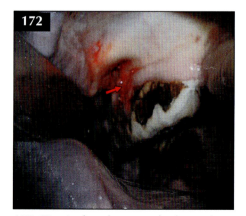

172 Gingival and mucosal trauma (arrow) can result from exuberant attempts to reduce buccal cusps to the gingival margin.

Complications include gingivitis, severe periodontal disease, and local and regional infections. Clinically the patient may display pain during bitting or mastication, or may have local swelling or abscess formation. These complications are obviously to be avoided.

Instrumentation used in floating is the same as in odontoplasty. Many choose to use hand instruments to finish rounding edges, since hand instruments are more easily controlled and maneuvered between the arcade and surrounding soft tissue, and in and around curvatures in the arcade (see Chapter 3: Anatomical characteristics of equine dentition).

BIT SEAT

The mesial borders of all 6s, or second premolars, are rounded as in figure **173**. This is the bit seat.

The purpose of the bit seat is patient comfort. It also aids the practitioner in complete removal of hooks and ramps. Comfort is provided as the bit and cheek pieces of the bridle pull or push the tongue, cheeks, and lips on to a smooth, rounded tooth edge. If sharp, these edges can cause bitting discomfort (**174**).

Since the purpose is rounding and smoothing edges, aggressive reduction of these teeth is unnecessary (**175**). The pulp horn in the mesial cusp should not be exposed. If iatrogenic pulp exposure occurs, vital pulpotomy should be performed (see Chapter 17: Principles of endodontics).

Many burs fitting in in-line rotary instrument handpieces work well for this procedure. Some are round, others are bullet-shaped, while still others are hourglass-shaped (**176**).

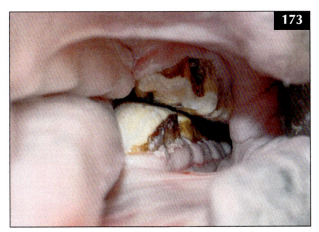

173 Bit seats are rounded mesial edges of the upper and lower 6s.

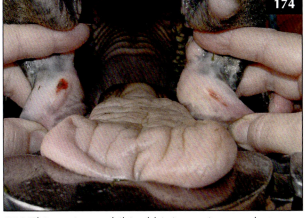

174 This patient exhibited bitting resistance that was alleviated by placement of a bit seat.

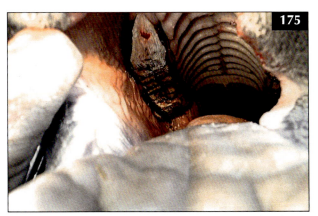

175 Excessive reduction of the mesial 6 can lead to direct or indirect pulp exposure.

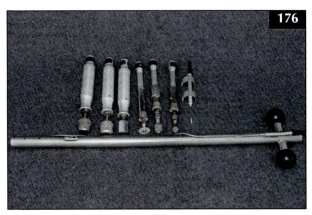

176 Examples of burs used for various procedures including application of a bit seat.

During this procedure, soft tissue is guarded and gingiva is preserved. Water irrigation assists in both cooling and cleaning the bur. Excessive heat can harm the pulp. Studies show that continuous application of a bur for 30 s can result in temperature increase of a degree sufficient to harm the pulp.[3] For this reason it is advisable to limit application of a bur to 30 s or less and to use water irrigation to cool all burs.

OCCLUSAL ANGLE

Occlusal angle is determined by comparing the occlusal surface with a line perpendicular to the patient's sagittal plane (see Chapter 3: Anatomical characteristics of equine dentition). This angle is evaluated during the examination process and is maintained throughout the dental procedure (see Chapter 2: Dental examination). After occlusal equilibration is finished, this angle is evaluated again.

The angle of occlusion should be the same or slightly flatter going distally on the arcade. Pathological angles should be corrected. Patients may have single teeth or entire arcades with incorrect angles. The only abnormal angle that should not be changed is the angle found in the patient with 'shear mouth'.

One of the advantages of reciprocating instruments is the ease with which occlusal angle can be corrected or maintained. One of the difficulties with any of the rotary instruments is the ease with which abnormal angles can be accidentally created during odontoplasty of single teeth. With rotary instruments, careful attention must be focused on maintenance of correct occlusal angle.

WOLF TEETH

The 'wolf teeth' (5s in Triadan) lie near the mesial border of the 6s. In many cases the bit seat procedure cannot be performed adequately without their removal. Many veterinarians routinely remove wolf teeth, while others do not. Wolf tooth removal is believed by many to facilitate bitting comfort. Their position, shape, and crown length are highly variable (see Chapter 3: Anatomical characteristics of equine dentition).

Some wolf teeth do not fully erupt, but migrate mesially 1–2 cm. The result is a subgingival nodule called an 'unerupted tooth' (also referred to by the slang term 'blind wolf tooth').

All extractions begin with submucosal infiltration anesthesia (see Chapter 11: Regional and local anesthesia). A small bleb of local anesthetic is placed submucosally (not subgingivally) medially and laterally to the tooth. It takes several minutes for the anesthetic to diffuse through the bone to anesthetize the PDL and pulp. In most cases, infiltration anesthesia is performed prior to odontoplasty. This allows sufficient time for anesthesia to occur.

Once anesthetized the teeth are elevated and removed. Unerupted teeth require an incision and gingival elevation before tooth elevation. Incisions are closed with 3 metric (2/0 USP) gut used in simple interrupted pattern. Usually one to two sutures are sufficient.

Many different types of elevators and gouges exist. Practitioners use the instruments with which they are comfortable.

DECIDUOUS TOOTH EXTRACTIONS

Two indications exist for removal of deciduous teeth:
- The visible presence of the crown of the adult tooth.
- Loose deciduous tooth.

The calendar age of the patient is not an indicator for deciduous tooth removal.

Infiltration anesthesia facilitates efficient extraction of deciduous teeth. For premolar extraction, correct procedure involves the use of molar forceps to rock the tooth from side to side followed by lifting the tooth out of its position. Incisor extraction is also facilitated with infiltration anesthesia. Elevation and extraction are similar to those employed in wolf tooth extraction. For further discussion please refer to Chapter 8: Eruption and shedding of teeth.

CANINE TEETH

The purpose of canine teeth in wild horses is to inflict damage on an opponent. Horses in captivity do not have this requirement. However, in domestic horses, canine teeth can damage hands of those administering oral medications. Insertion and removal of bridles can cause traumatic contact of the bit with the canine teeth. For these reasons, canine teeth are shortened and rounded. The process is referred to as canine odontoplasty. Figures **177** and **178** demonstrate conservative canine reduction.

Canine teeth do not fully erupt in until the horse is 4–5 years of age. Some teeth in normal patients require an additional year or two to fully erupt. When erupted, the pulp canal is large and close to the occlusal surface. Therefore minimal odontoplasty should be performed in young horses. In aging horses canine teeth are reduced by about one-third, and never more than half, leaving occlusal crown above the level of the gingiva. Reduction to the level of the gingiva is not necessary and can result in direct or indirect pulp exposure.

Canine tooth reduction is done with a diamond wheel and/or a bur used in a rotary handpiece. Edges are rounded and smoothed with round or bullet-shaped burs. Sharp instruments facilitate rapid reduction and minimize potential thermal trauma.

INCISORS

Incisor malocclusions are most commonly secondary to cheek tooth malocclusions. The exception is when incisor malocclusions occur secondary to fractures or displacements of teeth in either arcade or in class 2 or 3 malocclusions (parrot mouth and sow mouth) (refer to Chapter 18: Principles of orthodontics).

The degree of correction of diagonal or curvature malocclusions is determined by evaluating the POC (see Chapter 6: Principles of mastication biomechanics). As a general rule, incisor reduction is limited to only that amount needed to return the POC to the original measurement. If the original POC was half, and post-odontoplasty the POC is two-thirds, then incisor reduction can return POC to half. In general, reduction of 1 mm of incisor will move the POC 3–4 mm palatally.[4] Such reduction may not be adequate to correct fully an incisor malocclusion. In these cases, partial correction is indicated, and further staging of correction can be done on an annual basis.

The angle of occlusion of the incisors occurs on a line that if continued intersects the base if the ears (**179**). This angle should be maintained if normal and corrected if abnormal. It should be noted that this line is not parallel to the occlusal surface of the cheek teeth.

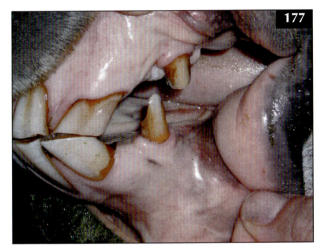

177 Canine teeth are long and sharp and can cause lacerations to the patient, other horses, or to one who administers medications.

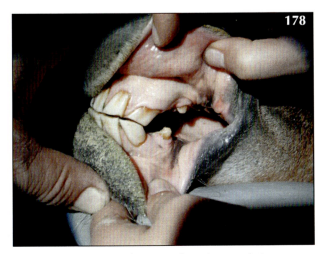

178 Conservative reduction of canine teeth improves safety considerations for the patient and owner.

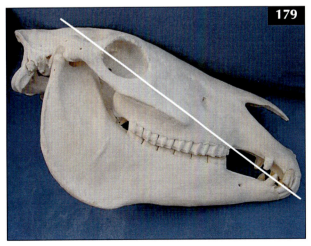

179 The angle of incisor occlusion is on a line that intersects the base of the ears.

A survey[5] of extracted incisors from horses ranging widely in age found that the average distance from occlusal surface to pulp was 8 mm, with a low of 4 mm and a high of 12 mm. Armed with such information, the dental practitioner should limit incisor reduction to the above parameters.

SUMMARY

The first step in occlusal equilibration is recognition and understanding of normal. The goal of occlusal equilibration is re-establishment of normal. It should be the aim of the practitioner to provide efficient, thorough services with minimal sedation. Efficient delivery of services is facilitated by restraint, access, a complete range equipment, and proper training.

Equine patients need dental care for the same reasons as other species. These reasons are:
• Immediate pain relief.
• Proper arcade alignment.
• Longevity of the arcade.

Treatment can be staged. Large overgrowths can be reduced in small increments at frequently repeated sessions. However, it must be kept in mind that partial reduction of overlong teeth does not return to normal the abnormal forces and pathological events that lead to creation of the malocclusion. Only complete reduction (when possible) of the malocclusion can return forces to normal.

There are several reasons for post-treatment problems. The most common problem encountered by the author is failure to balance or equilibrate arcades adequately. This stems from failure to understand, recognize, and reproduce normal anatomical relationships. Dysmastication may result from:
• Inadequate equilibration. Treatment is as above.
• Temporomandibular joint or muscular pain from prolonged time in a speculum. This problem can be avoided with efficient use of instrumentation and minimal delays in technique. In some patients periodic closure of the speculum is helpful. Treatment is with anti-inflammatories.

• Dentinal pain from exposure of odontoblastic processes: treatment is with light-cured dentinal bonding agents (see Chapter 17: Principles of endodontics for further discussion).
• Proprioception of change in occlusion. Adaptive period is a few days.

In the author's opinion, proprioceptive changes post-treatment are the most common reason for an adaptive period for mastication motion during the first few days after a patient has been correctly treated. This adaptive period is minimized or not present if close attention is paid to achieving equilibrium of forces, contact, and range of motion while performing a correct occlusal equilibration.

REFERENCES

1. Dacre IT. *A Pathological Study of Equine Dental Disorders*. PhD thesis, The University of Edinburgh, 2003.
2. Torneck CD. Dentin-pulp complex. In: Ten Cate AR, (ed). *Oral Histology: Development, Structure, and Function*, 5th edition. St. Louis: Mosby, 1998; pp. 150–196.
3. Dacre IT, Uttely L, Dixon PM. Thermal changes in equine dental pulp associated with mechanical grinding. In press.
4. Rucker BA. Incisor and molar occlusion: normal ranges and indications for incisor reduction. *Proceedings 50th Annual Convention American Association of Equine Practitioners* 2004; pp. 7–12.
5. Klugh DO. Equine incisor pulp canals: a closer look. *Conference Proceedings 17th Annual Veterinary Dental Forum* 2003; pp. 200–202.

ERUPTION AND SHEDDING OF TEETH

David O Klugh   Chapter 8

Tooth eruption is the movement of the developing tooth through the bone and soft tissue of the jaw and into mastication position. It has three parts. The first part is *pre-eruptive tooth movement*. In this stage, the deciduous or permanent tooth germs move within the jaw before penetrating the gingiva. The second part is *eruptive tooth movement*. In this stage, the tooth moves into mastication position. This stage is divided into the creation of a pathway for tooth movement, and tooth movement itself. The third stage of tooth movement is *posteruptive tooth movement*. In this phase, the normal functional masticating position of the tooth is maintained while the jaw grows, the tooth undergoes attrition, and normal age-related orthodontic movement occurs.

PRE-ERUPTIVE TOOTH MOVEMENT

In pre-eruptive tooth movement, the teeth are placed in a position within the jaw for correctly aligned

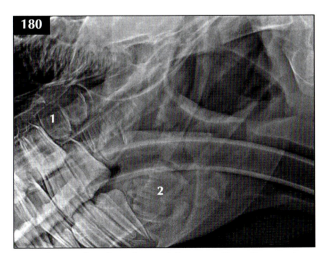

180 The occlusal surface of the maxillary first molar is directed ventrally while that of the mandibular first molar is angled mesially. **1.** Developing M1 facing ventrally; **2.** Developing M1 with occlusal surface angled mesially.

eruptive movement. Two factors are important: total bodily movement and growth of the tooth germ. The occlusal surface of a developing tooth must remain in a specific relation to the oral mucosa as both the tooth and the surrounding tissue grows. In order to maintain this spatial relation, the crypt in which the tooth develops must be remodeled by osteoclastic and osteoblastic activity as the jaw grows.

Brachydont permanent molar teeth develop within the maxilla with their occlusal surfaces facing distally and in the mandible with their occlusal surfaces facing mesially.[1] From this position, they rotate into the normal position as the jaw grows in length. While the same appears to be the case in the equine mandible, a different process occurs in the equine maxilla, where the permanent molar appears to develop only after sufficient bone is present so that the occlusal surface may face ventrally as in figure **180**.

Angulation of mandibular molars during pre-eruptive tooth movement remains directed mesially as the mandible grows in length until sufficient room is present to allow it to become straighter. If growth in length of the mandible is limited, tooth angulation remains directed mesially. This occurs in some short-headed breeds and individuals or as a pathological event in horses with class 2 malocclusions (parrot mouth). This principle is further discussed in Chapter 18: Principles of orthodontics.

ERUPTIVE TOOTH MOVEMENT

PATHWAY PREPARATION IN ADULT TEETH

Eruptive tooth movement is a two-part process. The creation of a pathway for movement of the tooth into mastication position is followed by the actual movement of the tooth.

Permanent equine incisors develop lingually to the deciduous teeth, while permanent equine premolars are situated between the roots of their deciduous counterparts. Eruptive movement of the permanent incisors is directed occlusally and labially, while that of the premolars and molars is directed occlusally (**181**).

Eruptive movement of the permanent incisor involves resorption of the lingual surface of the deciduous tooth root (**182**). The labial direction of incisor eruption is demonstrated in figures **183** and **184** where the erupting adult tooth is moving occlusally and labially. In this case the adult tooth has developed too far in the lingual direction. The root of the deciduous tooth is not dissolved adequately and requires extraction. The adjacent incisor required interproximal reduction to provide adequate space for the erupting tooth. Figure **184** demonstrates the follow-up of the procedure. The primary problem is that the position of embryological development of the adult tooth is abnormal. The eruption pathway created for the adult tooth results in its erupted position lingual to the deciduous tooth. Once the deciduous tooth is removed, the posteruptive movement of the adult tooth results in normal alignment. If the deciduous tooth was not removed, the adult tooth would not assume its normal position.

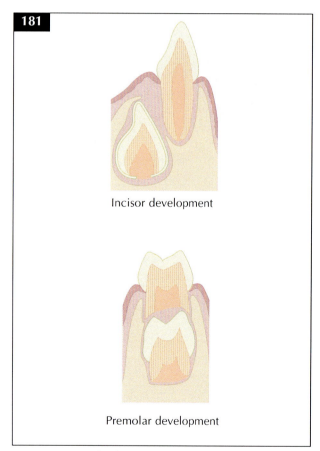

Incisor development

Premolar development

181 Diagram of relative eruption positions of incisors and premolars and molars. Incisors erupt from a lingual position. Premolars and molars erupt directly under the deciduous teeth.

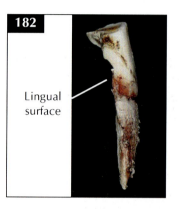

Lingual surface

182 Lateral view of a deciduous incisor demonstrating resorption of only the lingual surface of the tooth root.

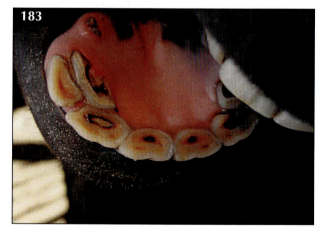

183 Eruptive movement of incisors is demonstrated by the position of the right lower third incisor (403). Its eruption pathway is directed labially and occlusally. In this case the adult tooth was positioned too far lingually and the deciduous tooth root had not resorbed. The deciduous tooth required extraction.

Eruptive movement of molars and premolars involves resorption of the apical aspect of the deciduous tooth (**185**). Most of the roots and part of the crown are broken down during this process.

The pathway of eruption of the permanent equine incisor follows the *gubernacular canal*. This is a fibrocellular remnant of the dental lamina connecting the dental follicle to the lamina propria of the oral mucosa. These foramina are identified on a dried skull lingually to the deciduous teeth in figure **186**.

PATHWAY PREPARATION IN DECIDUOUS TEETH

In Chapter 4, the development of the embryonic tooth germ is described as composed of the dental follicle, dental organ, and dental papilla. The external dental epithelium of the dental organ overlies the developing crown. As development of the crown enlarges, the stellate reticulum is reduced in size, placing the external dental epithelium in close proximity to the ameloblast layer of cells (**187**). This layer becomes known as the *reduced dental epithelium*.

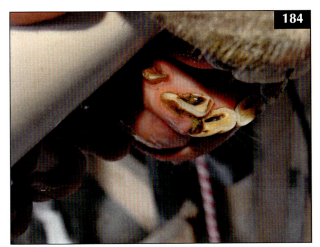

184 Photograph of the case in figure **183**, 6 months after treatment, demonstrating movement of adult incisor toward normal position.

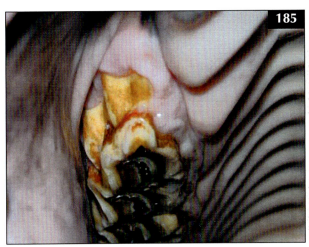

185 Occlusal direction of eruption of adult premolar.

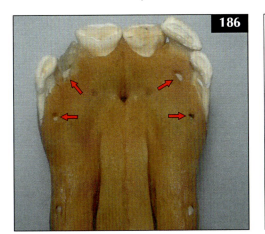

186 Gubernacular canal foramina (arrows) in a 2½-year-old Thoroughbred.

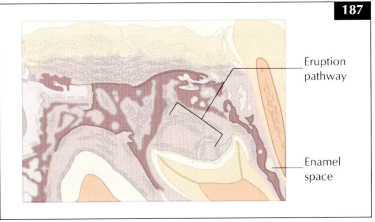

187 Condensation of the external dental epithelium, stellate reticulum, and the ameloblast layer into the reduced dental epithelium.

Eruption pathway

Enamel space

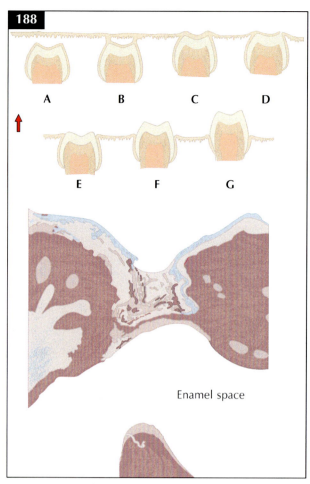

188 Eruption of the tooth into the oral cavity.
A. Crown penetrating bone and connective tissue;
B. Contact of crown with oral epithelium; **C**. Fusion of epithelia; **D**. Thinning of epithelium; **E**. Rupture of the epithelium; **F**. Crown emergence; **G**. Occlusal contact.

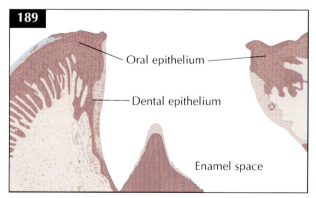

189 Oral epithelium and dental epithelium merge to form gingival epithelium. Attachment of the dental epithelium to the tooth creates the junctional epithelium. The space between the newly formed gingiva and the tooth is the gingival sulcus.

Bone and connective tissue lie between the reduced dental epithelium and the oral cavity. Breakdown of connective tissue is initiated by cytokines from the reduced dental epithelium. These messengers trigger chemotactic signals from the dental follicle cells that attract osteoclasts. Breakdown of bone and connective tissue creates a pathway for eruption. The reduced dental epithelium also secretes proteases that assist tissue breakdown.

As the overlying tissue becomes thinner, the oral epithelium and the dental epithelium fuse, creating the *epithelial plug*. The tooth enters the oral cavity by destruction of this tissue (**188**). Attachment of the fused epithelial layers to the tooth creates the gingiva, gingival sulcus, and junctional epithelium (**189**).

MOVEMENT OF THE ADULT TOOTH

Eruption is the movement of the tooth into mastication position. Responsibility for eruption lies with the PDL.[2] Its constituents are listed in *Table 5*.

Collagen fibers comprise the majority of the connective tissue. They are arranged in bundles called principal fibers. When they terminate in the cementum they are called Sharpey's fibers. The collagen fibers are produced by PDL fibroblasts.

The hypsodont PDL also contains elastic fibers in the form of oxytalan fibers. These fibers are arranged in two groups. One group is associated with blood

Table 5 Periodontal ligament composition
Connective tissue fibers:
Collagen
Oxytalan
Cells:
Fibroblasts
Cementoblasts and cementocytes
Osteoblasts
Epithelial cell rests of Malassez
Immune system cells
Ground substance:
Glycosaminoglycans
Glucosamine
Water

vessels and the other group is independent. The independent fibers are arranged as individual fibers diffusely distributed in random patterns and directions. All oxytalan fibers are located in the longitudinal half of the PDL near the cementum. Their primary function is stabilization of blood vessels during mastication.[3]

The principal fibers of mandibular cheek teeth in equines are arranged with horizontal and oblique fibers. The PDL is much thicker lingually than buccally.[4]

The PDL has many functions:
- Mechanical:
  - Shock absorption for occlusal forces.
  - Transmission of forces to bone.
  - Support of gingival tissue.
  - Protection of nerves and vessels.
- Remodeling.
- Nutritive and sensory.
- Eruption.

Microscopic measurements of alveolar bone under occlusal pressure demonstrate that tooth compression into the socket results in outward displacement of alveolar bone. If the PDL fibers alone were responsible for shock absorption, direct tooth pressure would result in inward movement of alveolar bone, pulled by PDL fibers. The outward movement of bone in shock absorption is explained by the viscoelastic system theory.[5,6] This theory suggests that fluid movement absorbs shock and transmits the force to the surrounding bone.

When tipping forces are applied, the tooth rotates on its longitudinal axis. One side of the PDL is compressed and the other side is stretched.[7] Forces applied to the bone are compensated by various remodeling patterns (see Chapter 18: Principles of orthodontics). The direction, frequency, duration, and size of the forces determine the pattern of bone remodeling.[8]

Blood vessels of the PDL supply its fibers, cells, cementum, bone, and gingiva. PDL nerves sense tactile, pressure, and pain stimuli via the trigeminal nerve.[9]

Hypsodont eruption is complex. Some older theories have been disproved. Root formation forcing upward crown movement is not a factor, since teeth continue to erupt after root removal. Other factors in eruption complicate the picture. Changes in hydrostatic pressure resulting from external stimuli are difficult to evaluate. Isolation of one part of the vasculature affects function of another. Bone remodeling is important in pre-eruptive tooth movement, but not in posteruptive tooth movement.

The force of eruption is provided by the fibroblasts associated with the collagen of principal fiber bundles. Several ingenious experiments demonstrate this.[10] *In vitro* studies show that the arrangement of PDL fibers can be altered by disrupting collagen synthesis. The result is a slowing or halting of eruption. If a tooth is cut into apical and coronal halves and a barrier is placed between the two, the coronal half continues to erupt. Since it has lost vasculature of the pulp, the only tissue with which it is associated is the PDL. This demonstrates that the PDL is responsible for tooth eruption.

Fibroblasts placed on silicone rubber are able to crawl and create wrinkles in the medium. Disrupting the cytoskeleton of the fibroblast removes this ability. PDL fibroblasts embedded in a collagen gel will convert the fibers into a three-dimensional tissue-like substance. By placing the PDL-derived fibroblasts in a perforated collagen mesh containing a slice of root dentin, the fibroblasts arrange themselves in a network and raise the slice of root from the bottom of the cup to the top. The slice of root is passed from cell to cell. Chemically disrupting the cytoskeleton of the fibroblasts prevents movement of the root slice. No movement of fibroblast cells occurs. Thus, it is concluded that fibroblasts provide the force necessary for eruption.

POSTERUPTIVE TOOTH MOVEMENT

Posteruptive tooth movements occur after the tooth reaches occlusion. The tooth adjusts within the alveolar socket by bone remodeling and replenishes worn tooth substance by eruption. These movements can be divided into three categories: accommodation for growth; compensation for occlusal wear; and accommodation for interproximal wear and maintenance of the tight-fitting dental battery.

As the jaw increases in size, teeth must remain in mastication position. They do so by adjusting within the socket. This requires remodeling of alveolar bone and addition of new bone at the floor of the socket. This accommodation for growth is not a force that significantly contributes to the eruptive process.

Compensation for occlusal wear is the major reason for the eruptive mechanism of hypsodont teeth. As forces of mastication are compensated for, wear and eruption patterns develop into malocclusions.

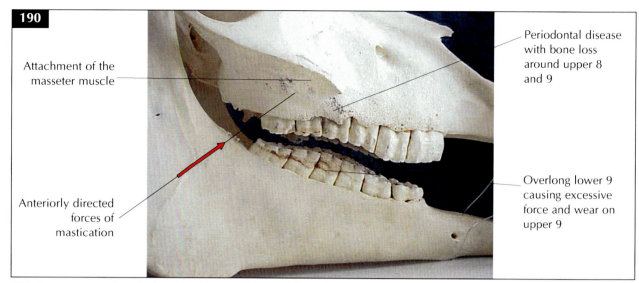

190

Attachment of the masseter muscle

Periodontal disease with bone loss around upper 8 and 9

Anteriorly directed forces of mastication

Overlong lower 9 causing excessive force and wear on upper 9

190 In a wave malocclusion, the forces of the overlong lower 9 are directed dorsally and anteriorly to the upper 9. In many cases periodontal disease results.

The pathophysiology of the development of malocclusions is discussed at length in Chapter 7: Principles of occlusal equilibration.

Compensatory eruption involves adaptation to forces delivered to the PDL. As mastication forces increase, attrition rates also increase. Lost crown is replaced by eruption. In its state of continual repair and remodeling, cementum, bone, and collagen respond to occlusal forces; in injury repair; and in physiological tooth movement. The PDL responds to physiological needs[11] and external stimuli[12] of mastication forces by increasing the size[13] and number of fiber bundles.[14] Consequently, fibroblastic activity also increases. Increased rates of attrition are in part balanced by increasing rates of eruption.

The eruption rate of equine teeth is generally thought to be about 2–3 mm per year. This represents an approximate average of eruption rates throughout the life of the tooth. It is a calculated based on scientific observations, and includes assumptions that all permanent equine cheek teeth are in wear by 5 years of age, and a 75 mm long tooth should be fully worn by 30–35 years of age.[15]

In clinical practice rates of eruption vary. Newly erupting adult teeth undergo the same *posteruption spurt* as brachydont teeth. This eruption rate continues until occlusion is reached. As the horse ages, the rate of eruption slows until, in a geriatric horse, the rate is quite slow.

Rates of eruption vary with other factors. When measuring second premolars, eruption rates varied with numerous factors, such as age, diet, and frequency of occlusal equilibration. Specifically, eruption rates of ramps on lower second premolars were measured at 5 mm per year as compared to 4 mm per year for all second premolars. This rate was reduced to 3 mm per year after three occlusal equilibrations were performed at 1-year intervals.[16] The reduction in rate of eruption is explained by the concept of even distribution of forces of mastication over a larger area on the arcade. By removing a protuberance, the mandible is allowed to have increased range of motion. Mastication forces are spread out over a larger area of the arcade. Since forces are not focused on one spot on the arcade, the rates of attrition and eruption become normal.

The tight-fitting dental battery and interproximal wear are accommodated by mesial drift of teeth. Mechanisms involved in the horse include:
- Anteriorly directed occlusal forces.
- Trans-septal PDL fibers.
- Mesially inclined eruption of posterior teeth.
- Soft tissue pressures.

The anterior direction of mastication forces is demonstrated by the commonly encountered 'wave'. In this condition the overlong lower first molar (Triadan system number 9) is directed anteriorly into the upper arcade (**190**). The wedge-shaped mandible

191 Distal teeth are angled mesially so that eruptive forces crowd teeth together.

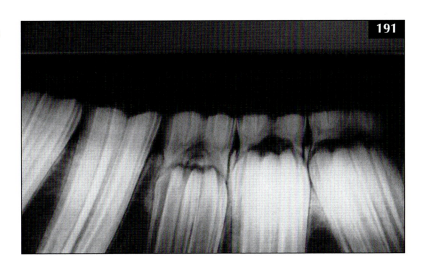

is pulled dorsally and rostrally during mastication by the massive masseter, temporalis, and other muscles. These forces are focused on the upper first molar (9 in the Triadan system). The results are demonstrated as periodontal disease with bone loss around the upper 9.

Trans-septal PDL fibers connect adjacent teeth and function to keep the teeth fitting closely together. The summation of their forces assist teeth in mesial drift.

In both the maxillary and mandibular arcades eruptive forces direct the teeth mesially. Tooth angulation is demonstrated in figure **191**. The combination of eruptive force and angulation directs teeth mesially. As the horse ages, these mechanisms maintain the tight proximity of the teeth.

Soft tissue pressure maintains tooth position, but has minimal effect on mesial drift. More likely, soft tissue forces keep the teeth in correct alignment. Tongue pressure may contribute to anteriorly directed occlusal forces.

TOOTH SHEDDING

Incisors erupt in a labial and occlusal direction. The result is that resorption of deciduous incisors begins on the lingual border of the root. Premolar adult teeth erupt in an occlusal direction, with resorption beginning primarily on the apical aspect of the deciduous tooth.

Hard tissues are resorbed by odontoclasts. These cells are derived from migrating monocytes of the bloodstream and tissue and break down root structure. After root resorption is almost complete, odontoblasts in the pulp degenerate. Pulp remains

viable, as a blood supply must exist from which monocytes invade. Odontoclasts continue to break down dental structure until the tooth is sufficiently loose for exfoliation to occur.

PDL breakdown has two features of change in cell function. Some fibroblasts cease secretion of collagen, and it accumulates intracellularly. Other fibroblasts undergo apoptosis. This phenomenon is an important function of embryogenesis in all tissues and is recognized as genetically programmed. When all processes are considered, tooth shedding is recognized as a programmed event.

Mastication pressure assists in tissue breakdown. It is not a primary mechanism of deciduous exfoliation. This is demonstrated by the fact that deciduous teeth exfoliate even in cases where there is no underlying adult tooth. These deciduous teeth shed more slowly. Increased mastication force applied to a deciduous tooth can speed up its resorption. The combination of pressure and mastication force causes loss of supporting soft tissue, so the tooth is less able to withstand mastication and exfoliation is hastened.

PATTERN OF ERUPTION AND EXFOLIATION

Exfoliation time of deciduous premolars varies. A pilot study was done involving 16 horses.[17] Nine of these horses had no prior dental care, and seven had at least one occlusal equilibration. Deciduous third and fourth premolars were extracted from all of these patients. In seven of the nine with no prior care, the lower premolars were gone and adult teeth had erupted above the normal occlusal level of the rest of the arcade. The

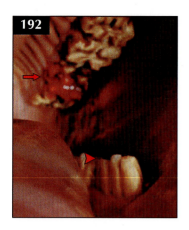

192 Uneven exfoliation of deciduous teeth results in uneven eruption of adult teeth. In this case the lower 8 has a step malocclusion. The arrow indicates freshly extracted deciduous upper left fourth premolar (708). The occlusal surface of the adult tooth is just above the gingival margin. The arrowhead indicates the level of the occlusal surface of the left lower fourth premolar (308). The 308 will erupt further before the 208 reaches a normal mastication position. The result will be a step malocclusion.

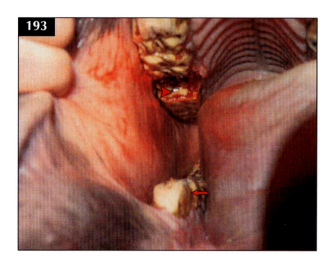

193 All four deciduous teeth exfoliate at the same time resulting in even occlusal surfaces of all four erupting adult teeth. The arrow indicates occlusal level of 408; the arrowhead indicates occlusal level of 108.

upper deciduous premolars were extracted with the underlying adult teeth situated with the occlusal surface well apical to the level of the occlusal surface of the rest of the arcade. The arcade was encumbered with a step malocclusion (**192**). This step was reduced. Left untreated this step would become a wave over time, and result in premature wear on portions of the arcade.

In six of seven of those having received occlusal equilibration on at least one occasion, the deciduous premolars were extracted as a group of four (**193**). Determination for extraction was made by either the presence of a loose deciduous tooth or visual presence of the adult tooth. All four were easily removed. All the underlying adult teeth were erupted to approximately the same level. No significant malocclusions were present.

It is hypothesized that the reason for the more even exfoliation of deciduous premolars and the even eruption of adult teeth lies in the concept of even distribution of forces of mastication over a larger portion of the arcade that results from occlusal equilibration. More even force distribution results in even eruptive rates of adult teeth, and normal rates of resorption of deciduous teeth resulting in balanced exfoliation of deciduous premolars.

Important features of eruption and exfoliation are included in *Table 6*. The following are clinically relevant:

• The first adult tooth to erupt is the first molar (9 in the Triadan system).
• The fourth premolar (Triadan 8) is the only adult

Table 6 Approximate eruption times[18]

TEETH		ERUPTION
A. Deciduous:		
1st incisor	(Di 1)	Birth of first week
2nd incisor	(Di 2)	4–6 weeks
3rd incisor	(Di 3)	6–9 months
Canine	(Dc)	
2nd premolar	(Dp 2)	Birth or first
3rd premolar	(Dp 3)	two weeks
4th premolar	(Dp 4)	
B. Permanent:	**Number***	
1st incisor	101 .... (I1)	2½ years
2nd incisor	102 .... (I2)	3½ years
3rd incisor	103 .... (I3)	4½ years
Canine	104 .... (C)	4–5 years
1st premolar (or wolf-tooth)	105 .... (P1)	5–6 months
2nd premolar	106 .... (P2)	2½ years
3rd premolar	107 .... (P3)	3 years
4th premolar	108 .... (P4)	4 years
1st molar	109 .... (M1)	9–12 months
2nd molar	110 .... (M2)	2 years
3rd molar	111 .... (M3)	3½–4 years

* Modified Triadan Numbering System

tooth that erupts between two previously erupted adult teeth. This tooth commonly suffers inflammatory eruption reactions at its apex visible radiographically as a lucent area.

- The last adult tooth to erupt is the canine tooth (Triadan 4).

SUMMARY

Pre-eruptive tooth movement is characterized by growth of the tooth germ while it maintains its spatial relation to the oral cavity and positions itself within the jaw for eruptive movement. Eruptive movement involves preparation of a pathway by resorption of tissue, and tooth movement. Incisors move labially and occlusally while premolars and molars move occlusally. Posteruptive tooth movement involves accommodation for growth, compensation for wear, and accommodation for mesial drift and interproximal wear. The rate at which worn tooth is replenished varies. The force of eruption is provided by fibroblasts. Mastication forces are compensated for by alterations in eruption rate. Interproximal wear is compensated for by mesial drift. Forces involved are elastic trans-septal fibers, mesially directed occlusal forces and eruption forces and, to some degree, soft tissue forces.

Tooth shedding is a programmed event. Root resorption occurs whether the adult tooth is present or not. Mastication forces can hasten the rate of exfoliation. Patterns of eruption and exfoliation vary, but generally follow standard times closely.

REFERENCES

1. Bhaskar SN (ed) *Orban's Oral Histology and Embryology.* St. Louis: Mosby, 1991.

2. Ten Cate AR. Physiologic tooth movement: eruption and shedding. In: *Oral Histology, Development, Structure and Function.* St. Louis: Mosby, 1994; p. 321.

3. Staszyk C, Gasse H. Oxytalan fibres in the periodontal ligament of equine molar cheek teeth. *Anatomia, Histologia, Embryologia* 2004: **33**; 17–22.

4. Kempson SA. The periodontium of the mandibular teeth of the horse. *17th Annual Veterinary Dental Forum* 2003.

5. Bien SM. Hydrodynamic damping of tooth movement. *Journal of Dental Research* 1966: **45**; 907.

6. Boyle PE. Tooth suspension: a comparative study of the paradental tissues of man and of the guinea pig. *Journal of Dental Research* 1938: **17**; 37.

7. Davies WI, Picton DC. Dimensional changes in the periodontal membrane of monkey's teeth with horizontal thrusts. *Journal of Dental Research* 1967: **46**; 114.

8. Beertsen W, McCulloch CG, Sodek J. The periodontal ligament: a unique, multifunctional connective tissue. *Peridontology* 1997: **13**; 20–40.

9. Bernick S. Innervation of the teeth and periodontium. *Dental Clinics of North America* 1959: 503.

10. Ten Cate AR. Physiologic tooth movement. In: Ten Cate AR (ed) *Oral Histology. Development, Structure, and Function*, 5th edition. St. Louis: Mosby, 1998; pp. 294–295.

11. Ten Cate AR, Deporter DA. The degradative role of the fibroblast in the remodeling and turnover of collagen in soft connective tissue. *Anatomical Record* 1975: **182**; 1.

12. Ubios AM, Cabrini RL. Tritiated thiamine uptake in periodontal tissues subjected to orthodontic movement. *Journal of Dental Research* 1971: **50**; 1160.

13. Freeman E. Periodontium. In: Ten Cate AR (ed) *Oral Histology: Development, Structure and Function* 4th edition. St. Louis: Mosby, 1994; pp. 277–312.

14. Harvey CE, Emily PP. *Small Animal Dentistry.* St. Louis: Mosby, 1993; 91—92.

15. Baker GJ. Oral examination and diagnosis: Management of oral diseases. In: CE Harvey (ed) *Veterinary Dentistry.* Philadelphia: WB Saunders, 1985; 217–228.

16. Klugh DO. Measurement of rates of eruption in equine 2nd premolars. *Conference Proceedings 15th Annual Veterinary Dental Forum* 2001; pp. 178–183.

17. Klugh DO. Unpublished data.

18. Martin M. *Guide to Determining the Age of the Horse*, 6th edition. Lexington: American Association of Equine Practitioners, 2002.

DENTAL RADIOGRAPHY

David O Klugh   Chapter 9

Radiography is an essential part of equine dentistry. Diagnosis, treatment, and prognosis for dental problems related to periodontal disease, extractions, endodontics, and orthodontics, among others, cannot always be performed adequately without information provided by quality radiographic images. Many practitioners are reluctant to radiograph dental structures because of the difficulties of interpreting overlying tissue layers that can obscure details. Contrasting air and mineral densities overlie dental structures, and while providing contrast to dental structures, can create images that are challenging to interpret. Isolation of specific anatomical structures facilitates radiograph interpretation.

Extraoral techniques have been developed to address some of these concerns. In addition to standard lateral, dorsoventral, dorsal oblique, and ventral oblique views, techniques have been described for open-mouth oblique and offset dorsoventral views.[1,2] These techniques assist in isolating arcades for improved visualization of details of apical anatomy, and reserve and clinical crown, such as for analysis of topography of malocclusions.

Intraoral techniques have previously been described.[3] The occlusal films used in human and small animal dentistry necessitate extended exposure time in the equine patient because they use nonscreen film. Since the largest size of film is 5.7 × 7.6 cm (2¼" × 3"), they present the additional complication of requiring very precise alignment of tube head, object, and film. A second technique was described by Gibbs,[4] using intensifying screens and film enclosed in light-proof plastic bags. Good-quality images were obtained with this method. The logistical problems associated with these techniques necessitate the use of general anesthesia in equine patients.

Extraoral radiography allows evaluation of the large anatomical structures of the head. It is used in taking survey films to evaluate size, position, shape, and number of teeth, general topography of arcades, along with abnormal conditions of bony structures and paranasal sinuses. Intraoral radiography provides evaluation of single teeth. This is appropriate for evaluation of diseases affecting the pulp, periodontium, crown, and apices of teeth.

X-RAY MACHINES

Most machines available in private practice can be used to produce quality dental films as long as they are properly calibrated, and the tube head can be raised, lowered, rotated, tilted, and moved from one side of the horse to the other. The large stationary machines commonly found in university and referral hospitals and the older model semi-portable machines produce excellent images with minimal exposure to radiation, but are cumbersome to manipulate.

Specifically designed dental x-ray machines can also be used. There are two significant differences between these machines and standard machines. The first major difference between x-ray units developed specifically for dentistry and others is that dental units are single phase machines. In single phase machines the kilovolt peak (kVp) setting is not adjustable. Most units are set at 60 or 70 kVp only. The time of exposure can be adjusted. Some can deliver up to 14 mA. Excellent images can be produced using these machines.

The second major difference between standard and dental x-ray machines is the size of the focal spot on the anode. Most standard machines have a larger focal spot (1–2 mm) than dental machines (usually <1 mm). This difference in size is an advantage in that it translates into less scatter of x-rays and a sharper image.

An additional benefit of dental x-ray machines in general is their ease of manipulation. They are lighter and more easily moved from one position to another.

FILMS AND SCREENS

The image seen on a piece of x-ray film is the result of the reduction of silver ions to metallic silver, thereby blackening the film. The chemical process involves a lattice of silver halide crystals or grains held in a gelatin emulsion. Prior to light or x-ray exposure, the silver ion is present in the lattice structure with various halide ions. Light or x-ray exposure causes the halide to be converted to the halide's atom phase by absorption of photon energy and release of an electron. This electron is trapped by sensitizing agents such as silver sulfide where it attracts and captures a silver ion. By combining with the silver ion, metallic silver is created. This silver atom then becomes an electron trap for a second electron. The negative charge will attract another silver ion. More and more metallic silver is formed in one or more spots on the silver halide crystal. The effect is to instigate the reduction of silver ions to metallic silver.

As a general rule film speed can be divided into three basic categories, each with its particular characteristics:[5]

- **Fast-speed film:**
  - Larger silver halide crystals.
  - Requires less exposure by x-rays or light from intensifying screens.
  - Produces a grainier image.
  - Has less latitude.
- **Medium-speed film:**
  - Is a compromise in size of silver halide crystals.
  - Medium latitude.
  - Most widely used film in veterinary medicine.
- **Slow-speed film:**
  - Smallest silver halide crystals.
  - Requires greater degree of light or x-ray exposure.
  - Produces an image with better definition and detail.
  - Wider latitude.

Radiographic contrast is a term that describes the difference in density between two spots on a film. Density refers to the degree of blackness of the film. If there is a large difference in blackness between the two spots, the contrast is high. When viewing films, one can see that the borders of the film are usually completely black, while the denser parts of the subject are completely white. In such an example the white areas have high x-ray absorption by tissue so that the film is clear. The black areas correspond to low tissue absorption.

The latitude of the film refers to the number of shades of gray visible between white and black. This correlates to the range of structures or densities that can be imaged. On a film, this characteristic is seen as numerous shades of gray. It is exemplified further by the stepped wedge image, where each separate step represents a different shade of gray. The number of steps required to go from black to white indicates the latitude of the film. A wide-latitude film will accept a significant variation in exposure without experiencing a great variation in density or blackness. Such a film is termed 'forgiving'. It shows densities in varying degrees of contrast. As latitude increases, contrast decreases.

Advances in film technology have been made by chemical and structural improvements in the crystal composition of the film emulsion. Silver halide crystal sizes are reduced, while light sensitivity is increased. The shape of the crystal has been made more regular. As a result, the degree of radiation absorbed by the emulsion is increased simply by reducing the open spaces between grains. This concept is demonstrated by considering the way grains of sand or rocks fit together loosely with many spaces between them owing to their irregular-shaped margins. Consider also the way triangles or blocks fit together with minimal spaces between them. As the open spaces are reduced, less x-radiation passes through the layer and thus reduces more of the silver halide. More efficient arrangement and character of the crystal result in the need for a thinner emulsion layer, since minimal radiation will pass between the more evenly matched crystals. By combining these benefits the result is maximum detail with a minimum of radiation exposure: the reduction of silver halide is more efficient and the detail produced by the smaller yet more efficient crystals is improved.

The film is exposed by light emitted from intensifying screens. Luminescent phosphor crystals are bound together and mounted on a cardboard or plastic base. When x-radiation hits the phosphor, it fluoresces and the light given off exposes the x-ray film.

Intensifying screens were developed for the purpose of reducing the amount of x-radiation required to produce an image. The ability of the phosphor to fluoresce in response to x-rays and the amount of light emitted by the phosphor is reflected in the speed of the screen.

Screen speed is a function of:[6]

- Ability of the phosphor to absorb radiation, or the *absorption coefficient*.
- Ability of the phosphor to convert x-rays to light, or the *conversion efficiency*.

Many physical and chemical factors affect these two properties.[7] The size of the phosphor crystal can affect absorption and conversion. The larger the crystal, the more light it gives off when irradiated. This makes the phosphor more sensitive and makes the speed faster. This phosphor produces an image when less radiation penetrates the subject, as when tissue is more dense or thicker. The trade off is that the image is grainy or less clear; detail of the image is sacrificed.

A smaller crystal gives off less energy when radiation impacts the screen. The effect is the production of a smaller point of light. A smaller point of light becomes a higher detail image. However, more radiation is required to create an image, such as when the tissue thickness or density is increased. Slower screen speeds tend to have smaller crystal sizes. Detail is improved, but the speed of the screen is reduced.

Phosphor layer thickness affects absorption and conversion by creating more medium to absorb radiation and emit light. Since these thicker layers are more sensitive to radiation energy, they can lose detail when exposed to higher energy. They are more efficient when used in areas of thicker tissue, where the amount of radiation penetrating to the screen is reduced. Speed is increased as phosphor layer thickness increases.

As a result of these considerations, it is understood that faster screens require less exposure, but provide images with less detail, while slower screens provide better detail, but require higher exposures.

Between the film and the phosphor is a reflective layer which increases the amount of radiation impacting the phosphor crystals. A more efficient reflective layer makes the screen speed faster. Dyes are included in the phosphor layer for the purpose of absorbing the laterally spreading light which would blur the image. More dyes result in slower screen speeds.

In summary, screen speed is inversely related to the amount of radiation required to create an exposure. Fast screens require less exposure, slow screens require more exposure. Image detail is inversely related to screen speed. Faster screens create less detail while slower screens create highly detailed images. It is screen speed that is the most important factor in the creation of a high-detail radiograph.

COMPUTERIZED RADIOGRAPHY

There are two types of computerized radiography systems. Digital radiography (DR) systems involve the use of a flat panel detector to create an image visible in a few seconds on a computer screen. Specific software allows image manipulation and enhancement. These sensors are rigid, fragile, and expensive. They are connected directly to the x-ray machine. Images can be visualized in seconds, rather than having to be transported to a second site for conversion. Image size is limited to the single size of sensors.

The second digital radiography system is computed radiography (CR). These systems use phosphor sensors like 'electronic film'. Sensors are scanned by a device that converts the phosphor image to a digital image that is visible on a computer screen. Sensors can be re-used after erasing for multiple repeated exposures. They are flexible and are available in multiple sizes.

There are two styles of CR systems. One uses flexible screens in vinyl cassettes. These screens are removed from the cassette after exposure and inserted into a drum-style reader. Sensing screens can be cut into any size. This system works well for intraoral radiography in horses.

The other style utilizes screens in cassettes. The entire cassette is inserted into the film reader, where the screen is removed by an automated system and replaced into the cassette. Screen sizes are limited to those of standard cassettes.

Currently available digital systems, both DR and CR, produce images comparable or superior in quality to film/screen systems. There is little difference in image quality between CR and DR.

All digital systems allow image manipulation and enhancement, simplified storage and retrieval, enhanced communication with colleagues and clients, and eliminate developing chemicals and their disposal. Their disadvantages include cost, training, and rapidly evolving technology.

EXTRAORAL RADIOGRAPHY

Many problems related to dentistry are effectively diagnosed with the aid of specific extraoral radiograph projections. Survey films give a view of multiple teeth, surrounding bone, and sinus detail. Several standard and recently introduced projections provide quality images.

Sedation of the patient is generally necessary for production of radiographs, as the cassette and x-ray machine are positioned close to the face. Frequently in veterinary practice, sedation is also necessary for the performance of diagnostic and treatment procedures related to the problem requiring radiographs.

Lateral projections are used for evaluation of sinus problems (**194**). Fluid lines, bony, and soft tissue abnormalities are identified. The lateral projection creates overlying densities precluding effective diagnosis of specific dental problems.

Oblique views demonstrate apical and reserve crown detail of teeth and related bone lesions. For maxillary teeth, a 30° oblique angle is used. The dorsal oblique view used for imaging maxillary teeth is more correctly referred to as a lateral-to-lateral dorsoventral oblique or laterodorsal to lateral oblique. This view highlights apices and reserve crowns and is used frequently to identify specific tooth disease related to sinus problems. Figure **195** demonstrates the view.

The ventral oblique view demonstrates mandibular teeth. It is more correctly termed a lateral-to-lateral ventrodorsal or lateroventral to lateral projection. A 45° oblique angle is effective for imaging apical anatomy. For many patients with narrow mandibles, a 50° angle is used for 6s and 7s. Changing the angle of the machine to be slightly caudal allows imaging of 10s and 11s. In such cases there are two angles considered. The first is the ventral oblique angle. The second is projecting the beam from slightly caudal to rostral and centering the beam near the apices of the teeth of interest. Figure **196** demonstrates the image created.

Open-mouth oblique projections demonstrate the topography of malocclusions and other abnormalities of the clinical crown. Reserve crown and apical anatomy can also be visualized. A mouth gag of plastic pipe is used for these projections. For a view of the roots and reserve crowns, the standard oblique angles are used. For viewing the topography of the malocclusion, the views projected are opposite. Maxillary teeth are imaged with a 15° ventral oblique angle. This creates the lateral-to-lateral ventrodorsal projection (**197**, **198**). Mandibular teeth are imaged with a 10° lateral-to-lateral dorsoventral projection (**199**, **200**).

Dorsoventral projections are used to produce images of midline problems. Deviation of nasal passages and tipping of specific teeth can be identified along with other site-specific lesions. Figure **201** demonstrates the angle used. Figure **202** shows a radiograph obtained with this projection.

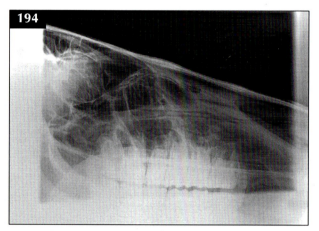

194 A lateral projection of normal sinus anatomy.

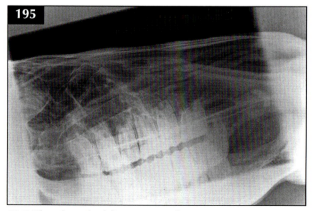

195 The dorsal oblique view demonstrates sinuses and apical and reserve crown anatomy of maxillary teeth.

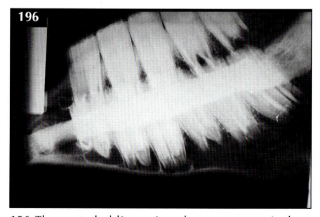

196 The ventral oblique view demonstrates apical and reserve crown detail of teeth and surrounding bone of mandibular teeth. This image is taken of a dried skull.

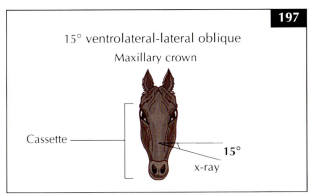

197 The open-mouth lateral-to-lateral ventrodorsal oblique angle for imaging the occlusal surface of the contralateral maxillary teeth.

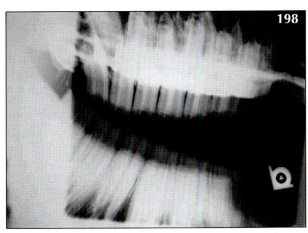

198 Radiograph of open-mouth ventral oblique projection of contralateral maxillary teeth. This image of a dried skull demonstrates the view.

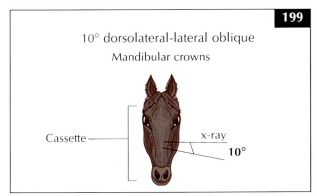

199 The open-mouth lateral-to-lateral dorsoventral oblique angle for imaging the occlusal surface of the contralateral mandibular teeth.

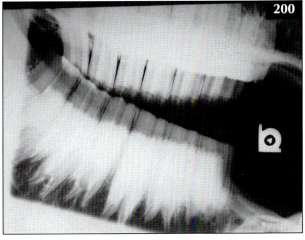

200 Radiograph of open-mouth dorsal oblique projection of contralateral mandibular teeth. This image of a dried skull demonstrates the view.

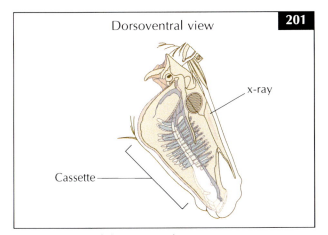

201 Diagram of dorsoventral projection.

202 Dorsoventral radiograph demonstrating the midline anatomy. This is a weanling with several fragments of fractured 606 and 607, indicated by the arrow.

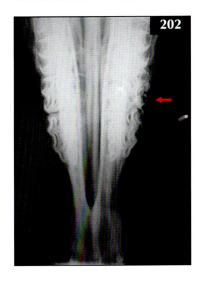

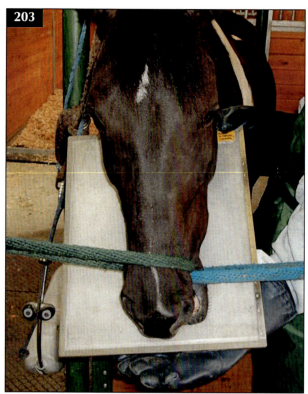

203 The open-mouth dorsoventral projection is demonstrated. The mandible is displaced laterally in a sedated patient.

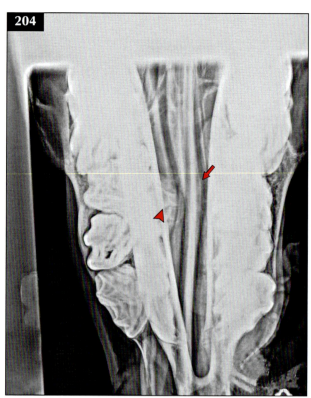

204 The open-mouth image is taken with the mandible displaced to the left side. This image of an abnormally positioned tooth (arrowhead) causing midline displacement (arrow) demonstrates the view.

Open-mouth dorsoventral projections of arcades are taken with the mandible displaced laterally (**203**). This allows imaging of the buccal and lingual or palatal aspects of the teeth and alveolus (**204**).

INTRAORAL RADIOGRAPHY

In intraoral radiography a single arcade is imaged, therefore tissue thickness and the requirement for x-ray penetration are reduced. Slow-speed, high-detail systems with minimal exposures can therefore be employed. Images of single teeth are effectively created for evaluation of:
• Periodontal disease.
• Fractures of teeth, including those with pulp exposures.
• Pulpitis, bony swellings, sinusitis, and draining tracts.
• Monitoring of surgical procedures.

FILMS AND SCREENS

Most x-ray films have the emulsion on both sides of the film. Single-emulsion films have the emulsion on only one side. They are also known as detail films. They create improved detail by reducing the amount of background and scatter radiation that interacts with the silver halide crystal. Most single-emulsion films are used with single-screen system cassettes. These films are best used with the slow-speed or detail screens.

Some films allow the light produced by a screen on double-screen cassettes with double-emulsion film to cross over to the opposite side of the film and add to the amount of light exposing the emulsion on the other side. This allows for the use of slightly lower exposures, resulting in a faster-speed system. Since the system speed is faster, images can be produced in areas of thicker tissue. The drawback is loss of detail, since an image is created by light from sources on each side of the film. Other films have an anticrossover layer that prevents light from one side from exposing the film emulsion on the other side. This film has improved detail.

A wide-latitude film will accept a variation in exposure without experiencing a great variation in contrast. This is beneficial in equine dentistry, as adjustment of machine technique settings is minimized for varying tissue thickness.

The film used is wide-latitude, medium-speed film with an anticrossover layer that functions like a single-emulsion, high-detail film. The system used for equine intraoral dental radiology utilizes this film in combination with a single screen, thus resulting in detail similar to a single-emulsion film. Two screen speeds are used: 100 speed and 200 speed. Vinyl cassettes with a paper liner are used with a single card-mounted intensifying screen attached to the liner.

The importance of film and screen in radiology can be exemplified by visualizing the stars at night. In a perfect match of screen and film as on a dark night in the country, all the tiniest stars can be seen. In the city, there is more background glare, as though the screen is picking up more light either because it is a faster screen, i.e. more phosphor layers, larger crystal size, or more x-rays are reaching the screen, as in too much kVp or mAs. When seen in daylight the stars are still present, but the glare from the sun obscures them. The type of film is insignificant if the screen doesn't match the needs of the exposure.

The slower-speed screens create small points of light like the stars in the sky. If the screen is too fast there will be glare and detail will be obscured.

As tissue thickness increases two changes can be made. If the same screen is used the exposure must be increased, since x-rays are absorbed by the tissue thus preventing them from activating the intensifying screen. Two complications arise with increased exposure. The first is the increased brightness of the light which risks glare. The second is the increased time which risks movement. The alternative change is to minimize the changes in the technique and use a faster screen. The compromise maintains good detail with minimal increase in exposure.

For example, compare two systems, both with a system speed of 200. The first system uses 400 speed screens and half-speed, or detail film. The second system uses 200 speed screens and regular film. The first system utilizes a screen whose speed creates more light at a given exposure. The points of light are larger and brighter. The smaller crystal size of the film in this system reacts to the brighter light and creates an image that is less sharp. The second system uses a screen speed that emits small points of light that are converted into better detail images on the film. The detail of the second system will be best. The speed of the screen has the most influence on detail.

PHYSICS OF RADIOLOGY AS RELATED TO INTRAORAL RADIOGRAPHY

The 40 cm film focal distance (FFD) technique can be modified. When doing so it is important to know the characteristics of the beam. For most machines, the beam becomes parallel at about 30–40 cm from the source. Closer to the source the beam is too divergent. Therefore the shortest FFD possible would be 30–40 cm.

It is also helpful to remember the inverse square law which states that beam intensity diminishes with distance in a predictable fashion. The formula is as follows:

$$\frac{\text{Old exposure time}}{\text{New exposure time}} = \frac{(\text{Old distance})^2}{(\text{New distance})^2}$$

When the FFD is doubled the original exposure time should be multiplied by 4.

When the FFD is halved the exposure time should be reduced to quarter the original time.

The kVp is the the peak accelerating voltage applied in an x-ray tube between the cathode and anode. It measures the kinetic energy of the radiation output. The kVp setting used in this technique is simplified so that a quality image can be created in a variety of head sizes. In most cases 50 kVp is used for premolars and 60 kVp is used for molars.

Milliampere-seconds (mAs) is the product of the x-ray tube current in milliamperes and the duration of the x-ray exposure in seconds. For a given kilovolt peak kVp, the mAs is directly proportional to the total number of x-ray photons produced and thus to the x-ray dose to the patient for that exposure.

The mAs settings for this technique are simplified so that a quality image can be produced in a variety of head sizes: 0.5 mAs is used for premolars and 0.6 mAs is used for molars.

FILM AND CASSETTE PREPARATION

Cassettes open by unfolding (**205**). Reinforcement of edges with radiolucent tape provides adequate seal against light and moisture. The cassette is constructed so that the image can be produced from only one direction. The folds of the vinyl and paper block the opposite side. The cassette is marked on the tube side. Loaded cassettes should be stored in a dark location. Prolonged exposure of the loaded cassette to direct sunlight will fog the film.

It is important to maintain good film-to-screen contact. Failure to do so results in blurred images. Good contact can be achieved by bending the cassette slightly by wrapping it with a rubber band. When stored in such a manner for extended periods, the cassettes will become permanently curved. Image quality is maximized.

The film size used is 10.1 × 20.2 cm (4" × 8"). This size can easily be created by cutting standard 20.2 × 25.3 cm (8" × 10") film down to size. A standard office paper cutter is used to cut the film (**206**). The use of scissors will cause disruption of the film emulsion and create artifacts.

When cutting the film a fast guillotine stroke is used to slice the film quickly. This procedure will minimize artifacts. Accurate measurement and cutting of film is necessary; making the film too large will result in a size that will not fit into the cassettes. Approximately 20 sheets of cut, unused film can be stored in a standard cassette. The cassette can be marked for identification purposes as holding intraoral films. The films are thus protected from light and moisture. The cassette can be transported as necessary, and individual films placed into intraoral cassettes as needed.

After exposure and removal from the vinyl cassette the film can be developed in any standard automatic processor.

DENTAL INTRAORAL RADIOLOGY TECHNIQUE USING A PORTABLE X-RAY MACHINE

When first learning the technique, multiple views and exposures should be taken. The first view taken of the arcade in question can be considered a survey view. The technique used can be adjusted to fit the needs of the problem or patient. In general, less penetration is required for detail of apical and more occlusally oriented periodontal anatomy, while increased penetration is required for details of pulp structures. The 100 speed single-screen cassette provides excellent detail of less dense tissues at low settings for radiation exposure. For more dense tissues, such as pulp detail of all teeth and for apical detail of molars where dense or thick tissue overlies the objects, the 200 speed screen is used. All exposures are taken at a 40 cm FFD. This technique provides sufficient exposure to penetrate the denser tissue while providing excellent detail. Mixing techniques and film/screen combinations will provide solutions to differing detail needs. For example, the technique used to image the pulp areas of premolars in some patients uses 60 kVp and up to 0.6 mAs with 100 speed screens for adequate exposure.

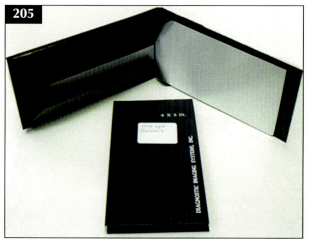

205 Intraoral equine dental cassettes with rare earth screens.

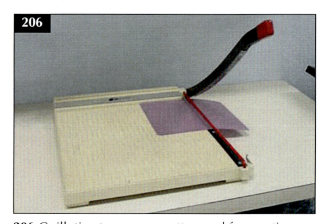

206 Guillotine-type paper cutter used for creating 10.1 × 20.2 cm (4" × 8") x-ray film.

Table 7 Tips for improving exposures

- Reducing the FFD by one-quarter doubles the penetration/film density. For example, reduce a 40 cm FFD by 10 cm to double the exposure
- Increasing the FFD by one-quarter halves the penetration/film density. For example, increase a 40 cm FFD by 10 cm to halve the exposure
- For each 1 cm increase or decrease in thickness add or subtract 2 kV
- Increasing the kVp by 10 doubles the penetration of the beam
- Halving the mAs will reduce the exposure by half, while doubling the mAs will double the exposure
- For every 5 cm of thickness double the mAs

Table 8 Specific settings are used for objects identified

Screen speed	Tissue density	Examples	kVp setting	mAs setting
100	Less dense	Premolars	50	0.5
	Canines			
	Incisors			
	Periodontium of molars			
200	More dense	Pulps of all teeth	60	0.6
	Apical details of molars			

Table 7 lists several suggestions for troubleshooting images that may be either too light or too dark.

STEP-BY-STEP PROCEDURE FOR INTRAORAL RADIOGRAPHY

The decision to radiograph is based either on knowledge of the patient's condition before examination or on clinical findings during a dental procedure. The sedation protocol is adjusted accordingly.

1. *Sedation protocol (first stage).* The author uses a two-stage sedation protocol. The first sedative is administered by intravenous injection of detomidine at 0.02 mg/kg[8] in combination with xylazine at 0.2 mg/kg.[8]

2. *General position of the x-ray machine and setting of exposure.* FFD is 40 cm in all projections. The collimator is opened to its maximum aperture. The settings for the x-ray machine vary depending on the location of the area of interest. *Table 8* summarizes these exposure techniques.
   - **Maxillary projections:** the cassette will be inserted into the mouth and placed over the tongue at an angle in order to capture an image of the maxillary arcade. The x-ray machine is positioned similarly to that used in a dorsal oblique technique for maxillary teeth.
   - **Mandibular projections:** images of more occlusally oriented anatomy of equine cheek teeth are best obtained with intraoral projections. This includes images of the clinical crown and of occlusally oriented periodontal structures. These projections are taken with the parallel technique. For best views of apical anatomy in young and mature horses, the lateral oblique extraoral technique at 45° remains the technique of choice. Apical anatomy of horses over 20 years of age can be imaged in some cases with intraoral projections approximating the parallel technique.

3. *Position patient's head.* It is necessary to use a speculum with lateral components that do not obstruct the x-ray beam: the author prefers a speculum with elastic side straps (**207**). When images are taken that include the second premolars, the poll strap and lateral brackets

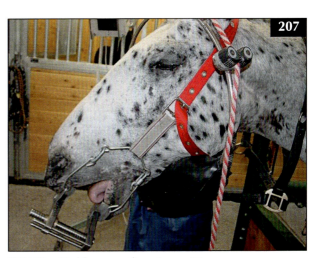

207 The Stubbs speculum in position.

are retracted away from the path of the x-ray beam. Alternatively, a McPherson speculum can be used for maxillary projections. However, the presence of the speculum in the radiograph will cause x-ray scatter and may blur the image.

The patient's head is placed in a support device. A head ring or head stand can be used for this purpose (**208**).

4. *Sedation protocol (second stage).* After 3–5 minutes, a second intravenous injection is administered of xylazine at 0.2 mg/kg together with butorphanol at 0.01 mg/kg.[9]

5. *Intraoral lidocaine.* After initial sedation, 5–10 ml of lidocaine can be sprayed topically on to the oral mucosa. This desensitizes the tongue, palate, and buccal mucosa to help limit motion caused by sensitivity of these soft tissues. The effect is very temporary, lasting a few minutes and is not necessary in all patients.

6. *Protective aprons and gloves and other safety equipment.* A protective lead apron, glasses, and other safety equipment should be donned prior to exposure. Radiation monitoring badges should be provided.

7. *Cassette holder.* The cassette holder (**209**) can be made from a 50 cm (20") length of 13 mm (½") plastic pipe. A slot is cut into the end of the pipe for holding the cassette. A handle is made from a 45° connector and an additional 15 cm (6") length of the same pipe.

8. *Set angles and final position of x-ray machine.* Radiographs of the maxillary cheek teeth are obtained utilizing the bisecting angle technique.[10,11] The vinyl cassette is placed on

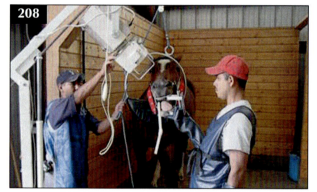

208 The patient's head is supported and the x-ray machine is positioned.

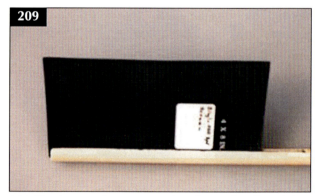

209 The intraoral cassette is fitted into the slot of the cassette holder.

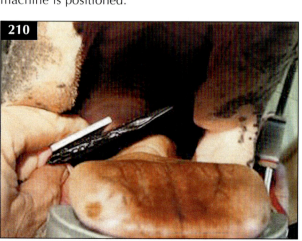

210 Approximate position of film in patient's mouth.

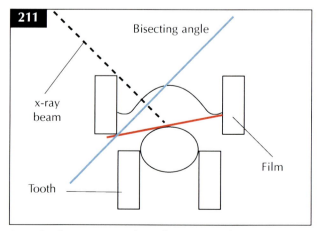

211 The bisecting angle technique used in imaging equine maxillary teeth.

top of the tongue and against the palate in as flat a position as possible (**210**). The film is slightly angled so that it extends from the occlusal surface of the side being radiographed to the gingival margin on the opposite side. To understand the bisecting angle technique, visualization of the positions of the teeth and film is necessary. The angle formed by intersecting planes of the long axes of the tooth (the object) and the film is bisected. The tube head is positioned perpendicular to the bisected angle. The resulting image closely approximates the actual size and orientation of the tooth and surrounding structures. Figures **211–214** demonstrate the bisecting angle technique. The bisecting angle technique is shown with

the x-ray beam projected perpendicular to the line that bisects the angle made by the film and object (the tooth root). This procedure produces a parallel projection of the object on to the film.

9. *Insert cassette*. The cassette should be inserted after the x-ray machine is set and positioned as in figure **215**. The tube side of the cassette should be noted and the cassette placed appropriately.
10. *Take exposure.*
11. *Remove and develop film.* Any processing system is appropriate for film developing. Rapid processors can handle film of this size and reduce the processing time.
12. *View image.*

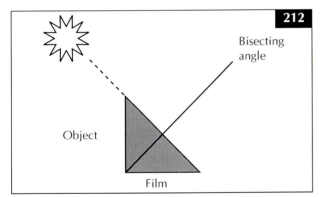

212 Correct angulation for the bisecting angle technique.

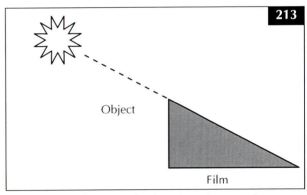

213 Elongated view. Tube head too low, angle too flat.

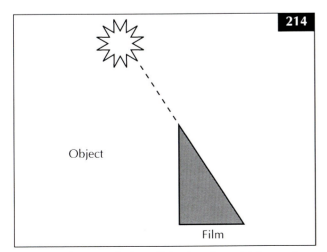

214 Foreshortened view. Tube head too high, angle too steep.

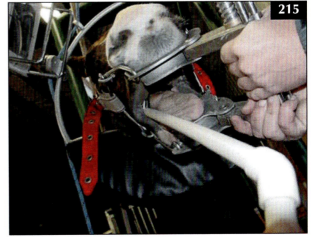

215 Intraoral cassette inserted in the patient's mouth using the cassette holder.

RADIOGRAPHIC INTERPRETATION

Interpretation of radiographic findings follows principles similar to those used for other species. Recognition of normal and abnormal anatomy on a radiograph begins with knowledge of and composition of the structures. The relevant terms are as follows:

- **Alveolar crest:** the projection of alveolar bone whose termination between proximal teeth is usually shaped in a point.
- **Apex/apices:** the terminal point(s) of the root tip(s).
- **Apical orifice:** the opening of the root tip where neurovascular supply enters the pulp. The size of this orifice decreases with age as the cementum and dentin of the root fill in the root canal.
- **Cementum:** the outer covering of the root, reserve, and clinical crown of the equine tooth. Also fills in the outside of the enamel folds of teeth.
- **Cortical bone:** the dense layer of bone at the periphery of the structure.
- **Dentin:** the dental tissue that fills in the pulp chamber and root canals. This tissue is less dense than enamel.
- **Enamel:** the most dense dental tissue. Enamel forms the layer under cementum and the lines seen on lateral views of the internal tooth structure.
- **Lamina dura:** denser bone, also known as the cribriform plate, which lines the alveolar socket. This structure is denser than trabecular bone but less dense then cortical bone. It serves as the attachment of the PDL.
- **PDL space:** the radiolucent line between the tooth and the lamina dura.
- **Pulp:** the less dense almost radiolucent internal portion of the tooth. Comprised of the pulp chamber and pulp horn in the crown part of the tooth and the root canal in the apical area of the tooth.
- **Trabeculae:** medullary bone.

When visualizing a radiograph, the practitioner should develop the technique of looking at the image in the same way as the patient is visualized. When looking at images of the right side of the horse, the radiograph should have the nose directed to the right; radiographs of problems on the left side of the patient are visualized with the nose directed to the left. When one becomes accustomed to this method, radiographic findings are more easily projected accurately to the patient.

This is most important when several images involving different projections are needed to arrive at an accurate diagnosis. For example, images such as extraoral survey films, intraoral views, and open-mouth oblique projections are created from both sides of the patient. Consistent visualization is important in correct diagnosis. This visualization is independent of the direction of projection of the x-ray generator or position of the film when taking the radiograph. It is, therefore, helpful to visualize these images as if one is looking at the patient.

In veterinary dentistry the basis of reference for dental radiography is the small animal patient. Therefore, recognition of normal structures begins there. Figure **216** is a radiograph of a mandibular tooth in a dog. Tissues and structure in equine dental anatomy vary somewhat from those of small animals:

- Enamel is folded into a complex pattern on both mandibular and maxillary arcades which can be seen as lines throughout the tooth.

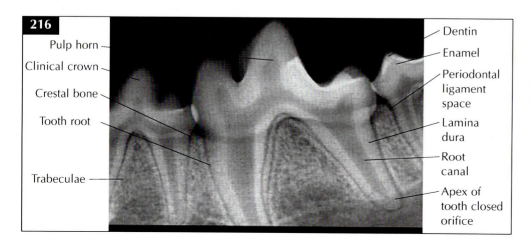

216 Normal radiographic anatomy of a dog tooth. (Courtesy of Dr. Randi Brannan.)

- Dentin and cementum closure of the apex is slower, so the orifice remains open for several years.
- The lamina dura is somewhat less regular in both mandibular and maxillary teeth.
- Cementum forms the outer layer of equine teeth.
- The pulp canal takes longer to fill.
- Equine teeth are radicular hypsodont: they have continually erupting crowns that suffer attrition on their occlusal surface. Root formation also

continues. The overall length of the tooth remains constant for many years, but is composed of less and less crown and more and more root. The result is a decrease in the overall mass of the tooth and entire arcade as the horse ages. Less mass means less exposure is necessary as the patient ages.

Radiographs of normal horse mandibular and maxillary cheek teeth are shown in figures **217**–**219**.

217 Normal anatomy of a horse's mandibular cheek tooth.

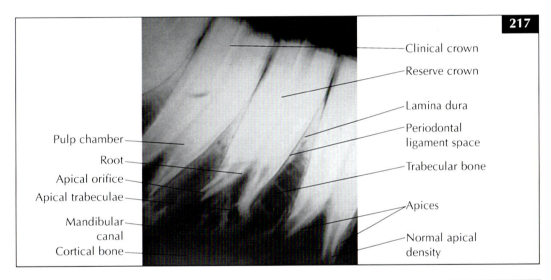

Clinical crown
Reserve crown
Lamina dura
Periodontal ligament space
Trabecular bone
Apices
Normal apical density

Pulp chamber
Root
Apical orifice
Apical trabeculae
Mandibular canal
Cortical bone

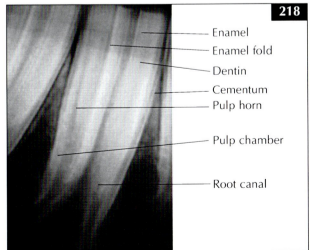

Enamel
Enamel fold
Dentin
Cementum
Pulp horn
Pulp chamber
Root canal

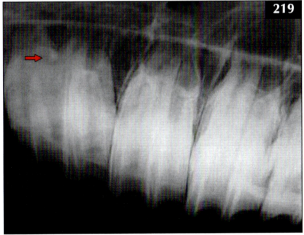

218 Normal radiographic anatomy of a horse's mandibular cheek tooth. The radiograph was taken at higher exposure than figure **217**.

219 Normal radiographic anatomy of a horse maxillary cheek tooth (arrow).

ARTIFACTS

Film-screen contact must be complete. Loss of contact will result in blurring of the image (**220**). Folding of the film or screen will create a line in the image (**221**).

RADIOGRAPHIC FINDINGS

The following pictures and descriptions include examples of specific pathological findings. The list of abnormalities includes some of the more common findings. An understanding of dental anatomy and physiology is necessary to interpret the films. Pathological conditions are described and compared to normal anatomy.

WIDENED PERIODONTAL LIGAMENT SPACE

The PDL space should be a consistent width from the area of the root apex to the crest of the alveolar bone (**222**). Suspected widening can be compared to another portion of the same tooth or to another tooth. Widened PDL space (**223**) is interpreted as an

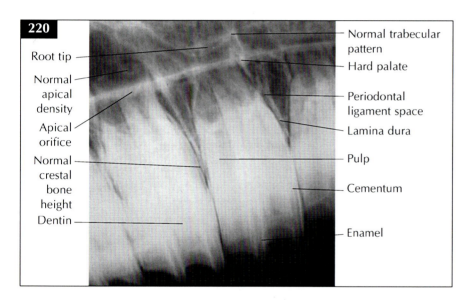

Labels (left): Root tip, Normal apical density, Apical orifice, Normal crestal bone height, Dentin

Labels (right): Normal trabecular pattern, Hard palate, Periodontal ligament space, Lamina dura, Pulp, Cementum, Enamel

220 Blurring artifact on left is due to poor film-screen contact.

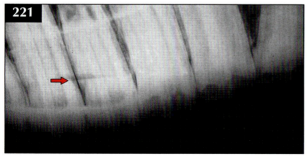

221 Folding the film or screen results in a line on the film (arrow).

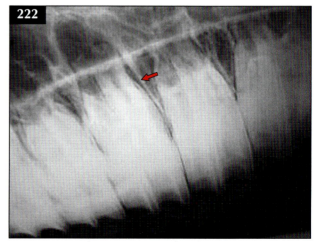

222 Arrow indicates a normal PDL space.

inflammatory remodeling of the periodontium or bone destruction from an apical abscess, cyst, or granuloma.

PULPITIS

The pulp chamber of cheek teeth can be visualized on higher exposures. In the normal tooth the radiolucent pulp has sharp margins at its borders (**224**). The more radiopaque dentin surrounding the pulp and the enamel of the apical margin of the infundibulum are very distinct. In pulpal disease the sharpness of these margins is lost and radiolucency of the area is increased (**225**).

ROUGHENED SURFACES

The surface of both the tooth and lamina dura should be relatively smooth and parallel (**226**). Roughened tooth and lamina dura surfaces are indications of

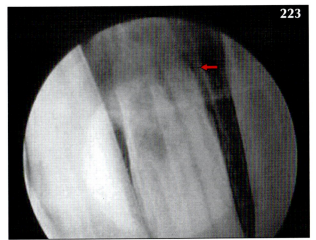

223 Arrow points to widened PDL space resulting from pulpitis extending from apex to surrounding tissue.

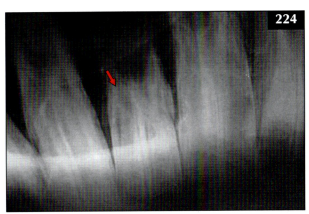

224 Arrow indicates sharp margins of pulp and surrounding structures in a normal 109.

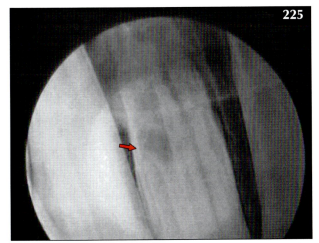

225 Arrow indicates loss of sharpness of margins of pulp with increased radiolucency in a case of severe pulpitis.

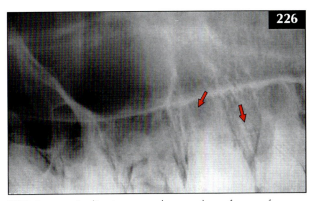

226 Arrows indicate normal smooth surfaces of hypsodont tooth.

inflammatory remodeling of the tissues as part of either the condition of periodontal disease (**227**) or the extension of pulpitis to involve periodontal structures.

REDUCED CRESTAL BONE HEIGHT

The alveolar bone surrounding each tooth terminates in its occlusal border in what is seen radiographically as a sharp point. This terminus is referred to as the alveolar crest (**228**). Inflammation related to periodontal disease results in lysis of bone in this location. The reduction of crestal bone height (**229**) is a hallmark of periodontal disease since it represents loss of attachment of the bony alveolus to the tooth.

BLUNTED APICES

In advancing periodontal disease and pulpitis, tooth and bone remodeling occur at the root apex. Apices become blunted by inflammatory remodeling. Normal and blunted apices can be compared in figures **230–233**.

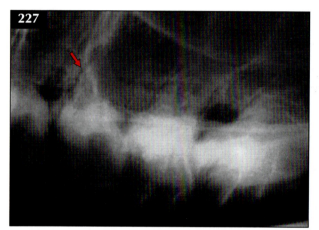

227 Arrow indicates roughened alveolar bone and lamina dura coincident with periodontal disease of the left upper first molar (209).

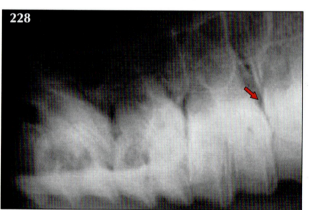

228 Arrow indicates normal crestal bone height in a geriatric patient.

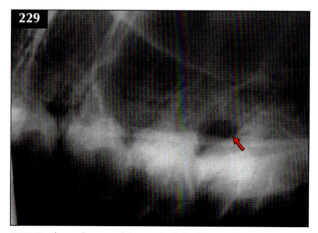

229 Reduced crestal bone height (arrow).

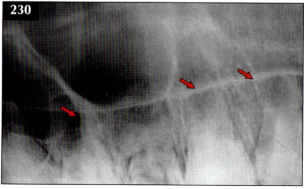

230 Normal apices in a geriatric maxillary arcade (arrows).

ALVEOLAR SCLEROSIS

Sclerosis of alveolar bone is an indication of long-standing inflammation. It is commonly encountered in periodontal disease of older patients (**234**).

APICAL LUCENCY

Commonly referred to as apical abscess, an apical lucency is an indication of active inflammation of the tissue at the root apex (**235**). Pulpal inflammation of varying degrees is associated with apical lucency and may be severe enough to cause pulp necrosis. Extension of apical disease may result in sinusitis or draining tracts.

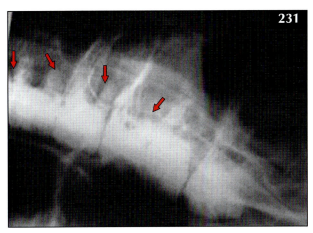

231 Arrows indicate blunted apices in a geriatric patient.

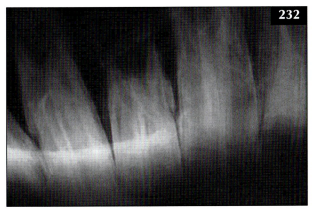

232 Normal apices in an 8-year-old Quarterhorse.

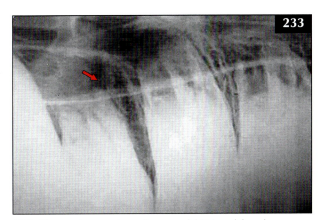

233 Blunted apex in a 6-year-old Warmblood (arrow).

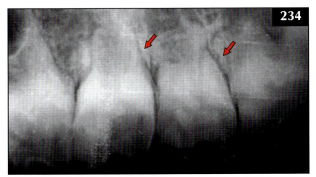

234 Alveolar sclerosis in a 22-year-old patient with periodontal disease (arrows).

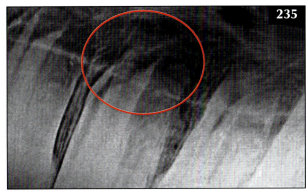

235 The circle indicates an apical lucency as seen on an intraoral radiograph.

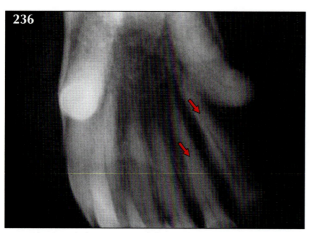

236 The apical portion of the pulps of 302 and 303 (arrows) are filled with tertiary dentin. These canals are obliterated. The same process occurs in canines and cheek teeth and can best be visualized with intraoral radiographs.

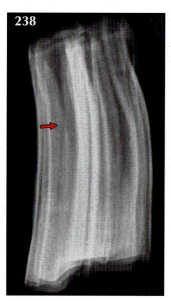

238 Dentin bridge formation is shown in this extracted tooth. The arrow indicates the closed pulp canal. Above the arrow the canal opened to the apical section of the tooth, and contained viable pulp. Below the arrow, the pulp was necrotic.

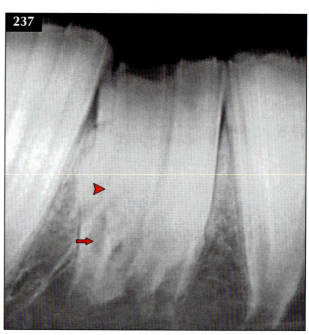

237 The hazy density (arrowhead) that obscures the pulp canal is dentin forming a bridge that walls off the normal pulp. The arrow indicates a viable normal pulp. This fractured tooth was extracted.

PULP CANAL OBLITERATION

The hypsodont pulp is very reactive and responsive to outside insult. In mild to moderate cases of insult the pulp may respond by filling the canal with tertiary dentin (**236–238**). In some cases the entire canal is filled, resulting in pulp canal obliteration.

DISCUSSION

Intraoral radiographs produced with rare earth systems create quality films of dental structures while minimizing the confusion of overlying densities. The visualization of greater detail of dental structures aids in diagnosis, treatment, and prognosis of dental problems. As equine dental procedures continue to advance, diagnostic detail of radiographs must improve. Intraoral radiographs provide this improved detail.

The use of intraoral radiographs in diagnosis, prognosis, and treatment of periodontal disease cannot be overemphasized. Determination of the extent of attachment loss of the periodontium is facilitated. When clinical examination fails to define the extent of a periodontal pocket, intraoral radiographs provide necessary information regarding the detail of structures surrounding the tooth.

Intraoral radiographs are practical when the following goals are achieved:
- Maximum efficiency.
- Maximum detail of the image.
- Minimum radiation exposure times.

Efficient production of radiographs is important for the practicality of the clinical application of the technique to routine equine practice. Minimal technique change is important when taking multiple films. In general only two different machine settings are used. The FFD is 40 cm. For less dense structures such as premolars, the setting used is 50 kVp at 0.5 mAs. For denser structures, such as molars, the settings used are 60 kVp and 0.6 mAs. The use of two different screen speeds effectively creates a total of four techniques that can be used interchangeably.

Detail is maximized by the use of slow-speed rare earth screens (100 and 200 speed) together with wide-latitude medium-speed film. A single screen is used. The film used employs the concept of an anticrossover layer within the film that blocks the light from one side exposing the emulsion of the other side of the film. The effective result is a single emulsion film.

Patient movement is minimized by sedation. Employment of a rare earth system with the use of wide-latitude film of medium speed allows for the shortest exposure times. This further reduces the potential for blurring of the film by slight motion.

The technique of intraoral radiography adds to the diagnostic arsenal for the equine veterinarian practicing dentistry. Interpretation is facilitated by increased detail resulting from isolation of each arcade. While the procedure for obtaining quality films may seem cumbersome at first, efficiency improves with practice.

Problems such as periodontal disease cannot be adequately characterized without intraoral radiographs. Improved radiographic detail aids in diagnosis, treatment, and prognosis of pulp disease. Fractures and surgical treatments can be evaluated and monitored easily. Diagnosis of dental disease and evaluation of surgical intervention becomes black and white with the use of intraoral radiography.

SUMMARY

Extraoral radiography provides wide-angle views of multiple teeth, sinuses, and bones of the head. Specific projections provide specialized views of various anatomical locations.

Intraoral radiography provides more focused and detailed views of specific teeth. The use of rare earth detail screens and specific film facilitates production of quality images in a variety of tissue thicknesses while minimizing technique changes.

New radiographic techniques provide the practitioner with more tools for better medicine.

REFERENCES

1. Easley J. A new look at dental radiology. *Proceedings 48th Annual Convention of the American Association of Equine Practitioners* 2002; pp. 412–420.
2. Barakzai SZ, Dixon PM. A study of open-mouthed oblique radiographic projections for evaluating lesions of the erupted (clinical) crown. *Equine Veterinary Education* 2003: **15**(3); 143–148.
3. O'Brien RT. Intraoral dental radiography: experimental study and clinical use in two horses and a llama. *Veterinary Radiology & Ultrasound* 1996: **37**(6); 412–416.
4. Gibbs C. Dental imaging. In: Baker GJ, Easley J (eds) *Equine Dentistry*. London: WB Saunders, 1999; 139–169.
5. Lavin L. Image receptors. In: *Radiography for Veterinary Technology*. Philadelphia: WB Saunders, 1994; 55–68.
6. Pettersson H, Allison DJ. (eds) *The Encyclopaedia of Medical Imaging*. Oxford: ISIS Medical Media, 2002.
7. Pizzutiello R, Culligan R. *Introduction to Medical Radiographic Imaging*. Rochester: Eastman Kodak Company, 1993.
8. Baker GJ, Kirkland KD. Sedation for dental prophylaxis in horses: a comparison between detomidine and xylazine. *Proceedings 41st Annual Convention of the American Association of Equine Practitioners* 1995; pp. 40–41.
9. Orsini JA. Butorphanol tartrate: pharmacology and clinical indications. *Compendium on Continuing Education for the Practicing Veterinarian* 1988: **10**(7); 849–854.
10. Eisner ER. Oral dental radiographic technique. *Veterinary Clinics of North America: Small Animal Practice* 1998: **28**(5); 1063–1087.
11. Mulligan T, Aller M, Williams C. *Atlas of Canine and Feline Dental Radiography*. Trenton: Veterinary Learning Systems, 1998.

STANDING CHEMICAL RESTRAINT IN THE EQUINE DENTAL PATIENT

Jane Quandt   Chapter 10

Equine dental procedures require that a horse is adequately sedated and has appropriate analgesia. One single agent is rarely sufficient to provide the necessary sedation and analgesia, for the required duration, and to provide a smooth recovery. Therefore two to three agents are commonly used in combination. Use of a balanced sedation technique minimizes the side-effects of a single agent and utilizes the synergistic effect of multiple agents. When doing standing restraint it is advisable to have an intravenous catheter in place. This will make drug administration easier and prevent the administration of the drug perivascularly or even intra-arterially. If a crisis should arise an intravenous catheter can be life-saving for the administration of reversal drugs or intravenous fluid therapy. Veins can be hard to raise or puncture in the event of cardiovascular collapse. An intravenous catheter is mandatory if a constant rate infusion (CRI) is used for the sedation technique.

Sedative agents will have a better effect if the horse is in a calm and quiet environment, and is kept undisturbed.[1] Adequate time must be allowed for the sedatives to have their maximum effect.[1]

Monitoring should consist of noting respiratory rate, heart rate, mucous membrane color, and pulse strength. Monitoring equipment such as electrocardiograph (ECG) and blood pressure may not be available or practical in the field situation. A pulse oximeter may not be accurate in the moving animal.

There are various classes of drugs that may be used for standing sedation. It is important to realize that all the agents used will have a central nervous system (CNS) effect in addition to peripheral actions.[2]

Tranquilizers produce calming and behavior modification, but do not have analgesic properties.[2] Sedatives are similar to tranquilizers in that they reduce excitement and induce calming, but in addition provide analgesia.[2] Sedatives include the alpha 2 agonists. Opioids provide analgesia but are rarely used alone as they may create excitement. They are often used in combination with a tranquilizer or a sedative. Some agents can be reversed by the use of specific reversal agents. This can result in a quicker recovery but will remove the sedation as well as any analgesic effect.

Table 9 shows drug doses for use of sedatives, tranquilizers, reversal agents, combinations, and CRIs.

TRANQUILIZERS

ACEPROMAZINE

Acepromazine (**239**) is a phenothiazine and has very low toxicity. It will induce calming, alter behavior patterns, produce loss of interest in the environment, but maintain arousability especially following a painful stimulus. It decreases mental alertness by depressing the reticular activation center of the CNS.[3] The mechanism of action is centrally mediated via antagonism of the dopamine-mediated synaptic transmission.[4] This leads to depression in the

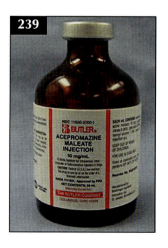

239 Acepromazine.

Table 9 Drug dosages[2,29]

Agents for chemical restraint and reversal agents	Suggested dose range
Doses will need to be adjusted based on the horse's response.	

Tranquilizers

Acepromazine	0.01–0.088 mg/kg IV
Diazepam	0.02 mg/kg IV
Flumazenil	0.04 mg/kg IV

Alpha 2 agonists

Xylazine	0.3–1.1 mg/kg IV
Detomidine	0.005–0.04 mg/kg IV
Medetomidine	0.0035–0.01 mg/kg IV
Romifidine	0.03–0.12 mg/kg IV

Alpha 2 antagonists

Yohimbine	0.04–0.2 mg/kg
Tolazoline	4 mg/kg slow IV
Atipamazole	0.15 mg/kg IV

Opioids

Morphine	0.02–0.1 mg/kg slow IV
Meperidine	0.2–1.0 mg/kg slow IV
Butorphanol	0.01–0.02 mg/kg IV
Buprenorphine	0.003–0.02 mg/kg IV

Opioid reversal

Naloxone	0.005–0.02 mg/kg IV

Drug combinations with suggested doses

Xylazine 0.55 mg/kg with acepromazine 0.05 mg/kg IV
Xylazine 0.66 mg/kg with acepromazine 0.02 mg/kg IV

Xylazine 0.66 mg/kg with morphine 0.3–0.66 mg/kg IV
Xylazine 0.5 mg/kg with butorphanol 0.05 mg/kg IV
Xylazine 0.66 mg/kg with butorphanol 0.03 mg/kg IV
Xylazine 0.6 mg/kg with buprenorphine 0.01 mg/kg IV

Detomidine 0.01 mg/kg with butorphanol 0.02 mg/kg IV
Detomidine 0.01 mg/kg with butorphanol 0.05 mg/kg IV

Romifidine 0.045 mg/kg with butorphanol 0.017 mg/kg IV
Romifidine 0.1 mg/kg with butorphanol 0.05 mg/kg IV
Romifidine 0.1 mg/kg with morphine 0.1 mg/kg IV

Acepromazine 0.02 mg/kg with buprenorphine 0.004 mg/kg IV
Acepromazine 0.02–0.05 mg/kg with detomidine 0.005–0.01 mg/kg IV

Infusions: infusion rate will require adjustment based on the horse's response

Detomidine: IV loading dose of 0.0075 mg/kg followed by an infusion of 0.00187 mg/kg/min IV
Detomidine: 0.0084 mg/kg IV loading dose, then 0.0005 mg/kg/min IV for 15 minutes, then 0.0003 mg/kg/min IV for 15 minutes, and thereafter 0.00015 mg/kg/min IV
Detomidine: 0.01 mg/kg with buprenorphine 0.006 mg/kg IV then detomidine infusion of 0.00016 mg/kg/min IV
Butorphanol: 0.0178 mg/kg IV loading dose and then 0.00038 mg/kg/min IV
Ketamine: 0.4–0.8 mg/kg/hr IV

brainstem and connections to the cerebral cortex, and will also block the CNS activity of norepinephrine and epinephrine. This blockade of dopamine and catecholamines explains how acepromazine can inhibit opioid-induced excitement as opioids will enhance the release of dopamine and norepinephrine in the CNS.[2] The release of dopamine and norepinephrine causes increased motor activity and excitement.

Large doses of acepromazine can produce extrapyramidal effects which can cause a reluctance to move, mild rigidity, muscle tremor, and restlessness. Peripherally acepromazine blocks cholinergic, adrenergic, and ganglionic activity. It is the alpha adrenergic blocking effect which produces antihistamine, antiarrhythmic, antifibrillatory, antipyretic, and antishock effects.

Hypotension is produced by the depression of the hypothalamus, peripheral alpha adrenoceptor blockade, and a direct vasodilatory effect on the blood vessels. This reduction in blood pressure is dose dependent and may produce reflex tachycardia, especially in horses with increased catecholamines as may occur with fear or stress. The blood pressure may decrease by 15–20 mmHg with clinical doses.[2] Due to the decrease in blood pressure acepromazine should probably be avoided in the hypovolemic horse as the hypotension could be severe.[1] Hypotension may cause ataxia, sweating, hyperpnea, weakness, tachycardia, and possibly excitement which should be treated with intravenous fluid therapy to prevent collapse.[2,3]

The use of this drug may be contraindicated in the excited or stressed horse due to the potential for epinephrine reversal. The acepromazine alpha blocking effect allows the vasodilating beta 2 effects of epinephrine to predominate. This will lead to a profound hypotensive effect. Treatment is through the rapid administration of intravenous fluids, such as lactated Ringers at 10 mL/kg/hr.[3]

The alpha adrenolytic activity along with the depression of the vasomotor center will cause splenic relaxation with consequent erythrocyte sequestration leading to a decrease in the hematocrit. The decrease in hematocrit can be as profound as a 20% decrease, with a gradual onset and the lowest value may take 6 hours to occur with a duration of up to 12 hours.[2,4] The decrease in the packed cell volume (PCV) and total protein (TP) concentration is dose dependent. There is also a dilutional effect of interstitial water entering the vascular compartment secondary to hypotension.

Acepromazine has little effect on blood gas tensions or pH and no effect on respiratory rate.[4] Acepromazine is metabolized by the liver and excreted in the urine. It has 90% plasma protein binding which could lead to a prolonged duration of action in a horse with hypoproteinemia.

Flaccid paralysis of the retractor penis muscle resulting in priapism and paraphimosis has been referred to as a side-effect of acepromazine. This effect is unpredictable and not dose related.[2,3]

The toxicity of organophosphate pesticides and antihelmintics is increased by acepromazine, as they both inhibit acetylcholinesterase and pseudocholinesterase.

If acepromazine is inadvertently given intracarotid, the horse will become excited, collapse, and develop uncontrollable paddling followed by seizures. The horse may 'fall off the needle'. Treatment consists of protecting the horse and giving an anticonvulsant, such as diazepam 0.01 mg/kg IV.[2]

When given IV the peak drug effect is seen within 10–20 minutes and within 20–30 minutes if given intramuscularly (IM).[1,2,4] Duration can be as long as 6 hours. There are no antagonists for acepromazine. Not all horses will respond to acepromazine. Re-administration or increasing the dose does not improve sedation and will only enhance the side-effects.

Acepromazine is compatible with alpha 2 agonists and opioids, and is frequently used in combination with these agents. Acepromazine does not produce analgesia, so it must be combined with an analgesic if a painful procedure is to be done.[3]

DIAZEPAM

Diazepam (**240**), is a benzodiazepine tranquilizer. It potentiates gamma-aminobutyric acid (GABA)-mediated inhibition in the CNS.[5] GABA is a major inhibitory neurotransmitter in the brain. The principal action is in the brainstem reticular formation and it produces hypnotic, sedative, anxiolytic, anticonvulsant, and skeletal muscle-relaxant effects. It also has the potential to cause CNS excitement, and doses higher than 0.2 mg/kg IV may induce recumbency due to the muscle relaxant effects and CNS depression. It is highly protein bound, 87%, and is metabolized by the liver with urinary elimination. The elimination half-life is 6.94–13.2 hours. There are minimal depressant effects on the respiratory and cardiovascular systems. Diazepam has no analgesic effects. Diazepam is commonly used in

240 Diazepam.

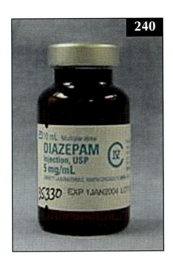

240

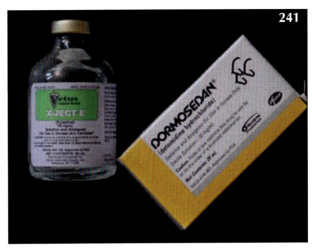

241

241 Examples of alpha 2 agonists include xylazine (left) and detomidine (right).

combination with alpha 2 agonists and dissociatives as part of an induction technique. It has been used in combination with alpha 2 agonists and opioids as a one-time injection to enhance relaxation and sedation for standing restraint. A one-time dose of 0.02 mg/kg IV can be used.[5] The effects of diazepam can be reversed with intravenous flumazenil; a dose of 0.04 mg/kg IV has been used for benzodiazepine reversal in foals.[6]

ALPHA 2 ADRENOCEPTOR AGONISTS

The alpha 2 agonists activate the alpha 2 adrenoceptors in the CNS and the peripheral tissue. Examples are shown in figure **241**. This stimulation in the CNS hyperpolarizes neurons and inhibits norepinephrine and dopamine storage and release, leading to a decrease in the discharge rate of central and peripheral neurons causing sedation, analgesia, and muscle relaxation. There are currently four alpha 2 agonists available for use: xylazine, romifidine, medetomidine, and detomidine. They are equipotent at the following doses, 20 µg/kg detomidine, 80 µg/kg romifidine, and 1.0 mg/kg xylazine.[7,8] The equipotent sedative dose of intravenous medetomidine and detomidine compared to 1 mg/kg IV xylazine range from 5–10 µg/kg and 20–40 µg/kg respectively.[9] There is a suggested alpha 2 to alpha 1 selectivity ratio of 1620, 260, 160 for medetomidine, detomidine, and xylazine respectively.[9] The systemic half-life in horses after intravenous administration of detomidine is 1.19 hours, longer than medetomidine at 51.3 minutes, or xylazine at 50 minutes, which suggests that the longer elimination time of detomidine is one of the causes of its prolonged cardiovascular depression and sedative effects.[9] Romifidine is a potent selective alpha 2 agonist approved for use in the horse. It produces less ataxia than comparable doses of xylazine or detomidine with a longer duration of sedation. A dose of 80 µg/kg of romifidine produced sedation lasting 200 minutes.[10]

Alpha 2 agonists have their peak effect with in 1–5 minutes following intravenous administration and within 10–15 minutes after intramuscular administration. Clinically useful sedation and analgesia last approximately 45 minutes with a range of 30–60 minutes for xylazine and 60–150 minutes for detomidine depending on dose.[2,3] A single intravenous dose of detomidine may produce a subclinical CNS depression and mild behavioral changes, that can persist for as long as 24 hours.[3,10]

Alpha 2 agonists will also potentiate the effects of other sedative drugs. Alpha 2 agonists undergo liver metabolism and urinary excretion.

There will be dose-dependent decreases in respiratory rate and tidal volume which will decrease the minute volume leading to a decrease in oxygen partial pressure, PaO_2, values. There is a decrease in pulmonary dynamic compliance. There can also be marked relaxation of the nasal alar and laryngeal muscles predisposing to upper airway obstruction and respiratory stridor in some horses. The cough reflex is suppressed which can increase the danger of accumulation of foreign material in the trachea which is an important consideration in horses undergoing oral procedures. This respiratory depression can be enhanced when alpha 2 agonists are combined with other agents.

Alpha 2 agonists will have a dose-dependent effect on the cardiovascular system. Xylazine and detomidine produce a rapid and significant decrease in heart rate that is secondary to an increase in vagal tone and the decrease in CNS sympathetic output.[2,3] The vagal reflex is from baroreceptor response to hypertension.[11] This decrease in heart rate may lead to first- and second-degree heart block and third-degree block may also occur. The incidence of atrioventricular block is more persistent with detomidine.[12] The effect of xylazine and detomidine on atrioventricular conduction does not seem to exacerbate pre-existing second-degree atrioventricular block, therefore they can be safely administered to a healthy, athletic horse that is 'dropping beats'.[3] Stroke volume remains relatively unchanged but cardiac output decreases markedly.[1,2,12] Heart block occurrs at the time of maximum bradycardia, the lowest heart rate was 20 beats/min in one study.[8] Both sino-atrial and atrioventricular heart block have been reported.[8]

There will be initial increase in arterial blood pressure; this effect is transient with normal blood pressure returning within 15–20 minutes. This hypertension is related to the stimulation of alpha 1 and 2 receptors on the vascular smooth muscle, resulting in arteriolar and venular constriction, which is then followed by a more prolonged decrease in blood pressure.[2,12] Peripheral alpha 2 adrenoceptors mediate constriction of the vascular smooth muscle which, when stimulated by alpha 2 agonists, increases blood pressure.[13] Central alpha 2 adrenoceptors play a major role in the hypotensive effects of the alpha 2 agonists. This hypotension is due to vagally-mediated bradycardia, decrease in cardiac output, and CNS sympathetic tone. Transient hypertension peaks about 2–5 minutes after intravenous administration, after which blood pressure decreases and then may become lower than baseline values.[12]

Xylazine is known to potentiate and increase the sensitization of the myocardium to catecholamines during halothane anesthesia. Similar effects are expected from detomidine or any alpha 2 agonist that produces alpha 1 activation. Sudden death resulting from ventricular fibrillation has been reported after administration of xylazine. Death after administration of detomidine has been attributed to cardiac sensitization and the concurrent use of potentiated sulfonamides.[2,13]

Cardiopulmonary depression is most prominent for 15–30 minutes after intravenous detomidine administration but the sedative effects have a longer duration.[11] Analgesia from xylazine or detomidine generally lasts one-half to two-thirds the duration of sedation.[3]

Alpha 2 agonists will produce a reduction in propulsive motility in the jejunum, cecum, pelvic flexure, and right ventral colon for a long duration.[1,2] They will produce hyperglycemia in horses but not foals. Increased urine output occurs between 30 and 60 minutes post drug administration.[1,2,8] The mechanisms of alpha 2 agonist-induced diuresis include increased glomerular filtration rate, inhibited antidiuretic hormone release, inhibited antidiuretic hormone response by renal tubules, and increased release of atrial natriuretic factor.[11] Penile prolapse will be seen with these agents.[8] Alpha 2 agonists can produce anorexia in some horses.

Thermoregulation will be altered resulting in sweating and transient increases in body temperature. Muscle twitching may occur when sedation is deep. Sweating may be noted at the time sedation is diminishing.[14] Piloerection may also occur. With detomidine there are occasional urticarial reactions but these are self-limiting and regress without treatment.[15] Instability and ataxia were more pronounced with detomidine, with the depth and duration of sedation and analgesia being dose dependent.[7] Sweating is common especially in the head and flank region with detomidine.[11] Sweating and urination are noted with all of the alpha 2 agonists, including romifidine.[15]

All doses of alpha 2 agonists can produce ataxia. This is marked after high doses of xylazine and detomidine, but there is considerably less ataxia with romifidine.[1] Both detomidine and xylazine also produce greater lowering of the head than romifidine.[7,8] Horses may be ataxic but are still able to kick accurately and hard.[1,2,3,16]

The duration of sedation was longer with romifidine than with detomidine or xylazine. Romifidine induced a sedative effect that was less clearly dose-dependent.[7] Detomidine is a better analgesic than romifidine.

A study involving the rasping of horses teeth 30

minutes after either romifidine at 80 or 120 μg/kg or detomidine at 20 μg/kg had scores for the procedure that were not significantly different between the three groups but the 80 μg/kg romifidine was the most variable and therefore may be less reliable. The effects of romifidine at 120 μg/kg had the longest duration.[16] Five of the 30 horses stumbled or fell forward onto their knees when asked to walk over a wooden bar.[17] Romidfidine produces effects more like those of xylazine but it is effective for a longer period of time.[17]

The newest alpha 2 agonist is medetomidine; it is not currently approved for use in horses. In one equine study medetomidine at 10 μg/kg was similar to 1 mg/kg of xylazine in its sedative effect but produced more severe and more prolonged ataxia, and one horse fell down.[18] Medetomidine is more specific in alpha 2 receptor binding than detomidine and xylazine, and more potent than detomidine in both behavioral and neurochemical effects.[19] The maximum degree of ataxia occurs within 5 minutes after intravenous administration, and the sedation is dose related. The ataxia appears to be greater than that associated with xylazine or detomidine.[19] Medetomidine appears to be a more potent analgesic than detomidine in horses, but causes less severe physiological alterations.[20] Medetomidine produces identical effects to detomidine but it is effective for a shorter period of time.[18]

Atrioventricular block lasted for 40 minutes in horses administered medetomidine at 10 μg/kg. The incidence and duration of atrioventricular block was most pronounced with detomidine at 40 μg/kg, lasting for 80 minutes.[9] The hypotensive phase was not observed in medetomidine at 10 μg/kg, detomidine at 10 μg/kg, 20 μg/kg or 40 μg/kg.[9] Medetomidine had a greater negative effect on cardiac output and resulted in hypotension.

Repeated administration does not appear to produce adverse side-effects but the magnitude and duration of sedation will be prolonged. There may also be an increase in ataxia.

Accidental intracarotid injection produces excitement, disorientation, ataxia, recumbency, and paddling. Some horses may flip over backwards and develop seizures. Treatment is symptomatic and supportive, but may involve the administration of diazepam to control seizures.

Alpha 2 agonists are reversible. Yohimbine, tolazoline, and atipamazole are alpha 2 adrenoreceptor antagonists. Atipamazole, although marketed for small animal use, can be used in the horse to reverse sedation and ataxia.[1] Compared with atipamazole, yohimbine has much lower specificity for alpha 2 adrenergic receptors, the alpha 2 to alpha 1 selectivity ratio is 8526 for atipamazole and 40 for yohimbine.[11]

OPIOIDS

Opioid receptors are found throughout the brain, spinal cord, autonomic nervous system, and peripheral organs. Opioid agonists and agonist–antagonists produce their major effects on the CNS and gastrointestinal (GI) tract. The mu receptor is responsible for potent analgesic effects, supraspinal analgesia, for mediating respiratory depression, miosis, and sedation but also for side-effects such as excitement.[1,20] Morphine, meperidine, fentanyl, hydromorphone, and oxymorphone are mu agonists.

Kappa receptors mediate spinal analgesia, miosis, and sedation, and sigma receptors mediate dysporia, hallucinations, and respiratory and vasomotor stimulation.[21] Kappa receptors contribute less intense analgesic effects than mu agonists. Butorphanol is a high-affinity kappa receptor agonist and an antagonist at the mu receptor.[1,21] Adverse behavioral effects of butorphanol are much less severe than morphine or fentanyl and include ataxia and stimulation of locomotor activity. Effects are transient and dose related and are more likely seen following intravenous bolus injection of high doses, 0.1–0.5 mg/kg.[21] Heart and respiratory rates did not change significantly after administration of butorphanol.[21] Effects include analgesia, sedation or excitement, respiratory depression, cardiovascular depression, decreased GI propulsive motility, dose-dependent increases in locomotor activity, and mild increases in body temperature.

Opioid agonists produce analgesia at low doses but do not induce calming or sedation, and may increase the horse's response to sound, movement, and touch. Opioids are not useful alone because of their potential to cause CNS excitement. This excitement may be manifest as muscular twitching around the muzzle, uncontrollable walking, or violent reactions especially when they are given alone IV. This can be eliminated by giving sedatives or tranquilizers with opioids or prior to opioid administration.[1,3] It has been shown that opioid agonists produce their most profound effect when they are combined with sedatives and tranquilizers.[1,2]

Morphine and meperidine can cause histamine release when they are given rapidly IV. When used alone morphine and butophanol can each produce restlessness, shivering, increased motor activity, ataxia, and sedation.[21] These effects are less common when alpha 2 agonists or acepromazine are co-administered, but sudden head jerking and startle response can still occur.[22] Butorphanol given alone IV was associated with adverse behavioral and GI effects including ataxia, decreased borborygmi, and decreased defecation. Affected horses may stagger and remain ataxic for up to 20 minutes.[21] Most of the agents have the potential to be cumulative and repeated dosing or large doses could produce untoward side-effects such as hyper-responsiveness, hyperexcitability, defecation, increased locomotor activity, sweating, tachycardia, hyperventilation, vocalization, and increases in body temperature. These signs may persist for extended periods of time, but can be diminished or abolished by administering the opioid antagonist or a tranquilizer or sedative.

Butorphanol, an agonist–antagonist, produces minimal effect on intestinal transit time and will reverse the effect of a previously administered mu agonist. A partial reversal of the agonist occurs, as the mu effects are reversed but the kappa effects remain. This is done to eliminate the hyperexcitability that may occur with mu agonists but maintain some degree of analgesia.

Buprenorphine (**242**) has partial mu agonist effects. It has minimal effect on the cardiovascular system and appears not to cause sedation by itself so it has been used in combination with alpha 2 agonists.[22] It does not cause respiratory depression at clinical doses.[23] It can induce excitement when given to unsedated horses or those that do not have signs of pain.[23] Buprenorphine does not seem to induce severe respiratory depression in normal horses or those with chronic obstructive pulmonary disease (COPD) following a dose of 3 µg/kg given IV once.[24] When given alone, buprenorphine causes mild and transient signs of CNS stimulation. This is characterized by neck rigidity, occasional pawing, chewing, continuous head nodding, shaking, stiffness of the limbs, ataxia, and facial rictus. There may be violent reactions to minimal movements of the observer that are suggestive of hallucinations. These effects from this dose of 3 µg/kg were mild and lasted less than 30 minutes. There is also a marked and a lasting increase in the arterial blood pressure. The CNS stimulation could have contributed to the arterial hypertension.[24] CNS stimulation is considered more prevalent when the horse does not have signs of pain, and this suggests that opioids should not be given to nonpainful horses without prior use of a sedative agent.[24]

Opioid agonists can cause respiratory depression, but there can be tachypnea and hyperventilation if the agonist has been administered at a higher dose that leads to excitement. Agonists have the ability to reduce respiratory center responsiveness to carbon dioxide but to delay the response to increased blood concentrations of carbon dioxide. There can be marked hypoventilation in a heavily sedated horse. They are also potent cough suppressants and this could lead to accumulation of secretions in the trachea during oral procedures. Opioid agonists produce no major effect on heart rate, cardiac output, arterial blood pressure, or cardiac contractility.

Sweating is common after administration of opioids to horses. Antidiuresis resulting from opioid-induced antidiuretic hormone release and urinary retention can occur. Opioids are metabolized in the liver and excreted in the urine.

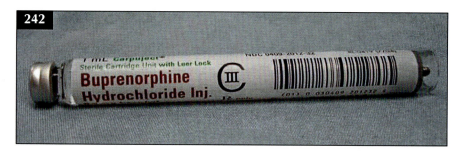

242 Buprenorphine hydrochloride.

The opioid antagonist is naloxone. Use of naloxone will reverse both the central and peripheral effects, including respiratory depression, locomotor activity, and analgesia. There will also be reversal of endogenous opiates such as enkephalins and endorphins which may lead to extreme pain and restlessness.

COMBINATIONS

Combinations of agents have been used in order to prevent some of the side-effects that can be seen with larger doses of a single agent. There are several possible combinations that can be used. The primary reason to combine two to three different drugs to achieve standing restraint should be to increase sedation or enhance analgesia, although increased muscle relaxation and prolonged duration of action could also occur.[1,2] Excessive CNS depression and concurrent effects on the respiratory and cardiovascular systems can be a potential hazard of drug combinations. Therefore, it is prudent to use small doses.

Neuroleptanalgesia refers to a combination of a tranquilizer or sedative combined with an opioid; it is characterized by two features, inattentiveness to the surrounding environment and profound analgesia.[3]

Xylazine and acepromazine
Xylazine and acepromazine is a common combination. Neither agent is controlled and they can be mixed in the same syringe. Acepromazine will enhance the effect of the alpha 2 agonists but without the profound effects of an opioid.[1] Xylazine at 0.55 mg/kg and acepromazine at 0.05 mg/kg has minimal hemodynamic and respiratory effects, and there is only mild ataxia. If this proves to be insufficient, the dose of xylazine may be increased or an opioid added.[3]

Alpha 2 agonist and opioid
Adding an opioid such as butorphanol to an alpha 2 agonist will produce profound and predictable sedation in standing horses. They are much less likely to kick in response to noxious stimulus or manipulation than when the alpha 2 agonist is used alone.[1] When using xylazine and morphine, give the morphine only after the horse is sedated from the xylazine.[1] The horse will have a 'saw horse' stance and may sway from side to side, so restraining stocks are useful to keep the horse from stumbling forward.[3]

Xylazine at 0.66 mg/kg and morphine at 0.66 mg/kg is a safely used combination. There will be a decrease in cardiac output lasting for 45 minutes.[3] Because xylazine does not last as long as morphine, as it wears off there may be some CNS excitement that can be treated with an additional dose of xylazine.[3] Detomidine lasts longer than xylazine so there is less likelihood of seeing excitement in a detomidine–opioid combination. Acepromazine can be added as it has a long duration of action and can reduce the opioid-induced dysphoria.[3] Acepromazine can be added to the alpha 2-opioid combination to increase the degree of sedation and to smooth the return to normal consciousness.[1]

There is less CNS depression when using xylazine at 1.1 mg/kg IV and butorphanol at 0.1 mg/kg IV.[3] There will be minimal and transient hemodynamic effects and no adverse respiratory effects. Lower doses, xylazine at 0.5 mg/kg and butorphanol at 0.05 mg/kg will produce even less CNS depression and ataxia and is suitable for minor procedures.[3]

The combination of detomidine 10 µg/kg and butorphanol 20 µg/kg IV will greatly minimize the adverse effects of butorphanol and accentuates the degree of sedation and analgesia.[24] It is best to let the effects of detomidine occur before the administration of butorphanol, with the dose of detomedine at 0.01 mg/kg and butorphanol 0.05 mg/kg IV. Horses receiving this combination did not sweat.[3] This combination was used in horses with COPD with no serious dysfunction.[25] This may in part be due to alpha 2 agonist effect of reduction of airway obstruction in people with asthma and ponies with COPD. Alpha 2 agonists and opioids inhibit cholinergic and noncholinergic airway constriction.[25] Ponies with COPD show a significant improvement in pulmonary function after intravenous administration of xylazine (0.5 mg/kg) and adult horses have no significant change in dynamic compliance of the lung after xylazine sedation (0.6 mg/kg). Dynamic compliance is reduced by 50% in horses sedated with detomidine at 0.04 mg/kg IV.[3] Xylazine appears to be safe for use in horses with lower airway disease.[3]

A combination of 45 µg/kg of romifidine and 17 µg/kg of butorphanol produced optimal sedation with minimal ataxia, and sedation of 60 minutes duration.[16]

Romifidine in combination with either morphine or butorphanol has been used as a preanesthetic combination in ponies undergoing castration.[25] Romifidine was used IV at 100 µg/kg with either butorphanol 50 µg/kg or morphine 0.1 mg/kg. The combinations were administered in the same syringe and given over 30 s. The combination of romifidine and butorphanol provided better sedation than the combination using morphine. Morphine could be a suitable alternative to butorphanol, but muscle twitching was observed when using morphine. Both combinations lead to a significant decrease in heart rate. Respiratory rates did not change significantly.[26]

It is unwise to antagonize the alpha 2 agonists, xylazine, detomidine, romifidine, or medetomidine, when they are used in combination with moderate to large doses of opioid analgesics. Reversal of their sedative effects could result in opioid-related CNS excitement, locomotor activity, and hyperthermia.

INFUSIONS

Procedures of a longer duration than 20 minutes may benefit from the use of a CRI to administer the sedative agents. The CRI facilitates the execution of longer, and perhaps more painful standing surgical procedures that require more than one drug bolus by allowing for a constant and consistent level of sedation and analgesia without the large fluctuations in sedation that occur with intermittent bolus injections.[26] The level of ataxia increases with each additional injection and large fluctuations of sedation make longer procedures difficult to complete. Providing sedation by CRI is one method of overcoming the negative side-effects of alpha 2 agonists.[27]

Restraint stocks are recommended when doing standing chemical restraint because some horses benefit from body support and their head may be more easily elevated to facilitate the procedure.[22]

If the horse is in stocks the halter should have foam padding where the side ropes attach to avoid iatrogenic facial nerve paralysis; in addition the horse's head should be supported under the mandible with padding. This technique has been used for dental procedures and is demonstrated in figure **243**.

DETOMIDINE

Detomidine has been used as a CRI for doing standing ophthalmic procedures in horses. An intravenous loading dose of 7.5 µg/kg is given followed by an infusion of 1.87 µg/kg/min to provide a constant depth of sedation, lasting up to 135 minutes.[22]

Another technique for the use of detomidine is to dilute it to 1 mg/mL, then a loading dose of 8.4 µg/kg IV is given followed by 0.5 µg/kg/min for 15 minutes, 0.3 µg/kg/min for 15 minutes, and thereafter 0.15 µg/kg/min until a few minutes before the procedure is complete.[27] The most accurate dosing is done using a syringe pump. If a syringe pump is not available, a 60 drop microdrip set and a 500 mL bag of 0.9% NaCl are used: 5 mL of NaCl is taken out of the bag and 5 mL of 10 mg/mL detomidine is added. This will result in a concentration of 100 µg/mL. After giving the 8.4 µg/kg bolus, the drip set is adjusted to a rate of 0.005 drops/kg/s for 15 minutes, then 0.003 drops/kg/s for 15 minutes and then 0.0015 drops/kg/s thereafter. The drip rate should be adjusted based on the level of sedation.

If more sedation and analgesia are desired, a butorphanol CRI can be piggybacked to the detomidine infusion.[27] Detomidine results in profound standing sedation and analgesia when combined with butorphanol. The loading dose of butorphanol is 17.8 µg/kg IV and the CRI rate is 0.38 µg/kg/min. Most horses can go back to their stall without significant levels of ataxia within

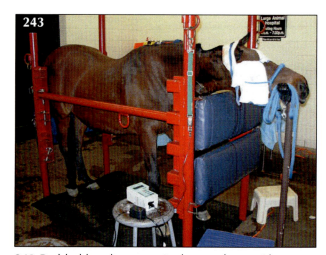

243 Padded head support is shown along with a syringe pump for CRI.

5–10 minutes of the drugs being discontinued. Food should be withheld for at least 4 hours after the procedure. This technique facilitates standing procedures of 20–30 minutes. Complications from detomidine and butorphanol CRIs may include temporary facial nerve paralysis from an unpadded halter, frequent urination, and cardiovascular depression.[27]

The combination of detomidine and buprenorphine has been used in horses and ponies for standing laparoscopic surgery. The initial drug combination was then maintained with a CRI of detomidine.[23] This combination and infusion can be used in procedures lasting up to 3 hours. The initial sedation was with detomidine (10 µg/kg) and buprenorphine (6 µg/kg) combined and given IV. When sedation had developed an infusion of detomidine was begun. This infusion was made up of 15 mg of detomidine in 3 L of Ringer's solution. The beginning infusion rate was 0.16 µg/kg/min and this was adjusted as needed based on clinical signs. The level of sedation/analgesia was easy to control by decreasing or increasing the infusion rate.[23] Deep sedation could lead to locomotor instability and this may be interpreted as inadequate sedation, which may cause the anesthetist to increase the infusion rate and actually worsen the ataxia. The appropriate level of sedation requires continuous monitoring of the patient and adjustment of the infusion rate. Profuse sweating and urination may occur with the detomidine infusion. Heart rate and respiratory rate decreased but remained stable during the procedure. At the end of the needed sedation detomidine was antagonized by atipamezole although this may not be necessary in all cases. Atipamezole was given IV at a dose equal to the total cumulative dose of detomidine each animal had received.[23] The sedative effects of the detomidine were reversed within 10 minutes after the atipamezole injection. Food and water were withheld for 1 hour after reversal.

KETAMINE

A ketamine infusion has recently been tested in equines for use as an analgesic technique.[27] Ketamine exerts its analgesic effects at central and peripheral sites mediated by multiple receptors, including n-methyl-D-asparatate (NMDA) receptors in the spinal cord. Ketamine is painful when given IM so it should be used IV. It may be a useful technique for pain management. The dose used was 0.4–0.8 mg/kg/hr. The method of delivery included adding 30 mL (3000 mg) of ketamine to a 1 L bag of saline to create a concentration of 3 mg/mL. The fluid rate can be altered depending on the desired dose of ketamine, but this concentration will give 8 hours of ketamine at 0.8 mg/kg/hr at 133 mL/hr.[28] A second method of administration is to place the ketamine in the maintenance fluids. Calculate the dose of ketamine wanted per hour, decide the fluid administration rate that is chosen for maintenance, multiply the calculated ketamine dose by the number of hours in the fluid bag and this will give the dose of ketamine to add.

Example: 500 kg horse at 0.4 mg/kg of ketamine = 200 mg of ketamine.

Fluid maintenance at 1 mL/kg/hr, so 500 mL/hr, a 5 L bag will last 10 hours.

200 mg of ketamine × 10 hours = 2000 mg of ketamine or 20 mL of ketamine added to the fluid bag.[28]

The use of a fluid pump is strongly encouraged to prevent accidental overdoses. Horses that have received ketamine for analgesia have appeared to be more comfortable and had improved appetites. Frequent monitoring is required when using CRIs. Adverse side-effects were noted when higher infusion rates of ketamine were used and included ataxia and sensitivity to sound.[28]

SUMMARY

Sedation of the equine dental patient is necessary in order to provide a quiet and manageable patient. In this way the dental procedure can be done safely and effectively. A through physical examination of the horse is required. Careful consideration of drug doses and the use of a balanced sedative technique will minimize potential complications. Diligent monitoring of the cardiovascular and respiratory systems will enhance the safety of sedation, and reversal agents and rescue therapy should be available. A suitable area to perform the sedation is also imperative; this would include appropriate stocks, head ties, solid footing, and secure halters. A planned and properly prepared standing sedation technique will result in dental repair that will greatly benefit our equine patients.

REFERENCES

1. Taylor PM, Clarke KW. Sedation, analgesia, and premedication. In: Taylor PM, Clarke KW (eds) *Handbook of Equine Anaesthesia*. London: WB Saunders, 1999; pp. 15–32.

2. Muir WW. Standing chemical resistant In: Muir WW, Hubbell JAE (eds) *Equine Anesthesia Monitoring and Emergency Therapy*. St. Louis: Mosby Year Book, 1991; pp. 247–280.

3. LeBlanc PH. Chemical restraint for surgery in the standing horse. *Veterinary Clinics of North America: Equine Practice* 1991: **7**(3); 521–533.

4. Marroum PJ, Webb AI, Aeschbacher G, Curry SH. Pharmacokinetics and pharmacodynamics of acepromazine in the horse. *American Journal of Veterinary Research* 1994: **55**(10); 1428–1433.

5. Shini S. A review of diazepam and its use in the horse. *Journal of Equine Veterinary Science* 2000: **20**(7); 443–449.

6. Doherty T, Valverde A. Pharmacology of drugs used in equine anesthesia. In: Doherty T, Valverde A (eds) *Manual of Equine Anesthesia & Analgesia*. Iowa: Blackwell Publishing, 2006; p. 128.

7. Hamm D, Turchi P, Jochle W. Sedative and analgesic effects of detomidine and romifidine in horses. *The Veterinary Record* 1995: **136**; 324–327.

8. England GCW, Clarke KW, Goossens L. A comparison of the sedative effects of three alpha 2-adrenoceptor agonists (romifidine, detomidine, and xylazine) in the horse. *Journal of Veterinary Pharmacology and Therapeutics* 1992: **15**; 194–201.

9. Yamashita K, Tsubakishita S, Futaoka S, *et al.* Cardiovascular effects of medetomidine, detomidine, and xylazine in horses. *Journal of Veterinary Medical Science* 2000; **62**(10): 1025–1032.

10. Diamond MJ, Young Le, Bartram DH, *et al.* Clinical evaluation of romifidine/ketamine/halothane anaesthesia in horses. *The Veterinary Record* 1993: **132**(23); 572–575.

11. Daunt DA. Detomidine in equine sedation and analgesia. *The Compendium for Continuing Education* 1995: **17**(11); 1405–1410.

12. Wagner AE, Muir WW, Hinchcliff KW. Cardiovascular effects of xylazine and detomidine in horses. *American Journal of Veterinary Research* 1991: **52**(5); 651–657.

13. Raekallio M, Vainio O, Karjalainen J. The influence of detomidine and epinephrine on heart rate, arterial blood pressure, and cardiac arrhythmia in horses. *Veterinary Surgery* 1991: **20**(6); 468–473.

14. Taylor PM, Rest RJ, Duckham TN, Wood EJP. Possible potentiated sulphonamide and detomidine interactions. *The Veterinary Record* 1988: **122**(6); 143.

15. Hall LW, Clarke KW, Trim CM. Anaesthesia of the horse. In: Hall LW, Clarke KW, Trim CM (eds) *Veterinary Anaesthesia* 10th edition. London: WB Saunders, 2001; p. 247.

16. Browning AP, Collins JA. Sedation of horses with romifidine and butorphanol. *The Veterinary Record* 1994: **134**; 90–91.

17. Freeman SL, England GCW. Investigation of romifidine and detomidine for the clinical sedation of horses. *The Veterinary Record* 2000: **147**; 507–511.

18. Muir WW. New perspectives on the drugs used to produce sedation, analgesia, and anesthesia in horses. *Proceedings 50th Annual Convention of the American Association of Equine Practitioners* 2004; 287–290.

19. Bryant CE, England GCW, Clarke KW. Comparison of the sedative effects of medetomidine and xylazine in horses. *The Veterinary Record* 1991: **129**; 421–423.

20. Bueno AC, Cornick-Seahorn J, Seahorn TL, *et al.* Cardiopulmonary and sedative effects of intravenous administration of low doses of medetomidine and xylazine to adult horses. *The American Journal of Veterinary Research* 1999: **60**(11); 1371–1376.

21. Sellon DE, Monroe VL, Roberts MC, Papich MG. Pharmacokinetics and adverse effects of butorphanol administered by single intravenous injection or continuous intravenous infusion in horses. *The American Journal of Veterinary Research* 2001: **62**(2); 183–189.

22. Robertson SA. Standing sedation and pain management for ophthalmic patients. *Veterinary Clinics of North America: Equine Practice* 2004: **20**; 485–497.

23. van Dijk P, Lankveld DPK, Rijkenhuizen ABM, Jonker FH. Hormonal, metabolic and physiological effects of laparoscopic surgery using a detomidine-buprenorphine combination in standing horses. *Veterinary Anaesthesia and Analgesia* 2003: **30**(2); 72–80.

24. Szoke MO, Blais D, Cuvelliez SG, Lavoie JP. Effects of buprenorphine on cardiovascular and pulmonary function in clinically normal horses and horses with chronic obstructive pulmonary disease. *The American Journal of Veterinary Research* 1998: **59**(10); 1287–1291.

25. Lavoie JP, Phan ST, Blais D. Effects of a combination of detomidine and butorphanol on respiratory function in horses with or without chronic obstructive pulmonary disease. *The American Journal of Veterinary Research* 1996: **57**(5); 705–709.

26. Corletto F, Raisis AA, Brearley JC. Comparison of morphine and butorphanol as pre-anaesthetic agents in combination with romfidine for field castration in ponies. *Veterinary Anaesthesia and Analgesia* 2005: **32**(1); 16–22.

27. Goodrich LR, Ludders JW. How to attain effective and consistent sedation for standing procedures in the horse using constant rate infusion. *Proceedings 50th Annual Convention of the American Association of Equine Practitioners* 2004; 229–232.

28. Mathews NS, Fielding CL, Swineboard E. How to use a ketamine constant rate infusion in horses for analgesia. *Proceedings 50th Annual Convention of the American Association of Equine Practitioners* 2004; 227–228.

29. Plumb DC. *Veterinary Drug Handbook* 4th edition. Ames: Iowa State Press, 2002.

REGIONAL AND LOCAL ANESTHESIA
David O Klugh   Chapter 11

Pain control is important in equine dentistry. It has obvious benefits for the patient. The practitioner also benefits from reduced motion, facilitating the efficiency of the procedure; and the patient benefits again from the reduced need for further sedation.

Regional anesthesia of various nerves supplying dental structures and local infiltration of tissues are practical methods of pain control. When used in a standing sedated patient, regional and local anesthesia affords the practitioner the ability to perform many surgical procedures without the inherent risks of general anesthesia. These procedures include, but are not limited to the following:

- Sinusotomy.
- Intraoral extraction.
- Repair of lacerations, tooth luxations, and fractures.
- Selected tooth repulsions (see Chapter 13: Standing repulsion of equine cheek teeth).

PHYSIOLOGY OF NERVE IMPLUSES

Depolarization of electrical resting potential conducts nerve impulses. The resting potential is −70 to −90 mV. The inside of the nerve fiber is negative relative to the outside, as a result of potassium ions held inside the cell membrane and sodium ions kept outside in the extracellular fluid. This is the resting state of a polarized membrane. The two ion pools are separated by a semi-permeable membrane, with its sodium and potassium channels regulating flow of the ions. On stimulation, these channels allow inflow of sodium ions and outflow of potassium ions, resulting in depolarization. At depolarization, the membrane potential is 40 mV. Repolarization occurs rapidly, and the membrane is ready for the next impulse.[1]

The method and speed of propagation of impulses varies with the type of nerve fiber. In unmyelinated fibers impulses propagate by progressing from channel to channel along the axon. The speed of propagation is relatively slow compared to that of myelinated fibers. In myelinated fibers, impulses skip from one node of Ranvier to the next, and the rate of transmission of impulse along the nerve fiber is faster.[1]

CHEMISTRY OF ANESTHETIC AGENTS

Local anesthetics consist chemically of a lipophilic group connected to a hydrophilic group by an intermediate chain. The lipophilic group is an aromatic hydrocarbon ring that provides lipid solubility. This allows the molecule to pass through the cell membrane. The hydrophilic end contains an amino group. The intermediate chain is either an amide or an ester.

Ester-type agents include cocaine, procaine, tetracaine, and others. Amide-type agents include lidocaine, mepivicaine, bupivicaine, and others.[2]

Most local anesthetic agents are weak bases that readily combine with acids to form water-soluble, usually hydrochloric acid, salts. They are dispensed in either water or saline solutions. In this form the chemical is relatively stable.

The chemical exists in both ionized and nonionized forms when in solution. The nonionized base form is necessary for penetration of the lipid-soluble nerve fiber cell membrane. Potency is increased as lipid solubility of the molecule increases. This potency is reduced in acidotic areas such as infected tissues, where the presence of local acidosis reduces the proportion of the nonionized base form that is available to penetrate the cell membrane.[2]

Ester local anesthetic agents are stabilized in more acidic solutions than amides. Therefore, in normal tissues, amides act faster and are more potent. Amides have longer duration of action because of greater protein binding. Allergic reactions to amides are rare. Esters are metabolized in the circulation while amides are metabolized in the liver. This may be a concern in patients with liver disease.[2]

Local anesthetics exert their action by blocking the flow of sodium ions through the cell membrane.[3]

PERIPHERAL NERVE ANATOMY

Nerve fibers are divided into three groups (A, B, and C) based on size, function, and degree of myelinization.[1] A-fibers are subdivided by decreasing size as alpha, beta, gamma, and delta. A-fibers are large myelinated fibers. A-alpha fibers have motor, proprioception, and reflex function. A-beta fibers have touch and pressure sensation functions. A-gamma fibers control muscle tone. A-delta fibers sense pain and temperature. B-fibers are myelinated preganglionic sympathetic fibers that manage vascular smooth muscle contraction. C-fibers are unmyelinated postganglionic fibers that sense pain and temperature.

The sequence of neural blockade correlates to the degree of myelinization and the thickness of the nerve fiber.[1] The first nerve fibers blocked are the B-fibers. The result is vasodilatation and increased skin temperature. A-delta and C-fibers are blocked next, resulting in pain blockage. The A-gamma, A-beta, and A-alpha fibers are blocked next in that order. Senses lost are proprioception, touch and pressure, and motor activity. Differential blockade of some fibers can occur while the function of others remains intact. Heavily myelinated nerve fibers are more difficult to block, and thin nerve fibers are more readily blocked. Both fiber types are contained within a single nerve. Thus it is possible a patient can respond to pressure sensation while unable to respond to pain,[1] possibly giving the impression of having inadequately blocked the nerve. This may require either additional anesthetic or additional time for chemical penetration of the heavier nerve fiber.

LOCAL INFILTRATION ANESTHETIC USE IN EQUINE DENTISTRY

The technique of infiltration anesthesia can be adapted for use in sedated equine patients for minor dental procedures such as extraction of deciduous incisors, deciduous premolars, and wolf teeth. In human dentistry, submucosal infiltration of various anesthetic agents results in sufficient anesthesia to allow pain-free endodontics[4] and extractions.[5]

Teeth are bordered by gingiva. The mucogingival junction connects the gingiva with the mucosa. The mucosa is identified by its looser attachment to underlying periosteum and bone. When tension on lips is relaxed, the mucosa can be identified by the small folds that result. The location of infiltration is submucosal, and therefore supraperiosteally, over the area of the root of the tooth to be addressed.

Anesthetic agents such as lidocaine and mepivicaine are widely used in equine medicine and surgery. These agents work well for dental infiltration anesthesia. A 3 mL syringe filled with 1–2 mL of anesthetic agent and connected to a 25 gauge 16 mm (⅝") needle suffices for the procedure. After appropriate sedation, a drop or two of anesthetic agent may be placed on the mucosa to desensitize the tissue for injection. Desensitization occurs within 1–2 minutes. Alternatively, topical anesthetic agents such as those used in human dentistry may be employed. These agents contain benzocaine and are applied with a cotton tipped applicator (**244**). The needle is inserted and up to 0.5 mL of drug is injected. This procedure is repeated until a sufficient area is infiltrated. The total volume injected is approximately 1 mL.

The site of injection is submucosal. The anesthetic agent is deposited supraperiosteally. This site is apical to the gingiva and adjacent to the point of attachment of the lip or cheek. The gingiva adheres tightly to the periosteum, therefore injection in this area is difficult

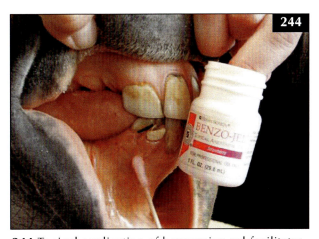

244 Topical application of benzocaine gel facilitates needle placement.

and frequently results in leakage of medication. There is a wide area of mucosa that is freely mobile and easily identified (**245**).

For the anesthetic to reach full effect, one must allow sufficient time for complete diffusion of the drug through all soft and bony tissues.[6] In horses the bone is somewhat thicker than in man and more time for complete diffusion is required. Usually 5–10 minutes is necessary for complete anesthesia of wolf teeth and deciduous teeth. This can be achieved by anesthetizing the appropriate sites first and then performing other dental procedures and extracting the anesthetized tooth (teeth) last.

SPECIFIC PROCEDURES

Deciduous incisors can be sufficiently anesthetized in many cases by a single injection on the labial surface apical to the tooth as in figure **245**. In some cases where the retained tooth root is wide or long and significant mucosal attachment on the palatal aspect remains, infiltration of the palatal mucosa is necessary. A small bleb of anesthetic agent is injected submucosally in the palate near the tooth to be extracted. It is necessary to wait 3–5 minutes for the palatal injection to have full effect.

Wolf teeth can be extracted quietly and safely after submucosal infiltration. The buccal mucosa is loose enough to allow easy injection. The anesthetic is injected just apical to the attached gingiva. When injecting palatally it is important that the site is in close proximity to the tooth and the palatine artery is avoided. An easy landmark for injection is the tip of the palatal fold (**246**).

Deciduous premolars can be anesthetized by the same method. Access to the injection site is more difficult as the tooth resides more distally in the

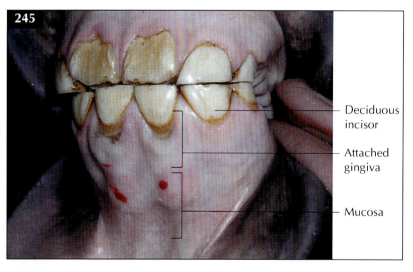

245 Submucosal injection site for supraperiosteal infiltration of local anesthetic agent. A bleb of anesthetic agent can be appreciated above the injection site.

Deciduous incisor

Attached gingiva

Mucosa

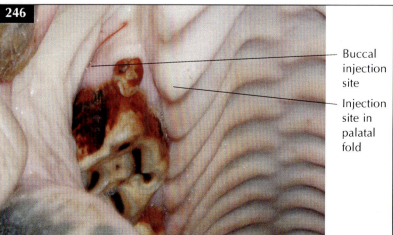

246 Palatal and buccal submucosal injection sites for infiltration of local anesthetic agent.

Buccal injection site

Injection site in palatal fold

arcade. In these cases, both the buccal and palatal or lingual sides of the tooth must be anesthetized. The anatomical landmarks are the same as in the other locations. Patience and practice allows one to become proficient in the procedure.

Selected cases of extractions in geriatric patients are facilitated by the infiltration of local anesthetic administered via subcutaneous injection. The site is determined by assessing the location of the apical aspect of the affected tooth (**247**) and injection of 5 mL of anesthetic agent (**248**). This requires 10–15 minutes for complete diffusion of anesthetic through bone to anesthetize the pulp and periodontium. This method is used for maxillary teeth whose roots are not contained in sinus cavities. For mandibular teeth,

this technique is not appropriate, as the thickness of bone requires much longer for diffusion of the chemical.

The syringe used in figure **248** is a dental syringe, or 'aspirating syringe'. This is the same syringe used in human dentistry for regional and local anesthesia. It uses 1.8 mL compules of anesthetic agent that are inserted in the open barrel of the syringe, as demonstrated in figures **249** and **250**. Many different anesthetic agents are available in this form. The harpoon tipped plunger is inserted into the rubber plug in the compule and twisted a quarter turn to secure the tip. A threaded dental needle is secured to the end of the syringe. The syringe is then ready for use.

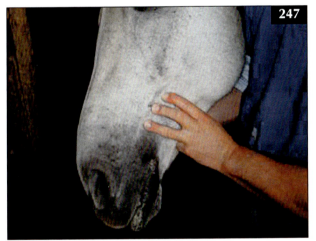

247 Subcutaneous injection of anesthetic can be used to desensitize teeth in geriatric patients. The dorsal reflection of the vestibule at the locations of the three premolars is identified.

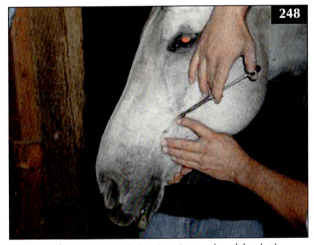

248 A subcutaneous injection is used to block the pulp and periodontium of the upper left fourth premolar (Triadan 208).

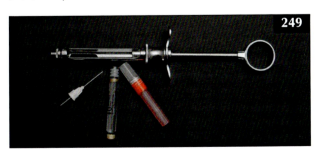

249 The components of the dental syringe include the open barrel syringes, a compule of anesthetic agent, and the threaded needle which attaches to the syringe tip.

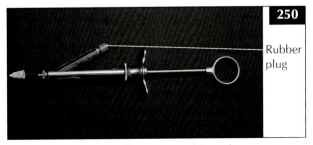

Rubber plug

250 The glass compule is inserted into the open syringe barrel. The sharp tip of the plunger inserts into the rubber plug in the compule.

REGIONAL NERVE BLOCKS

The primary sensory nerves for the head come from one of the three branches of the trigeminal nerve (cranial nerve V). These branches include ophthalmic, maxillary, and mandibular nerves. Dental structures are anesthetized by one of four nerve blocks:

- Maxillary.
- Infraorbital.
- Mandibular.
- Mental.

MAXILLARY NERVE BLOCK

The maxillary nerve[7] is entirely sensory and exits the cranium via the foramen rotundum and accompanies the maxillary artery through the pterygopalatine fossa to enter the maxillary foramen and the infraorbital canal as the infraorbital nerve. Figure **251** demonstrates these foramina on a dried skull. While in the infraorbital foramen it supplies branches to the premolars, molars, canines, and incisors. As it emerges from the infraorbital foramen, branches are supplied to the skin of the upper lips and face dorsal to the facial crest and rostral to the eye.

The maxillary teeth, maxilla, nose, and upper lip are anesthetized when blocking the maxillary nerve either as it emerges from the foramen rotundum or as the infraorbital nerve enters the maxillary foramen.[8] An 88 mm (3.5"), 20 gauge spinal needle is inserted through the skin immediately distal to the zygomatic process of the frontal bone, where it attaches to the zygomatic bone and there is a right angle formed by the zygomatic arch. The needle is angled 20° above horizontal and inserted as in figure **252** until it meets the dorsal aspect of the orbital part of the frontal bone. It is then stepped down the frontal bone by retracting and inserting. Each insertion results in advancement of the tip of the needle 1–2 cm ventrally (**253**). The final position of the needle is well dorsal to the maxillary nerve and optic bundle (**254**). After the third insertion 15–20 mL of anesthetic are deposited in the periorbital space. Tissue diffusion and gravity pull the anesthetic further ventrally to anesthetize the maxillary nerve. The danger of puncture of blood vessels is minimal. Anesthesia is achieved in about 20 minutes.

Complications include anesthesia of the optic nerve and relaxation of occulomotor muscles. Blindness, pupil dilation, and orbital protrusion result. Some complications are shown in figure **255**. Some patients develop a mild conjunctivitis. All signs return to normal when the anesthetic agent is metabolized. Management of complications requires the patient to be in a safe, familiar stall where injury potential is minimal. The use of topical ophthalmic ointments is necessary to prevent corneal dehydration. In the author's practice these blocks are always performed in a hospital and the patient is not released until all effects of the block are returned to normal.

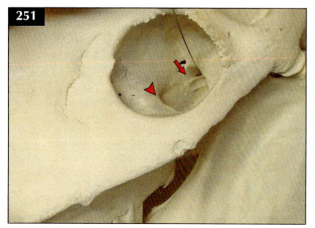

251 The foramen rotundum is identified by the arrow. The maxillary nerve passes along the pterygoid fossa and enters the maxillary foramen identified by the arrowhead.

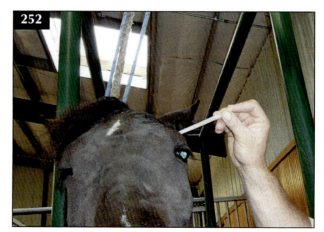

252 The location and angle of insertion of the needle for the maxillary nerve block.

INFRAORBITAL NERVE BLOCK

A second method of anesthesia for the upper arcade, lip, and nose is blocking the infraorbital nerve as it enters the maxillary foramen(as the maxillary nerve). A 76 mm (3") 18 gauge needle is inserted in a nearly horizontal position and directed rostromedially until it contacts the palatine bone (**256**). Anesthetic agent (10 mL) is deposited in the perineural space.

Complications include puncture of the maxillary artery, transverse facial vein, or internal carotid artery, making this a potentially dangerous procedure.[8]

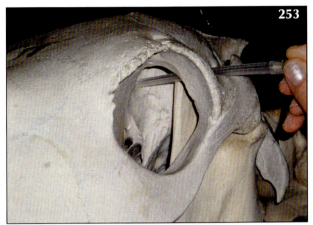

253 The needle is retracted, the tip of the needle is moved ventrally and the needle advanced until it contacts the pterygoid fossa.

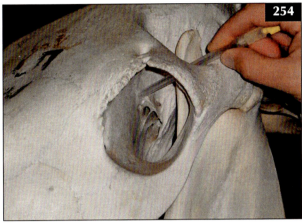

254 The final position of the needle is shown in relation to the foramen rotundum. The tip is well dorsal to the nerves and vasculature. The anesthetic agent is deposited and allowed to diffuse ventrally.

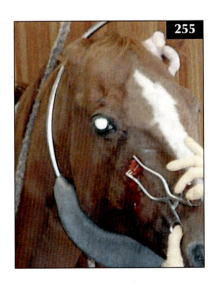

255 Pupil dilation and slight orbital protrusion are shown in this patient after performance of the maxillary nerve block.

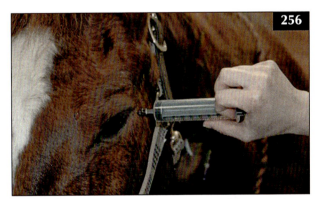

256 The position of the needle inserted for anesthesia of the maxillary nerve on its entrance into the maxillary foramen is demonstrated. (Courtesy of Dr. Mike Lowder.)

As the infraorbital nerve exits the infraorbital foramen dorsal and rostral to the facial crest, the nerve supplies the skin of the upper lip and nose. The foramen is located about half the distance from the nasomaxillary notch and the rostral border of the facial crest. This location is shown in a dried skull in figure **257** and in a live animal in figure **258**. The foramen lies about 2.5 cm dorsal to

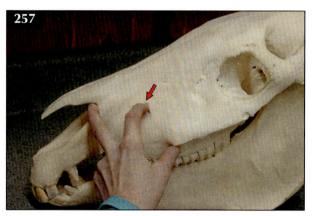

257 The location of the infraorbital foramen is shown on a dried skull (arrow).

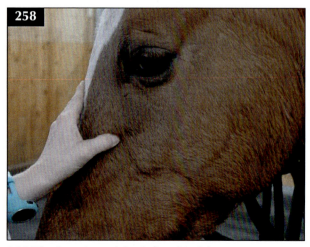

258 The location of the infraorbital foramen is demonstrated on a live patient. There is variation among individuals.

this point under the levator labii superioris. A needle can be inserted into the canal and 3–5 mL of anesthetic agent can be deposited. Digital pressure at the foramen will prevent extrusion of anesthetic agent. This block will anesthetize all teeth in the maxillary arcade back as far as the first molar in most cases.[8]

Complications include ventral diffusion of anesthetic agent and resulting facial nerve paralysis. Additionally, insertion of the needle may traumatize the nerve and result in a neuritis that may be longstanding or permanent.

MANDIBULAR NERVE BLOCK

Mandibular teeth, skin, and mucosa of the lower lip can be anesthetized by blocking the mandibular alveolar nerve as it enters the mandibular foramen on the medial aspect of the ramus of the mandible, shown in figure **259**.[9] The site of insertion of a 139 mm (5.5") 18 gauge stylet from an intravenous catheter is found on the ventral mandible. A line is drawn that parallels the angle of occlusion of the cheek teeth. This line intersects a line drawn ventrally from the lateral canthus of the eye. This measurement identifies the approximate location of the mandibular foramen, and represents the depth of insertion of the stylet. This distance and location is demonstrated in figure **260**. The needle is bent toward the operator and is inserted from the ventral border of the mandible, following the curvature of the bone until reaching the nerve. Anesthetic agent (15–20 mL) is fanned out in the region of the nerve. This block requires 15–20 minutes for complete diffusion.

Complications include failure to locate the mandibular foramen accurately and lack of anesthesia. In such a case, the procedure may be repeated.

MENTAL NERVE BLOCK

Insertion of a needle into the mental foramen and injection of anesthetic agent within the canal results in variable desensitization of the mandibular incisors and canine teeth.[9] The mental foramen is positioned under the tendon of the depressor labii inferioris on the lateral border of the mandible in the middle of the interdental space. The needle is inserted as far as possible into the space. Anesthetic (3–5 mL) is injected into the canal. Digital pressure helps prevent loss of anesthetic through the foramen. Figure **261** shows the location of insertion in a dried skull, while figure **262** demonstrates the block in a live patient.

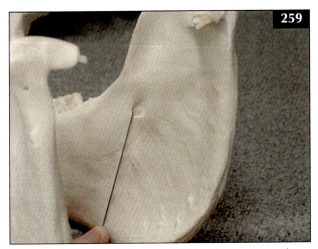

259 The location of the mandibular foramen on the medial aspect of the ramus of the mandible.

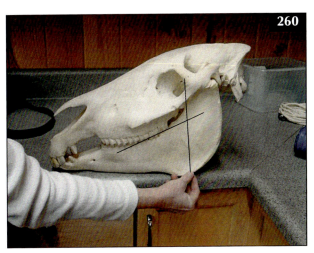

260 The mandibular foramen is identified as the intersection of a line paralleling the occlusal surfaces of the cheek teeth and a line ventrally from the lateral canthus. This distance is measured and marked on the needle.

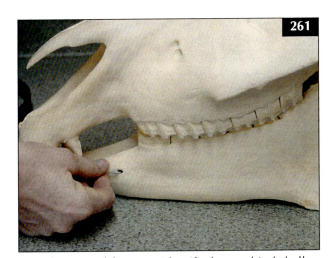

261 The mental foramen identified on a dried skull.

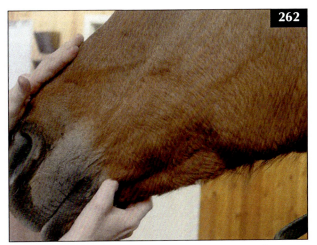

262 The location of the mental foramen on a live patient.

SUMMARY

Regional anesthesia requires knowledge of anatomical structures. It assists the veterinarian in efficiently performing various surgical procedures. It benefits the patient in relief of pain and reduction of sedation requirements. The techniques can be perfected with practice on cadavers.

REFERENCES

1. Day TK, Skarda RT. The pharmacology of local anesthetics. *Veterinary Clinics of North America: Equine Practice* 1991: **7**(3); 489–500.
2. Milam SB, Giovannitti JA Jr. Local anesthetics in dental practice. *Dental Clinics of North America* 1984: **28**(3); 493–508.
3. Butterworth JFT, Strichartz GR. Molecular mechanisms of local anesthesia: a review. *Anesthesiology* 1990: **72**(4); 711–734.
4. Meechan JG, Ledvinka JI. Pulpal anaesthesia for mandibular central incisor teeth: a comparison of infiltration and intraligamentary injections. *International Endodontic Journal* 2002: **35**(7); 629–634.
5. Mellor DJ, Mellor AH, McAteer EM. Local anaesthetic infiltration for surgical exodontia of third molar teeth: a double-blind study comparing bupivacaine infiltration with i.v. ketorolac. *British Journal of Anaesthesia* 1998: **81**(4); 511–514.
6. Yonchak T. Anesthetic efficacy of infiltrations in mandibular anterior teeth. *Anesthesia Progress* 2001: **48**(2); 55–60.
7. Godinho HP, Getty R. Peripheral nervous system. In: Getty R (ed) *Sisson and Grossman's: The Anatomy of the Domestic Animals*, 5th edition, Volume 1. Philadelphia: WB Saunders, 1975; pp. 650–664.
8. Skarda RT. Practical regional anesthesia. In: Mannsman RA, McAllister ES (eds) *Equine Medicine and Surgery*, 3rd edition, Volume 1. Santa Barbara: American Veterinary Publications, 1982; pp. 228–249.
9. Scrutchfield WL, Schumacher J, Martin MT. Correction of abnormalities of cheek teeth. *Proceeedings 42nd Annual Convention American Association of Equine Practitioners* 1996; pp. 11–21.

EXODONTICS OF EQUINE TEETH

Michael Lowder   Chapter 12

INTRODUCTION

The practice of veterinary medicine has historically included tooth extraction. While the techniques and equipment have changed little over time, the ability to diagnose which teeth need extraction and the level of pain management have greatly improved.[1–17]

Prior to extracting any tooth from a horse, the practitioner needs to be certain that he/she has the equipment and experience to perform the extraction with minimal complications. As with any disease process, the history of the patient and the management of the diseased tooth should be obtained in detail. Questions regarding disease duration, treatment duration and response, attempted extraction, and so on should be asked.

The area for performing the procedure should be secure and away from distracting noise and movement. A complete set of radiographs should be obtained prior to most extractions to augment the clinician's ability to determine the area of disease involvement, diseased tooth shape, size, and location. An exception might be the older horse with diseased teeth that are loosely attached, as these extractions should cause few, if any, potential complications. Postextraction radiographs are indicated in most cases to ensure complete extraction of the diseased tooth.

The age of the patient will determine the type and arsenal of instruments required by the practitioner for extraction of incisors, premolars, and molars. If the practitioner is going to limit his/her extraction cases to older horses, then the number of extraction instruments, e.g. forceps, will not have to be as extensive as someone whose cases include younger horses.

Exondontia of equine incisors will require a specific incisor forceps (both the short- and long-handled varieties), periosteal elevators, and maybe a high-speed headpiece or a flex-cable rotary tool, e.g. dremel, to remove the labial surface of the alveolar plate in some cases.

As noted, horse's teeth are asymmetrical (maxillary teeth are wider than the mandibular teeth), which will influence instrument selection for the extraction process. If the practitioner is going to be performing extractions on a routine basis, a complete set of upper and lower, i.e. maxillary and mandibular, extraction instruments should be purchased.

Few companies make a complete set of equine dental extraction forceps, and the practitioner should be discriminating in his/her purchase, as these instruments should last a lifetime in most cases.[18–20] One should be mindful of the quality of metal and the coating. Good instruments require careful selection. The length of the instrument must be sufficient, bearing in mind that a large Warmblood or draft horse may have an oral cavity that is 40–46 cm deep. The handles of the instrument must reach past the speculum and give enough working room for the practitioner's hands.

The degree of movement at the forceps's head does not correlate with the degree of movement of the handles. Depending upon the craftsmanship of the instruments, the amount of play at the end of the handles where the practitioner's hands hold the instrument is important. Too much play (movement) will only give a sense of false achievement and cause the practitioner to try premature extraction of a tooth. In addition, instruments with lots of play just function to tire out the practitioner.

A prerequisite to extraction of any tooth is a thorough knowledge of the exfoliation/eruption times of each tooth. Variation with breed should be noted. Large breeds and exotics mature slower and thus may exfoliate their teeth at a later date than normal-sized horses.

WOLF TEETH EXTRACTION

EQUIPMENT

Extraction of wolf teeth requires a limited number of tools.[5,21–26] In most cases a simple elevator and a pair of extraction forceps are all that is needed.

However, most practitioners have numerous tools for the extraction of wolf teeth. The author frequently uses a pair of ronguers as his extraction tool of choice after elevating the tooth.

Numerous types of elevators are on the market. The most important factor for an efficient effective tool is sharpness. A sharp elevator will hasten separation of the gingiva from the tooth and the underlying PDL. The reason to use the curved rongeurs is access to the wolf tooth from the side of the mouth and, if the tooth is broken, the rongeur can be used to extract/cut out the remaining root.

TECHNIQUE

Anesthesia is indicated in extracting any wolf tooth except in cases where a fragment or a very small residual tooth is in place. Infiltration anesthesia of the adjacent tissue was described in Chapter 11: Regional and local anesthesia.

All wolf teeth extraction tools perform the same basic principle of elevating the PDL away from the tooth and freeing the tooth from any attachment to the gingiva. Once the PDL has been elevated, the tooth is grasped with a pair of forceps and oscillated to augment its movement within the alveolar socket. It is important to take time and be patient in extraction, as many teeth have a large root.

Once the tooth is loosened, slow steady pressure should be applied away from the gingiva and the whole tooth will come out. If the tooth root fractures, the fragments should be extracted if possible. More elevation of the fragment may be necessary. If the fragment cannot be extracted, the practitioner may leave the fragment alone and recheck the horse at a later date. In some cases, the fragmented root will erupt more, due to an intact PDL. If the fragmented root is believed to cause discomfort to the horse, a pair of ronguers may be used to 'chip' away at the fragment and smooth out any sharp edges. Alternately, the horse can be placed under general field anesthesia for elevation and extraction of the root. In most cases, the remaining tooth fragments do not cause any mastication or riding problems.

The vacant socket needs no special attention post extraction.

INCISORS

Extraction techniques of deciduous incisors will vary with the maturity and length of the tooth.[22,26–31] The length is affected by the maturity of the tooth and the resorption of the deciduous tooth via eruption of the permanent tooth directly behind it. Any eruption of the permanent tooth other than the path of the deciduous is abnormal. Eruption of the permanent tooth in an aberrant pattern is frequently a genetic defect. Horses that have one aberrant erupted tooth or a persistent deciduous tooth (i.e. cap) usually will have more than one tooth affected (incisors or premolars). See Chapter 8: Eruption and shedding of teeth, for normal tooth eruption.

Infection of deciduous incisors is rare. Most extractions are due to trauma, aberrant eruption of a deciduous tooth or its permanent counterpart, eruption of the permanent distal tooth, delayed exfoliation or, in rare cases, a supernumerary incisor tooth.

EQUIPMENT

Extraction of mature-term deciduous incisors requires minimal equipment. A periosteal elevator and a small pair of dental forceps are all that are needed in most cases. Extraction of immature deciduous incisors will require the same arsenal as mature permanent incisors due to their length.

TECHNIQUE

The first step in extraction is to determine the age of the tooth. A deciduous tooth that is at term and ready to exfoliate will have a dome shape. A deciduous tooth that does not have a permanent tooth undermining its root structure may have the same shape as the permanent erupting/erupted tooth. The permanent tooth erupts palatally or lingually to the deciduous. Radiographs may be indicated to determine the length, size, and configuration of the deciduous tooth root.

A periosteal elevator is used to detach the labial gingiva from the deciduous incisor at term (ready to exfoliate) in the sedated horse. Infiltration anesthesia may be used if desired. There is minimal detachment to do and a pair of forceps is placed on the labial and palatal surfaces of the tooth. A sharp twist and pull will extract the tooth. Postextraction care of the surgical site is not necessary. In most cases the practitioner can either see or palpate the permanent tooth. Some cases may require postoperative pain medication.

The principle for any extraction should be adequat restraint and anesthesia.[32–36] The extraction procedure is dictated by the clinical examination, radiographic findings, and clinician's experience. Extraction may be done standing or under general anesthesia. Involved (long-rooted teeth) extractions should incorporate prior pain medication, and regional and infiltration anesthesia. In most cases, systemic antibiotics are indicated prior to the extraction procedure(s), due to the depth of the alveolus.

Extraction of deciduous incisors with an intact root involves the same techniques as permanent incisors (**263**, **264**). Radiographs are indicated in most cases prior to extraction to determine the length, size, and shape (direction) of the root (**265**).[37–41] Postextraction radiographs are indicated anytime pre-extraction radiographs were taken to ensure complete removal of the tooth and any tooth fragments.

First, the mucosa is incised along the lines that the practitioner desires to elevate it (usually down the center or edges of the tooth). One incised, a sharp periosteal elevator is used to free the mucosa. When elevating the mucosa, the type of closure should be kept in mind (primary *vs.* secondary).

Once incised and elevated, a retaining suture may be placed to hold the flap out of the way. To hold the lip out of the way in the standing horse, a bungee cord can be connected to one side of the halter positioned under the lip, and connected to the other side. Alternatively, a piece of 5 cm tape can be used to hold the lip up (**266**). It is imperative that a free airway is maintained if the upper lip is retracted.

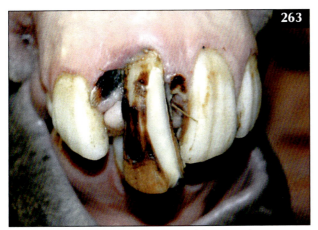

263 A diseased 101 in a 4-year-old. Note the fragments of 501.

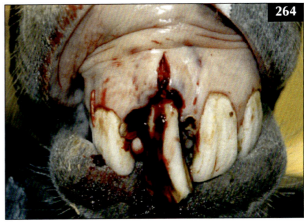

264 Note swelling of the gingiva of the diseased 101 in figure **263** due to infiltration anesthesia.

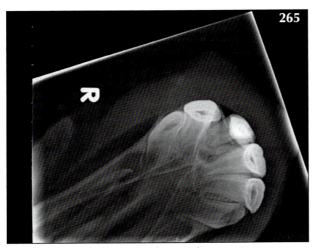

265 Radiograph showing diseased 101 prior to extraction.

266 A 5 cm wide piece of medical tape is used to hold the upper lip out of the surgical field in a standing extraction.

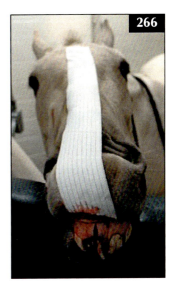

Next, the labial alveolar plate needs to be removed to free the distal end of the root. This is best done with a No. 8 round bur on a high-speed dental headpiece. A small flex-cable grinder with a proper head can also be used if a dental handpiece is not available. Water should be dripped on the grinding bur to minimize heat generation and dust if a flex-cable grinder is used.

The tooth should be grasped with a pair of medium-sized incisor forceps on the labial and palatal surfaces. The forceps should be oscillated slowly at first as the horse becomes accustomed to the pressure of the tooth movement. The practitioner should guard against any sudden movement of the head, especially sharp upward movements that might cause the tooth to fracture.

As the tooth is oscillated, the practitioner will note progress as the PDL is broken down and the socket distorted as foamy blood is noted around the gingiva tooth junction (**267**).

As the tooth begins to move freely within the alveolus, premature extraction should not be attempted. It is only when the tooth is extremely loose and little blood is seen that it is ready for extraction (**268**, **269**). Most often the extraction site is allowed to heal via secondary intention (**270**).

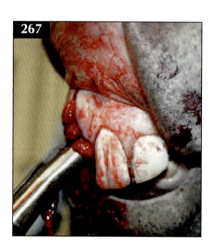

267 As a tooth becomes loosened, foamy blood will be noted around the base of the tooth.

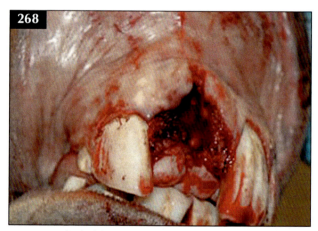

268 Note little bleeding of extraction site. This extraction site was left to heal by secondary intention.

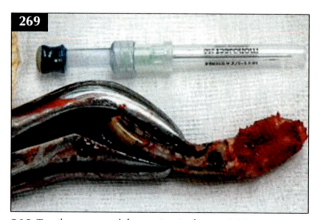

269 Tooth extracted from site in figure **268**.

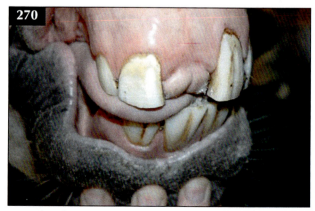

270 The diseased 101 extraction site (figure **268**) 6 months later.

During the extraction process, the anatomy of the tooth should be kept in mind. Depending upon the tooth and the age of the tooth, its length and shape may vary greatly. The clinical crown will change shape from rectangular to triangular with age. Concurrent changes are taking place in the tooth structure below the gingiva margin. In most middle-aged to older horses, the tooth changes shape from being wider in an abaxial-axial direction to a labial-distal direction.

PREMOLARS AND MOLARS: EQUIPMENT AND TECHNIQUE

No cheek tooth extraction can be done without the aid of a good mirror. The author prefers one that has a fixed mirror head. Two or three bent at varying angles are beneficial. Most can be bent for various mirror angles. The mirror should be about 46 cm long and have a large-diameter head (**271**).

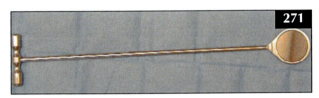

271 An equine dental mirror.

Dental picks are used to elevate the gingiva away from the diseased tooth (**272**). This is important to reduce discomfort to the horse during the extraction process and to allow proper placement of the forceps on the crown. Prior to elevating the gingiva from the diseased tooth, it is helpful to infiltrate the surrounding gingiva with mepivicaine using a butterfly catheter as shown in figure **273**. This will allow painless elevation of the gingiva. The forceps must be placed carefully so they do not slip. Any instrument improperly placed could lacerate the palate and/or the palatal artery.

Three-root molar forceps, like all forceps, were adapted from human dentistry. The three-root (claw) molar forceps is designed to enclose the crown of the tooth with the roots of the forceps. The upper cheek teeth have two buccal roots and one large palatal root. The single claw of the forceps is placed between the two lateral roots of the tooth and the two-clawed side of the forceps is placed on the medial side of the tooth to fit around the single medial root of the tooth.

The forceps are functionally best used on teeth that have short reserve crowns, i.e. old horses, but not in young horses. However, the three-root forceps often offer superior holding ability on some teeth. The practitioner is encouraged to purchase both an upper pair (left and right) and a lower pair (left and right). The upper pair of three-root forceps is wider

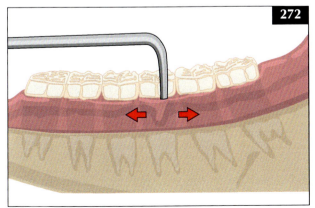

272 A dental pick is used to elevate the gingiva from both sides of the diseased tooth.

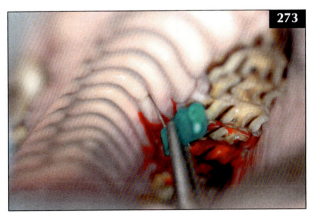

273 Local infiltration of mepivicaine via a butterfly catheter into the surrounding gingiva of the diseased tooth eliminates pain prior to elevating.

between the claws of the forceps than the lower pair (**274**).

Box-jaw molar forceps are the most commonly used molar forceps. They are called box-jaw because the claws are square to one another (**275**). It is important in selecting this pair of forceps to view the serrations of the teeth on the claws. They should not be too short or worn smooth; if they are, the head of the instrument should be re-milled or it should be replaced.

This is the often the instrument of choice in most extractions. The box-jaw is placed as far up on the clinical crown (close to the gingiva) of the tooth as possible. Once placed on the tooth, a bicycle tire inner tube should be placed around the handles of the forceps (**276**, **277**). To do this, a loop is made out

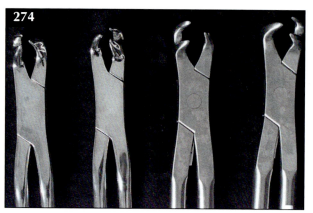

274 Lower pair on left and upper pair on right of three-root molar forceps. Note the increased distance between the claws of the pair on the right.

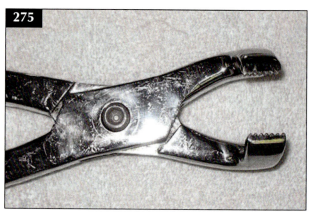

275 A pair of box-jaw forceps.

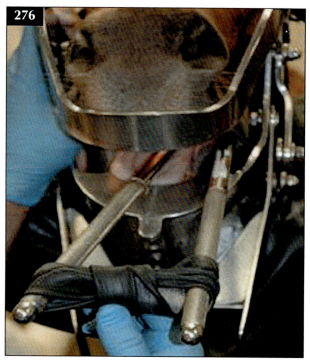

276 The inner tube is wrapped around the handles of the forceps.

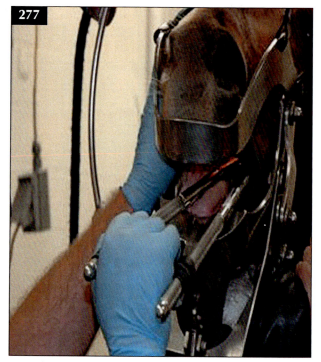

277 The inner tube is not tied, and should come loose if the practitioner's hand is released.

of one end of the inner tube and it is slid over one handle of the forceps. With one end looped around one handle of the forceps, the free end of the inner tube is pulled around the other handle of the forceps. It is wrapped around the handles a few times and then the free end of the inner tube is brought between the handles and wrapped around the section of inner tube between the handles and tucked between the practitioner's fingers so that the inner tube may be freed in case of emergency.

Once secured, the handles of the box-jaw forceps should be moved in a lateral-to-lateral oscillating movement (**278**). This is done to set the jaws of the forceps into the sides of the tooth. As the jaws work their way into the tooth, the inner tube will keep steady pressure on the tooth. Only after the forceps are set in the tooth (**279**) should the handles be rotated side to side (**280**). If this is done before the handles are set into the tooth, the forceps will make vertical grooves and slip off the tooth. The author prefers to oscillate the handles of the forceps for about 45–60 minutes before rotating them as oscillating takes less effort.

A leverage bar can be used to hasten the loosening of a tooth (**281**). The head of the leverage bar is slid over the handles of the forceps as close to the head of

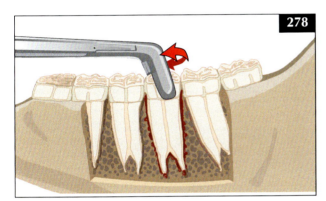

278 Forceps are rotated in an oscillating side-to-side motion.

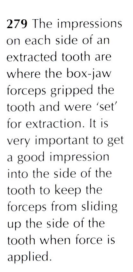

279 The impressions on each side of an extracted tooth are where the box-jaw forceps gripped the tooth and were 'set' for extraction. It is very important to get a good impression into the side of the tooth to keep the forceps from sliding up the side of the tooth when force is applied.

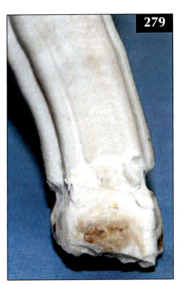

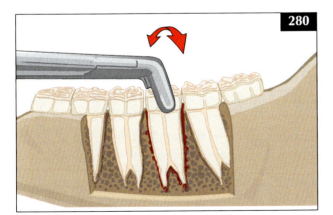

280 Forceps moving the diseased tooth from a buccal to lingual direction. The forceps are slowly moved to one side then held in position for 1–3 minutes and then moved to the opposite side. This process is repeated over and over to break down the attachment of the PDL and to eventually distort the socket.

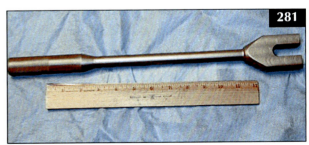

281 A leverage bar is applied to the handles of a pair of forceps to increase the amount of leverage applied to the distal end of the forceps. The bar should be constructed of one piece of solid stainless steel.

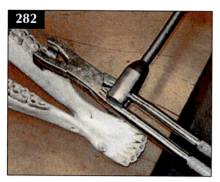

282 The leverage bar is slid over the handles of the forceps to increase the amount of leverage at the head of the forceps.

the forceps as possible (**282**, **283**). It is important that the leverage bar be constructed of one piece of solid stainless steel to add weight to the tool to reduce the amount of force needed by the practitioner. The head of the leverage bar *must* fit securely around the handles of the forceps to prevent any 'play' in the bar as it is used to apply leverage to the forceps head. A practitioner may need more than one leverage bar to fit different manufacturers' forceps.

Only moderate pressure should be applied with this tool. It is very easy to fracture the crown of a tooth if it is used improperly. The practitioner must allow the weight of the leverage bar to do the work. The leverage bar is only used when rotating the handles of the forceps and not when oscillating the handles.

Molar spreaders (separators) are used to move the diseased tooth in a mesial-distal direction (**284**, **285**).

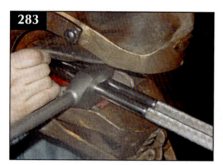

283 The leverage bar in use.

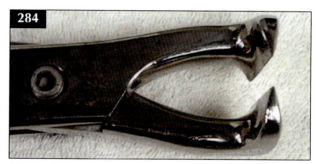

284 Molar spreader used to move a cheek tooth in a distal to rostral direction.

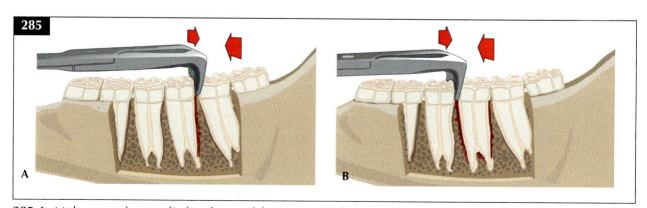

285 A. Molar spreaders applied to the caudal interproximal space of diseased first molar. **B.** Molar spreaders applied to the mesial space of diseased first molar.

There are several types of spreaders available, with variation in the jaw width and the angle of the jaws. The first spreader used in most cases is one with thin straight jaws. The selection is based on the fact that the interproximal space in a young to middle-aged and even in an older horse is very tight. Only in aged horses is there a true diastema that one may see.

In application of the molar spreaders, the practitioner has to keep in mind the natural curvature of the upper dental arch. What this implies is that the buccal jaw of the spreaders will be inserted into the interproximal space rostral to the palatal spreader jaw. The long handles of the spreaders will be projecting across the mid-plane of the horse's head pointing toward the contralateral arch. This is an extremely important thing to note. If the spreaders are applied in a straight line with the dental arcade, the buccal jaw will be closed on the tooth and may fracture the crown.

On the lower arcade, the spreader's jaws are inserted in alignment with each other as the lower dental arcade is in a straight line. Spreaders are not indicated in the caudal part of the lower dental arcade in horses with a Spee curve (upward curvature of the lower dental arcade as the last few molars are erupting at an angle at the transition between the vertical and horizontal ramus of the mandible) as the long handles of the spreader will prevent them from being inserted into the interproximal space.

An inner tube is applied to the handles as with any other forceps. The spreader is allowed to remain in place for 2–3 minutes then moved to the opposite side of the tooth (**283**). Repeated several times, this process aids in the breakdown of the PDL and distorts the alveolus. Once the jaws of the spreaders are closing within the interproximal space, a larger (thicker jaw) set of spreaders should be selected. The process of slowly closing the thicker spreaders is done as previously. The author finds that using the spreaders is as much an art as anything; he has broken more crowns and distal roots with spreaders than with any other dental forceps.

Spreaders with angled jaws should only be used in geriatric cases and with caution. The angle allows for much more pressure to be applied to the tooth, and the potential for tooth fracture is high.

Occasionally, the practitioner will come across two check teeth adjacent (side by side) to one another. Traditional forceps will not allow contact and special forceps that close front to back and not side to side are needed. If the affected tooth is an upper, the jaws of the tool should be angled forward and if a lower tooth, the jaws should be at a right angle to the tool handle (**286**). The tool can be made by simply putting a rod inside a pipe and having the end forged to the desired shape (**287**). The opposite end of the rod should be threaded and a large nut threaded into the rod to adjust the width of the head (**288**).

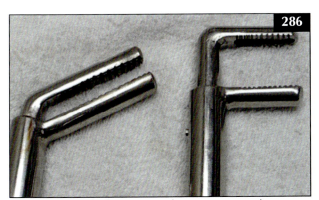

286 Homemade forceps used to remove teeth adjacent to one another. Upper tooth forceps on left and lower tooth forceps on right.

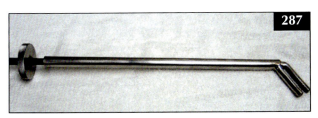

287 A homemade extraction forceps.

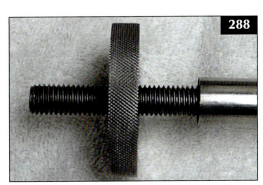

288 The threaded end of the rod is used to adjust distance between the jaws.

Fulcrums are used to apply leverage to the head of a forceps only when the diseased tooth is ready for extraction (**289–291**). The diseased tooth is only ready for extraction when the practitioner sees foamy blood around the tooth and the movement of the tooth makes a 'squishy' sound (like wet tennis shoes). This may not be the case in some older expired teeth.

Almost anything can be used as a fulcrum. It is helpful if more than one size of fulcrum is available. The author commonly uses a small piece of square wood. Pine is a soft wood that will give with pressure without splintering. In addition, small square pieces of rubber mats can be used and, if needed, can be stacked on top of one another to give more leverage. It is important that the fulcrum be placed close to the head of the forceps when attempting to extract the tooth (**292**).

Offset molar forceps are used most often to remove cheek teeth in the caudal aspect of the dental arcade when the diseased tooth is long, as in a young horse, and there is little room for extraction (**293**). These forceps may be mistaken for a pair of incisor forceps. Incisor forceps are of the same shape but about a third of the size.

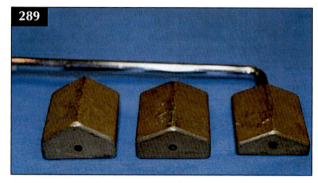

289 A metal fulcrum with various size heads.

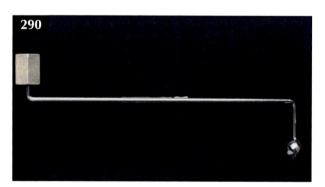

290 A short fulcrum with interchangeable heads. The fulcrum rotates to work on either side of the oral cavity.

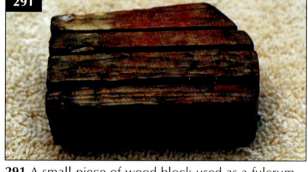

291 A small piece of wood block used as a fulcrum.

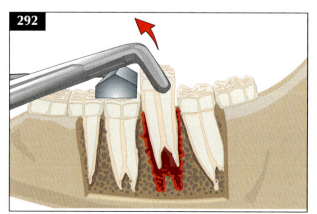

292 The fulcrum is placed close to the head of the forceps to aid in the extraction process.

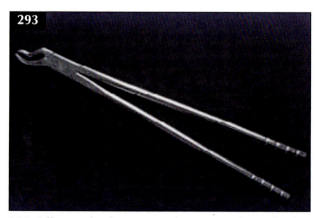

293 Offset molar forceps used to extract long cheek teeth.

The offset molar forceps are placed upon the crown of the diseased tooth once it is sufficiently loose and the tooth is extracted toward the medial plane of the head. It should be noted that extraction with these offset forceps should only be attempted once the diseased tooth has been partially extracted with a 'normal' pair of molar forceps. As the diseased tooth is partially extracted, the length of the tooth prevents it from being brought straight up out of the socket. Thus, the offset forceps are used to remove the tooth towards the medial plane.

The practitioner may try to cut the tooth in half in young horses with long teeth. This is not recommended. Warning! If the tooth is cut in half, it must be prevented from falling back into the socket by securing the bottom half of the tooth with umbilical tape. If the cut half of the tooth does fall into the socket, the practitioner can use a small Steinmann pin to repulse the tooth.

POST EXTRACTION CARE

The horse's head is taken out of the head support and the mouth is washed out with an antiseptic solution. The blood is allowed to set in the socket for a few minutes. In older horses with shallow alveoli, no treatment is necessary to prevent feed materials from entering the space. However, in young to middle-aged horses, it is necessary to use some type of material to cover the extraction site. It is very important *not* to put anything down into the alveolus (**294**). The author prefers to make a patch out of polymethylmethacrylate material. The deep socket is rinsed, dried with gauze, and then a patch is placed. Placement of some petroleum jelly on the practitioner's hand will help prevent the patching material from sticking. The patching material should be shaped to the form of an 'H' with the cross-arm of the 'H' over the hole (alveolus) and the legs of the 'H' on the sides of the teeth in front and behind. It is very important to keep the surface of the patch very smooth as it dries. The legs of the patch should be kept on the surface of the supporting teeth and off the gingiva. The 'patch' should cover the entire hole of the alveolus and be rounded over the edges. The depth of the patch should be no more than quarter the depth of the socket (**295**).

When patching the extraction site of a sinus maxillary tooth, a small sheet of dental wax is placed over the hole and then the patch is put in place. As the patching material cures, it will melt the wax, forming a tight seal to prevent migration of feed materials. This is especially important when placing a patch over a maxillary tooth with sinusitis or one that has an oral–nasal fistula.

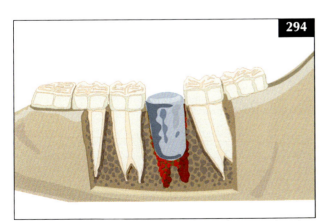

294 Material should not be used to 'plug' an alveolus post extraction. The only exception to this might be plaster of Paris but this material is very hard to work with in the standing horse.

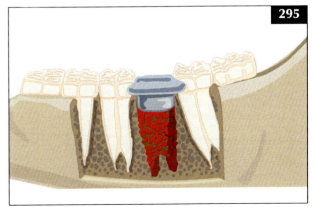

295 A correctly placed patch. Note it does not prevent granulation tissue from forming inside the alveolus and forms a tight bond to the mesial and distal tooth.

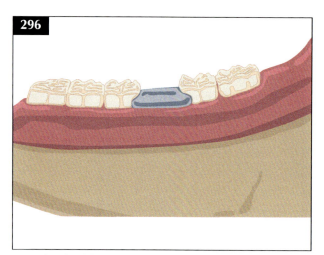

296 The final height of the patch should not exceed the height of the adjacent teeth to prevent the patch from being pulled out during mastication or causing discomfort to the horse. Poorly placed patches should be replaced.

It is beneficial to watch the horse eat later on that day to see if the height or shape of the patch is causing discomfort (**296**). The patch should always be checked the next day to ensure a tight fit. Depending upon the tooth location and disease state of the surrounding area, e.g. sinusitis, the patch should be removed in 2–4 weeks.

MANAGEMENT OF COMPLICATIONS

Things will go badly every now and then.[42–44] One way to minimize this is to select cases very well. The inexperienced practitioner should work with an experienced practitioner or attend an extensive 'hands-on' short course before attempting an extraction of a tooth in a middle-aged to younger horse.

The most common complication encountered is the inability to remove the tooth. There is nothing wrong with not being able to remove a tooth. If the practitioner is unable to remove a tooth, the case should be referred. The most common reasons for the inability to remove a tooth are not allowing sufficient time for the procedure, fracturing the crown of the diseased tooth, or not having the right equipment. If

the crown is fractured, the tooth should be repulsed.

Frequently, the practitioner will fracture a tooth into multiple fragments. If this occurs, the tooth can still be extracted. A pair of forceps with small jaws with little or no gap between the jaws is use to remove the fragments. If a fragment is lodged against the side of the socket, a dental pick is used to elevate the fragment away from the socket and extract it. If a fragment is below the depth of the pick, then the fragment will have to be repulsed with a Steinmann pin.

Occasionally, the author will see a horse with a fractured alveolus from an attempted extraction. If the alveolus is fractured, the fragment should be left *in situ* in most cases and allowed to heal.

ERRORS TO AVOID

A frequent complication is when a practitioner discovers a fractured tooth and grinds (floats) the fracture fragment(s) down. This does nothing to improve the immediate situation and only makes it harder to remove the diseased tooth.

Often, when performing a standing extraction, the horse is aware of his surroundings and quite comfortable if proper sedation and restraint have been administered. However, one must remember that once the initial stimulation of tooth extraction is over and the facial nerve blocks are working well, it will take less sedation to continue the working procedure of extraction and the level of sedation should be closely monitored.

It is important to be mindful of placing the extraction forceps on the correct tooth or loosening adjacent teeth. One should guard against bruising the tongue with the extraction forceps. The speculum should not be left on a horse for more than about 45 minutes at a time without giving the horse a chance to close its mouth for about 5 minutes. The horse's mouth should not be allowed to dry out during the extraction process.

Horses will urinate as a result of the sedation and may become dehydrated. An intravenous catheter should always be inserted for prolonged extractions, and hydration can be assured via intravenous fluids at 2–10 mL/kg/hr in these cases.

Postextraction radiographs should be taken to indicate all tooth fragments are removed. If a tumor is suspected, the extracted tooth should be submitted for histology.

In facial nerve blocks, the anesthetic must have enough time to work before the nerve block is repeated.[32,34–36,45] If a maxillary or mandibular nerve block is performed, the horse should be watched after the procedure and when back in the stall. A few horses will rub their face or chew on their tongue as the anesthetic is wearing off. If a horse becomes irritated as the nerve block is wearing off, the horse should be walked until the irritation is gone.

Geriatric horses may have special considerations.[25,46–49] Their liver and/or kidney function may be altered. Either could affect the blood clotting time post extraction, and the type of medication used. Blood chemistry analysis should be performed on geriatric horses with suspected disease.

SUMMARY

In conclusion, intraoral extraction of equine teeth can be rewarding but the practitioner should be prepared to handle the potential complications that come with this procedure. Having proper equipment, good patient selection, and allowing time for the procedure will increase the chances of positive outcome.

All owners should be informed that if intraoral extraction does not work that they should be prepared to have surgical repulsion of the diseased tooth, and that once a tooth has been disturbed, extraction should be completed.

REFERENCES

1. Dixon PM. Dental extraction in horses: indications and peroperative evaluation. *Compendium on Continuing Education for the Practicing Veterinarian* 1997: **19**(3); 366–375.
2. Duncanson GR. A case study of 125 horses presented to a general practitioner in the UK for cheek tooth removal. *Equine Veterinary Education* 2004: **6**(3); 212–216.
3. Easley J. Cheek tooth extraction: an old technique revisited. *Large Animal Practice* 1997: **18**(1); 22–24.
4. Easley J. Equine tooth removal (exodontia). *Veterinary Dental Forum 16th Annual Conference* 2002.
5. Easley J. Dental corrective procedures. *Veterinary Clinics of North American: Equine Practice* 1998: **14**(2); 411–432.
6. Easley J. Surgical procedures. *The Horse* 2007; 73–78.
7. Lowder MQ. How to perform oral extraction of equine cheek teeth. *Proceedings 45th Annual Convention of the American Association of Equine Practitioners* 1999.
8. Evans LH, Tate LP, LaDow CS. Extraction of the equine 4th upper premolar and 1st and 2nd upper molars throught a lateral buccotomy. *Proceedings 27th Annual Convention of the American Association of Equine Practitioners* 1981.
9. Gaughan EM. Dental surgery in horses. *Veterinary Clinics of North American: Equine Practice* 1998: **14**(2); 381–397.
10. Pavlica Z. Methods of teeth extraction in horses. *Prvi Slovenski Veterinarski Kongres* 1993: **18**(20); 267–271.
11. Vlaminck I.E, Steenhault M, Maes D, *et al.* Evaluation of periodontal changes following intra-alveolar prosthesis for maxillary cheek tooth extraction in ponies. *Journal of Veterinary Dentistry* 2007: **24**(2); 77–84.
12. Tremaine WH. Oral extraction of equine cheek teeth. *Equine Veterinary Education* 2004: **6**(3); 191–198.
13. Tremaine WH. Oral dental extraction in standing horses. *British Equine Veterinary Association 43rd Congress* 2004.
14. Hawkins JF, Dallap BL. Lateral buccotomy for removal of a supernumerary cheek tooth in a horse. *Journal of the American Veterinary Medical Association* 1997: **211**(3); 339–340.
15. Schumacher J, Honnas CM. Dental surgery. *Veterinary Clinics of North American: Equine Practice* 1993: **9**(1); 133–152.
16. Scott EA. Surgery of the oral cavity. *Veterinary Clinics of North American: Equine Practice* 1982: **4**(1); 3–31.
17. Gayle JM, Redding WR, Vacek JR, Bowman KF. Diagnosis and surgical treatment of periapical infection of the third mandibular molar in five horses. *Journal of the American Veterinary Medical Association* 1999: **215**(6); 829–832.

18. Foster DL, Blake Caddel L. Equine dental instruments. *Proceedings 37th Annual Convention of the American Association of Equine Practitioners* 1992.

19. Allen T. Know the drill when selecting tools. *DVM Newsmagazine* 2001; 4E–6E.

20. Dacre KJP, Dacre IT, Dixon PM. Motorised equine dental equipment. *Equine Veterinary Education* 2002: **14**(5); 263–266.

21. Dixon PM, Dacre I. A review of equine dental disorders. *Veterinary Journal* 2005: **169**(2); 165–187.

22. Dixon PM, Tremaine WH, Pickles K. Equine dental disease part 1: A long-term study of 400 cases: disorders of incisor, canine and first premolar teeth. *Equine Veterinary Journal* 1999: **31**(5); 369–377.

23. Easley J, Hodder A. Wolf teeth. *DVM Newsmagazine* 2000; 1E–2E.

24. Lane JG. A review of dental disorders of the horse, their treatment and possible fresh approaches to management. *Equine Veterinary Education* 1994: **6**(1); 13–21.

25. Scrutchfield L. Correction of abnormalities of the cheek teeth. *The North American Veterinary Conference* 1999.

26. Scrutchfield WL, Schumacher J. Examination of the oral cavity and routine dental care. *Veterinary Clinics of North American: Equine Practice* 1993: **9**(1); 123–131.

27. Barasa A, Dazia S, Canavese B, *et al.* Structure and vascularization of the dental pulp in horse incisors. *Bulletin de l'Association des Anatomistes* (Nancy) 1981: **65**(191); 367–381.

28. Easley J. Equine dentistry and oral disease. *Ocala Equine Conference* 1994.

29. Misk NA, Semieka MMA. Radiographic studies on the development of incisors and canine teeth in donkeys. *Equine Practice* 1997: **19**(7); 23–29.

30. Rucker BA. Incisor problems. *The North American Veterinary Conference* 1999.

31. Scrutchfield WL. *Incisors and canines. Proceedings 37th Annual Convention of the American Association of Equine Practitioners* 1991.

32. Lowder MQ. Straight from the horse's mouth: equine dental anesthesia. *Veterinary Technician* 1999: **20**(2); 66–72.

33. Ford TS. Standing surgery and procedures of the head. *Veterinary Clinics of North American: Equine Practice* 1991: **7**(3); 583–602.

34. Klugh DO. Infiltration anesthesia in equine dentistry. *Compendium on Continuing Education for the Practicing Veterinarian* 2004: **26**(8); 625–630.

35. Skarda RT. Local anesthetics and local anesthetic techniques in horses. In: Muir WW, Hubbell JAE (eds) *Equine Anesthesia.* Philadelphia: Mosby-Year Book, Inc, 1991; pp. 199–246.

36. Tremaine WH. Local analgesic techniques for the equine head. *Equine Veterinary Education* 2007: **19**(9); 495–503.

37. Barakzai SZ, Dixon PM. A study of open-mouthed oblique radiographic projections for evaluating lesions of the erupted (clinical) crown. *Equine Veterinary Education* 2003: **5**(3); 183–188.

38. Easley J. A new look at dental radiology. *Proceedings 48th Annual Convention American Association of Equine Practitioners* 2002.

39. Gibbs C, Lane JG. Radiographic examination of the facial, nasal and paranasal sinus regions of the horse. II. Radiological findings. *Equine Veterinary Journal* 1987: **19**(5); 474–482.

40. O'Brien RT. Intraoral dental radiography: experimental study and clinical use in two horses and a llama. *Radiology & Ultrasound* 1996: **37**(6); 412–416.

41. Verstraete FJM. Routine full-mouth radiographs as a teaching tool in veterinary dentistry. *Journal of Veterinary Medical Education* 1999: **25**(2); 28–31.

42. Pascoe JR, Blake Caddel L. Complications of dental surgery. *Proceedings 37th Annual Convention of the American Association of Equine Practitioners* 1992.

43. Prichard MA, Hackett RP, Erb HN. Tooth repulsion in horses: complications and long-term outcome. *Proceedings Annual Convention of the American Association of Equine Practitioners* 1990.

44. Prichard MA, Hackett RP, Erb HN. Long-term outcome of tooth repulsion in horses: a retrospective study of 61 cases. *Veterinary Surgery* 1992: **21**(2); 145–149.

45. Frank ER. Affections of the head and neck. In: *Veterinary Surgery*. Minneapolis: Burgess Publishing Company, 1964; pp. 128–177.

46. Briggs K. Long in the tooth. *The Horse* 2000; 101–108.

47. Lowder MQ. Dental disease in geriatric horses. *The Southern Horse Connection* 1999; 34.

48. Paradis MR. Demographics of health and disease in the geriatric horse. *Veterinary Clinics of North America: Equine Practice* 2002: **18**; 391–401.

49. Ralston SL, Breuer LH. Field evaluation of a feed formulated for geriatric horses. *Journal of Equine Veterinary Science* 1996: **16**(8); 334–338.

STANDING REPULSION OF EQUINE CHEEK TEETH

David O Klugh   Chapter 13

Most equine cheek tooth extractions[1] can be readily performed intraorally[2] in the standing, sedated patient after appropriate regional anesthesia. Some dental disease requires repulsion. Techniques for repulsion under general anesthesia have been described.[3,4] In selected cases, dental disease requiring extraction of premolars may be accessed via buccotomy.[5] The technique of standing repulsion of equine premolars and molars offers an alternative to general anesthesia and adds to the list of methods for removal of specific diseased teeth.

INDICATIONS

Any maxillary or mandibular molar or premolar can be removed by repulsion. Upper cheek teeth 8 through 10 (Triadan system)[6] are accessed via sinus trephination and are the teeth most readily removed via standing repulsion. Standing repulsion is indicated when intraoral extraction is not possible due to shortened or fractured crowns or when intraoral extraction has resulted in root tip fracture.

SEDATION

The patient is sedated with an intravenous injection of detomidine (0.02 mg/kg)[7] in combination with xylazine (0.2 mg/kg)[7] After 5 minutes, additional intravenous sedation is administered with xylazine (0.2 mg/kg) together with butorphanol (0.01 mg/kg).[8]

An alternative protocol is CRI sedation.[9] Several protocols are available for this procedure. See Chapter 10: Standing chemical restraint in the equine dental patient.

PAIN CONTROL

In addition to the analgesic effects of alpha adrenergics[10] and opoids,[11] pain control is maintained with nonsteroidal anti-inflammatory drugs (NSAIDs) administered IV prior to treatment.

Regional anesthesia to the tooth and surrounding structures is achieved by the use of a maxillary or mandibuar nerve block. Descriptions for these blocks are in Chapter 11: Regional and local anesthesia.

In addition to the tooth and bone, structures partially or completely anesthetized by the maxillary nerve block include the retractor bulbi muscle and the optic nerve. In some cases the globe will protrude. In most cases partial loss of vision occurs. All effects of anesthesia disappear as the anesthetic agent is metabolized, which takes 3–5 hours. It is critical to keep the patient in a safe environment until vision returns.

Palpebral movement is not affected, though the patient may undergo reduced tear production and reduced eyelid movement. Corneal dessication may occur unless the cornea is regularly moistened with ophthalmic ointment.

Anesthesia to the skin, submucosa, and periosteum of the bone overlying the site of tooth exposure is provided by local infiltration or an inverted 'L' block.

SURGICAL PROCEDURE

After sedation and local anesthesia, a skin flap is created and the bone is exposed overlying the root of the affected tooth. Blood vessels and muscles are retracted. The periosteum is incised and elevated.

In sinus access, it is helpful to use a trephine large enough to allow manipulation of the punch to all the tooth roots. A 12 mm or larger trephine is appropriate. In many cases the sinus must be flushed prior to tooth removal (**297**). Flushing via the trephine access with high volumes of sterile saline creates drainage via the nasal cavity and externally at the surgical site. This external drainage may contaminate the surgical site and must be thoroughly cleansed prior to wound closure.

Instrumentation for repulsion includes a variety of straight, offset, and curved punches, a mallet, and a bone chisel. A Steinman pin is used to repel retained tooth roots. The bone chisels are used to remove fragments and slivers of tooth that remain attached to the alveolus after tooth repulsion. Examples of instrumentation are shown in figures **298** and **299**.

Standing repulsion requires two operators. One person has a hand in the mouth to identify the tooth and to determine proper punch placement. This operator holds the punch, using proprioceptive abilities to direct and assure proper location of the punch. A second operator taps the punch to assure correct placement. Tapping is easily felt by the intraoral operator (**300**). Alternatively, the extraoral operator may hold the punch and tap while the intraoral operator determines correct placement.

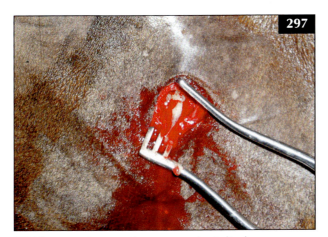

297 Large volumes of mucopurulent discharge require preoperative flushing.

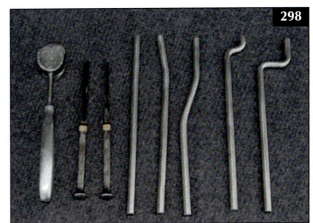

298 Surgical instrumentation including punches, osteotomes, and others are used in tooth repulsion.

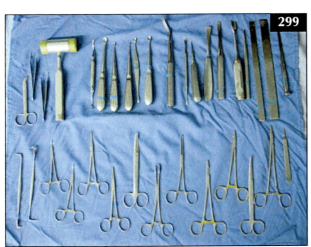

299 Surgical instrumentation for tooth repulsion.

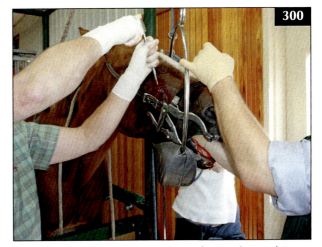

300 Two operators are necessary for tooth repulsion. One has a hand on the tooth to determine correct punch placement. The second operator repels the tooth.

Intraoral radiographs may be taken to assist in accurate punch placement.

After tooth repulsion, intraoral radiographs confirm complete removal. It is helpful to reduce exposure technique to image the retained fragment adequately. Further radiographs (**301**) are taken as fragment removal is confirmed.

After complete tooth removal, the sinus or other operative space is flushed to remove all mucopurulent material and remaining fragments of tooth and bone.

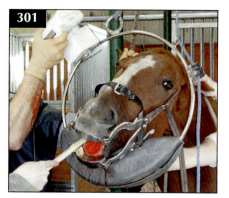

301
Postoperative intraoral radiographs are taken to determine complete removal of all fragments.

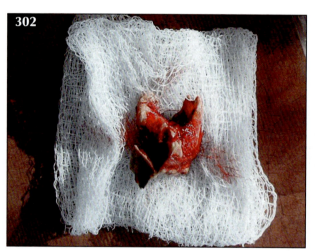

302 The patient shown in figures **300**, **301** had a fractured crown that precluded intraoral extraction. The repulsed tooth is shown here.

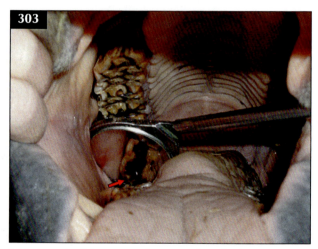

303 A sagittal fracture of 408 is identified.

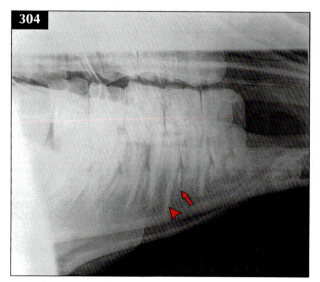

304 The preoperative radiograph demonstrates the long roots (arrowhead) of the affected tooth as well as moderate alveolar sclerosis (arrow).

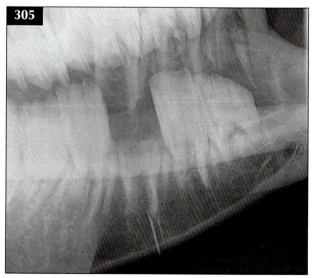

305 An intraoperative radiograph demonstrates fractured tooth roots that must be removed by repulsion. The needle is inserted to mark the position of the tooth.

The alveolus is patched with vinyl polysiloxane impression material. In most cases involving a sinus, a catheter is placed for continual postoperative flushing. Antibiotic and anti-inflammatory treatment is continued as needed. The result of the repulsion of a tooth with a fractured crown that precluded intraoral extraction is shown in figure **302**.

Figures **303–309** demonstrate the procedure in a mandibular tooth. The principles of the surgery are the same as in maxillary teeth.

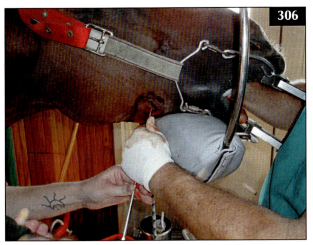

306 After exposing the tooth roots, the retained fragment is repulsed. As with maxillary tooth repulsion, one hand is in the mouth to assure proper placement of the punch.

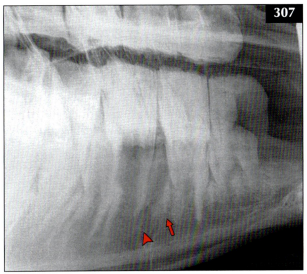

307 A postoperative radiograph shows complete removal of the tooth fragment (arrowhead). Sclerosis of the alveolus (arrow) can be mistaken as a retained tooth fragment. This film was taken after placement of an alveolar patch.

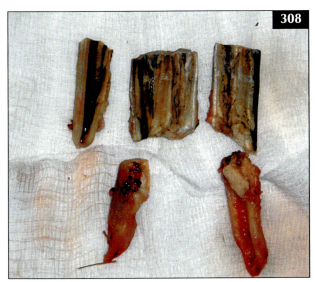

308 Visual inspection of the removed fragments confirms complete tooth removal.

309 The incision is closed.

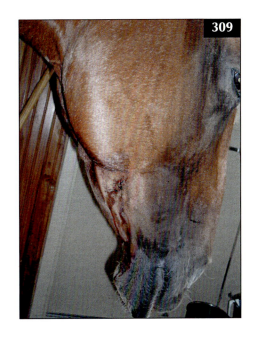

COMPLICATIONS

The maxillary nerve block can result in drying of the cornea, protrusion of the globe, and reduced eyelid movement. All effects return to normal when the anesthetic agent is metabolized. The patient must remain in a safe environment, free of objects that may cause injury since vision remains in only one eye. Global protrusion and corneal desiccation are prevented by intraoperative ophthalmic ointment. Sinusitis is treated by removal of the primary cause and by sinus flushing postoperatively.

During tooth repulsion punches may become wedged between teeth or within the alveolus. It is helpful to have a pair of pliers with which the punches may be removed. During the process of repulsion, it is critical that the operator never misses hitting the punch.

Occasionally a sequestrum of the alveolar bone creates a complication. It is to be suspected in delayed healing of the alveolus or in the development of a new draining tract. In most cases, the sequestrum is a result of loss of vascular supply to an alveolus which has undergone sclerosis. It is important to remember the principle of orthodontic tooth movement that sclerosis develops as the PDL is stretched and new bone is added. The new bone is supplied by the arteries of the PDL. When the tooth is removed and the PDL and its blood supply are disrupted, the sclerosed bone loses its nutritive supply. If this bone is not remodeled by the vasculature supplying the cortex of the bone the result is a sequestrum. Sequestrum removal, though challenging at times, is curative. The case seen in figures **310–312** demonstrates this problem and the resulting removal of the offending bone.

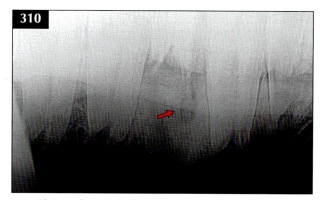

310 This radiograph shows the presence of a sequestrum (arrow).

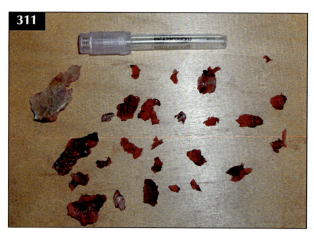

311 The sequestrum and associated bone fragments are removed.

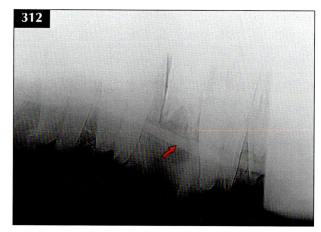

312 Postoperative radiograph demonstrates the clean alveolus (arrow).

SUMMARY

Standing repulsion provides an alternative to general anesthesia and surgical removal. It requires good regional nerve blocks and sedation. Intraoral radiographs assist in punch placement and complete tooth removal. This procedure is indicated when teeth are fractured or shortened due to excessive wear, or when fractured or retained root tips occur after intraoral tooth extraction.

REFERENCES

1. Lowder MQ. Oral extraction of equine teeth. *Compendium on Continuing Education for the Practicing Veterinarian* 1999: **21**(12); 1150–1157.
2. Dixon PM, Tremaine WH, Pickels K, Kuhns L, Hawe C. Equine dental disease Part 4: a long-term study of 400 cases: apical infections of cheek teeth. *Equine Veterinary Journal* 2000: **32**(3); 182–194.
3. Auer J. Extraction and repulsion of cheek teeth. In: *Atlas of Equine Surgery*. London: WB Saunders 2000; pp. 53–59.
4. Dixon PM. Dental extraction and endodontic techniques in horses. *Compendium on Continuing Education for the Practicing Veterinarian* 1997: **19**(5); 628–638.
5. Tremaine WH, Lane JG. Exodontia. In: Baker GJ, Easley J (eds) *Equine Dentistry*. Edinburgh: Elsevier Limited, 2005; pp. 267–294.
6. Floyd MR. The modified Triadan system: nomenclature for veterinary dentistry. *Journal of Veterinary Dentistry* 1991: **8**(4); 18–19.
7. Baker GJ, Kirkland KD. Sedation for dental prophylaxis in horses: a comparison between detomidine and xylazine. *Proceedings 41st Annual Convention of the American Association of Equine Practitioners* 1995; pp. 40–41.
8. Orsini JA. Butorphanol tartrate: pharmacology and clinical indications. *Compendium on Continuing Education for the Practicing Veterinarian* 1988: **10**(7); 849–854.
9. Goodrich LR, Clark-Price S, Ludders J. How to attain effective and consistent sedation for standing procedures in the horse using constant rate infusion. *Proceedings 50th Annual Convention American Association of Equine Practitioners* 2004; pp. 229–232.
10. Daunt DA, Steffey EP. Alpha-adrenergic agonists as analgesics in horses. *Veterinary Clinics of North America: Equine Practice* 2002: 18; 39–46.
11. LeBlanc PH. Chemical restraint in the standing horse. *Veterinary Clinics of North America: Equine Practice* 1991: **7**(3); 521–533.

HEAD TRAUMA IN HORSES

Henry Tremaine

Chapter 14

INTRODUCTION

Injuries to the equine head are common, especially in young horses, due to their inquisitive and excitable nature. Despite the apparently severe nature of many injuries, the good vascularity and relatively small mechanical loads placed on the structures of the head usually make the prognosis for a successful outcome good with only minor cosmetic blemishes remaining in most cases.[1,2]

Careful evaluation of soft tissue, osseous, and dental trauma is required before selecting the appropriate treatment. Skull injuries usually result from direct trauma and many fractures are open, involving communication to the skin, oral cavity, nasal cavity, or paranasal sinuses.

FRACTURES OF THE EQUINE MANDIBLE

The mandible is the most frequently fractured bone of the equine skull,[2] and mandibular injuries occur most commonly in young animals.[3] Most fractures result from kicks or as a result of entanglement of the incisors in steel fencing wire or other objects due to the inquisitive nature of the young horse.[4]

DIAGNOSIS OF MANDIBULAR FRACTURES

Horses with injuries to the mandible usually present with clinical signs including salivation, dysphagia, oral hemorrhage, halitosis, asymmetrical swellings over the mandibles, crepitus, abnormal incisor occlusion, or discharging tracts. A careful examination including digital palpation should be performed, with the horse sedated if necessary. Caution should be exercised before performing an oral examination with a full mouth speculum if a mandibular fracture is suspected.

Nondisplaced mandibular fractures may become displaced when loaded by opening a mouth speculum. Displaced factures can result in instability of the mandible and malocclusion of the incisors. Careful palpation within the mouth can reveal buccal communication with the fracture. The physical examination will reveal damage to adjacent soft tissue structures associated with the mandible such as the parotid salivary gland, linguo-facial artery and vein, mental nerve, and dorsal or ventral buccal nerves.

ANCILLARY DIAGNOSTIC EXAMINATIONS

The mandible should be radiographed with the horse sedated. Straight lateral, ventrolateral–dorsolateral oblique, and dorsoventral projections are advisable. In addition, intraoral, occlusal views are extremely useful for rostral mandibular fractures. Digital or computed radiographs offer good control over resolution and gray scale compared to conventional films. Radiopaque markers should be used to indicate the position of any discharging tracts. Although it is usually possible to diagnose the fracture from the clinical examination, radiography is required to clarify the configuration of the fracture, and possibly to identify comminution and additional dental fractures. Multiple projections with varying exposures may be needed to image the mandible and cheek teeth reserve crowns and apices. More recently computed tomography (CT) and magnetic resonance imaging (MRI) have been used to assist with the diagnosis of equine head lesions. These modalities, although not yet widespread, offer great promise in the configuration of head injuries in three dimensions. In almost all clinics general anesthesia will be necessary to obtain CT or MR images, and this may be undesirable in horses with severe acute injuries. A few centers have the facility for standing MRI.

MANAGEMENT OF MANDIBULAR FRACTURES

The most common configuration of mandibular fractures comprises an avulsion of the incisors and part of the rostral mandible, often occurring in young animals becoming snagged on objects such as wire fencing.[5] Other common fracture locations are in the interdental space (bars of the mouth) and in the horizontal ramus. Fractures of the caudal horizontal and vertical rami are less common, due to the extensive protection afforded these areas by the large *masseter* muscles.

First aid

Most mandibular fractures are open with communication with the skin or into the oral cavity. Extensive contamination with food material and external debris is often present. Gross debris can carefully be physically removed and this is followed by extensive lavage with isotonic fluid. Dilute (0.005–0.01%) chlorhexidine or povidone–iodine may be included. Effective lavage can be obtained with a hosepipe if polyionic fluids are unavailable. Broad-spectrum antimicrobial therapy is recommended. Food should be withheld until the injury is treated to avoid further gross contamination, provided that treatment is expedient.

Repair of mandibular fractures

Fractures of the rostral mandible, involving incisors

These fractures are very common especially in weanlings, which frequently present with fractures of the rostral mandible involving the corner incisors and a portion of the bone. Most rostral mandibular fractures can be repaired using a configuration of cerclage wires to reduce and stabilize the fracture fragments (**313**).

Damaged incisors should be salvaged where possible, although loose deciduous teeth or coronal dental fragments with no attachments may be devitalized and therefore require removal. Devitalized or contaminated soft tissues and the fracture line should be surgically debrided and lavaged before reduction of the fracture. The wires are passed through the rostral mandibular bone. In young animals with soft bone this can often be achieved under sedation by perforating the bone using a 16 gauge needle and subsequently threading the needle through it.[6] The use of mental and mandibular alveolar nerve blocks will desensitize the affected area. Rostral branches of the mandibular nerve may be damaged by the injury resulting in loss of sensation of the lower lip and rostral mandible. Older animals

313 The avulsion fracture of this foal's mandible has been reduced and stabilized using multiple surgical steel wires.

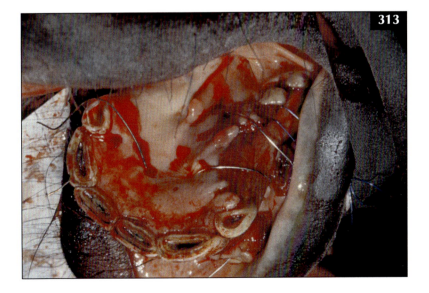

may require the holes to be drilled with a hand chuck or air drill. Cerclage wires are placed around the remaining incisors if their alveolar attachments are intact. Various patterns of cerclage wire application are shown in figure **314**.

If suitable stability and reduction are not achieved additional wires can be placed around the canine tooth if present (which may be grooved to prevent the wire slipping when tightened), through holes drilled in the interdental space, or around the first or second cheek tooth. Wires are preplaced and then tightened by twisting the ends or tightening loops in the interdental space. Sharp ends are twisted down on the labial aspect for ease of removal, and twisted flat to prevent trauma to the gums during eating, or are embedded in a material such as vinyl polysiloxane or methylmethacrylate. The skin and subcutaneous tissue should be closed where possible over the fracture repair. In addition to reducing the amount of contamination of the fracture line, closure of the soft tissue will accelerate healing and prevent excessive granulation tissue, which can become cosmetically undesirable.

Wires can be removed from the sedated horse after 4–8 weeks, depending on the degree of instability of the original fracture.

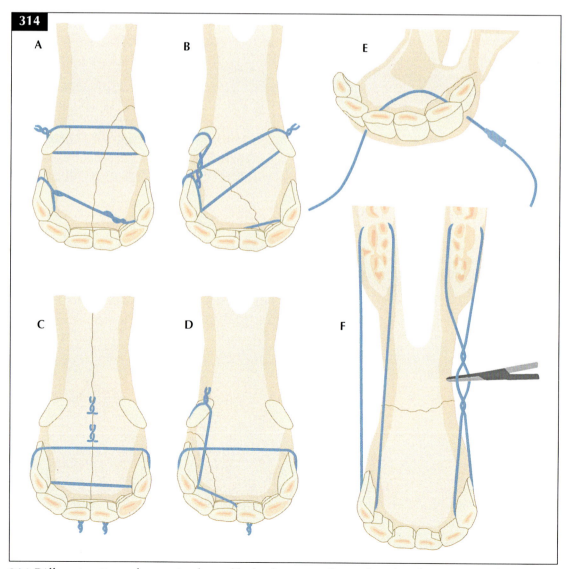

314 Different patterns for repair of mandibular fractures. (Reproduced with permission from EVJ Ltd, Newmarket, UK.)

Fractures of the rostral mandible or maxilla, involving all of the incisors

Fractures involving the complete row of incisors and the rostral maxilla or mandible are unstable (**315** and **316**). Such fractures require increased support, and may be fixed using wires placed around the pregrooved canine tooth, in the interdental space or around the first mandibular cheek tooth (306, 406). Examples are demonstrated in figures **317** and **318**.

The use of acrylic splinting devices or external fixators may be considered. The mandibular nerve, which emerges from the mental foramen on the lateral aspect of the mandible, caudal to the corner incisor (Triadan 303 or 403), should be preserved where possible.

Unilateral mandibular fractures of the interdental space

Many unilateral fractures involving the interdental space are stable, with splinting provided by the contralateral mandible. Such fractures may often be treated conservatively. More unstable or displaced fractures are usually repaired using tension band wires placed around the corner incisor and the first

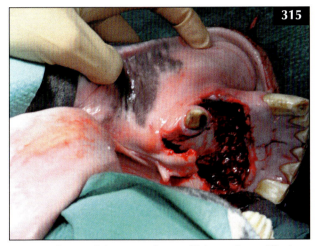

315 Avulsion of the rostral mandible and maxilla is a common injury in young horses. Careful debridement and accurate reduction enable a good prognosis for repair.

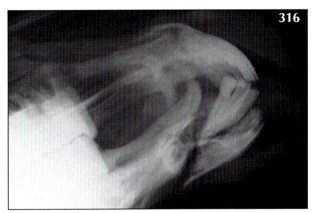

316 Radiographs of mandibular fractures should be taken in order to configure the fracture and plan the repair.

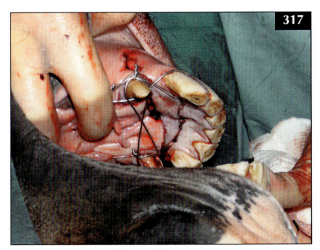

317 Stabilization of rostral fractures using stainless steel wiring is often possible and can be performed with the horse under general or regional anesthesia.

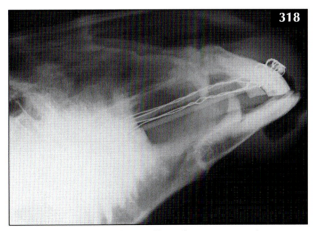

318 Unstable rostral maxillary fractures can be immobilized using wires arranged according to tension band principles and anchored around the cheek teeth.

mandibular cheek tooth. In this arrangement the splinting effect of the intact mandible is utilized and the wire is placed on the tension aspect of the fractured bone in accordance with standard internal fixation principles. Placement of the wire around the first cheek tooth is impeded by the (rostrally placed) commissures of the lip. A skin incision at the level of the site of wire placement allows introduction of a soft tissue protector to enable the hole to be drilled accurately between the apices of the first (306, 406) and second (307, 407) cheek teeth. After careful reduction of the fracture (if displaced), the wires are twisted and then tightened to achieve interfragmentary compression. For comminuted fractures or those not involving the incisors, lag screws, plating, and external fixators can also be used.

This area is also subject to bitting injuries (**319**). Many of these injures can be managed successfully with surgical curettage (**320**).

Bilateral fractures of the interdental space

Bilateral fractures of the interdental space are inherently less stable than unilateral ones, and nondisplaced fractures may become displaced if not sufficiently stabilized. Some fractures may be sufficiently stabilized using bilateral wire tension bands. Severely unstable fractures may require external support using a U-shaped external fixation device anchored with wires.[5] Some small movement

of the fractured mandible is often possible after placement of the U-bar, and accurate placement of the wires through predrilled holes in the wire can be frustrating. U-bars made from aluminium or brass have been used.

Alternatively intraoral splints may be prepared using methylmethacrylate (cold-curing orthopedic standard). Cerclage wires are preplaced around the incisors leaving large loops on the lingual aspect. Similar wires are placed through holes between mandibular cheek teeth 306 and 307 (or 406 and 407). Methylmethacrylate is now molded to the mandible so as to incorporate the wire loops. The wires can be tightened once the methacrylate has set hard. Care is taken to avoid the frenulum and sublingual caruncle when molding the methacrylate. The final prosthesis should not be so bulky as to impede eating.

External fixation devices have been used successfully to immobilize unstable bilateral fractures of the interdental space[7] and horizontal rami. The use of these devices is particularly suitable in open fractures. A proprietary device with the rigid sidebar fixed to the mandible using clamps has been reported.[8] Alternatively, threaded Steinmann pins can be inserted through both mandibles and then rigidly fixed to sidebars to immobilize the fracture. The sidebars can be manufactured from polypropylene tube filled with acrylic. Such a fixation is demonstrated sequentially in figures **321–323**. The pins and bars are usually removed in 4–6 weeks, and

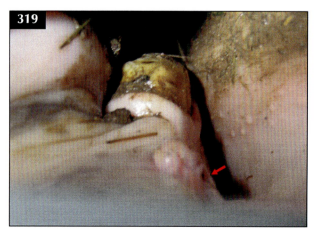

319 Injuries from bit trauma to the bars of the mouth are easily overlooked but can cause considerable discomfort and pain when the horse is ridden (arrow).

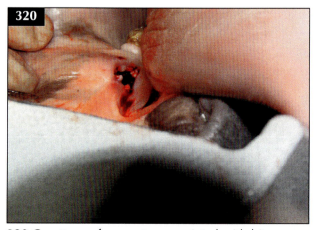

320 Curettage of sequestra associated with bit trauma, combined with 3–6 weeks of convalescence allows the lesions to heal by granulation.

some serous discharge from the pin holes is not uncommon.

Fractures of the horizontal or vertical mandibular rami

Fractures of the horizontal rami, such as in figure **324**, are usually unilateral, resulting from kicks. Frequently the cheek teeth may be involved with damage and contamination of the reserve crowns. Nondisplaced, stable fractures may be treated conservatively. Eventual extraction of damaged cheek teeth may be necessary but this is sometimes delayed until after stabilization of the callus. It is possible that attempts to remove the compromised cheek teeth in the acute stage may be complicated by further destabilization of the mandibular fracture, which may delay healing, especially in young horses, due to the difficulty of removing equine cheek teeth.

Comminuted open fractures of the rami, which are incomplete or nondisplaced, heal by conservative management after careful debridement to remove any contaminants of devitalized fracture fragments.

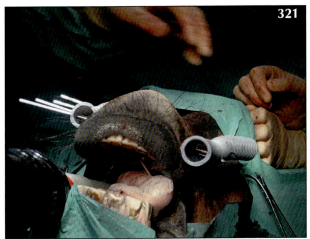

321 Bilateral unstable fractures of the interdental space are repaired using external fixation devices.

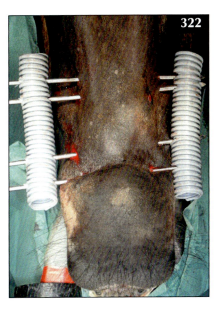

322 External fixation devices are well tolerated and enable a rapid return to eating; protection of the sidebars is advised to prevent their entanglement in stable fittings.

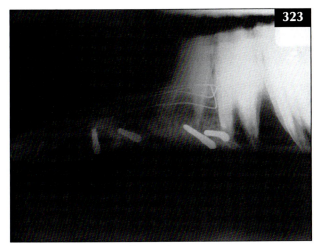

323 Postoperative radiographs are necessary to assess the degree of fracture reduction.

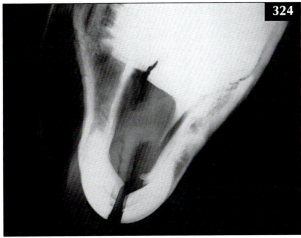

324 Radiograph of a displaced oblique fracture of the horizontal ramus.

Care must be taken to avoid iatrogenic trauma to the parotid duct and transverse facial vessels on the medial aspect of the caudal mandible.

Severe displaced fractures of the horizontal ramus may be repaired using half-pin splintage, placed through the skin and through the mandible and cut to 10–12 cm. These are then connected to a horizontal bar of methylmethacrylate incorporated into a plastic cylinder.

Dynamic compression plates placed on the ventral aspect of the mandible have also been used successfully. The caudal mandible is very thin except along its ventral border, which renders screw implantation difficult. Examples of injury to this area are shown in figures **325–328**.

Care must be taken to avoid damage to dental apices during screw placement. The parotid salivary duct and sublingual vessels must be avoided as they cross the ventral aspect of the mandible approximately at the level of the fourth cheek tooth. Mandibular fractures are almost invariably open and the oral cavity is a contaminated environment, and it is therefore advisable that all implants are removed after 6–12 weeks if the repair is stable, to avoid chronic sepsis.

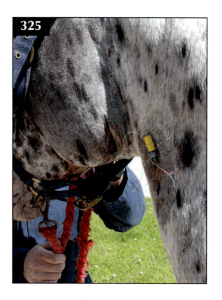

325 This Appaloosa has an open fracture of the vertical ramus accompanied by marked swelling.

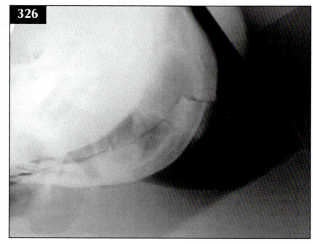

326 Radiograph showing comminuted vertical ramus fracture. These fractures are well protected by musculature and are difficult to immobilize accurately with implants.

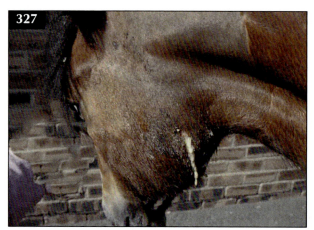

327 This mandiblar fracture is infected and discharging through a sinus tract.

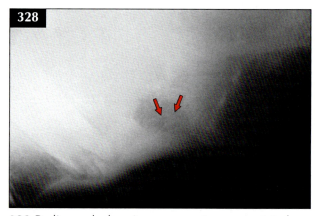

328 Radiograph showing a sequestrum associated with a mandibular fracture (arrows) which has resulted in a discharging tract.

MAXILLARY AND FRONTAL BONE FRACTURES

Depressed fractures of the facial bones occur sporadically usually as a result of kicks or when the horse rears and strikes the skull on an overhanging object (**329**).

Clinical signs vary with severity, and fractures without skin tearing may remain undetected for some time after the injury. Figure **330** demonstrates a long-standing depressed fracture that has healed with a sinus tract. Figure **331** shows the repair by advancing a skin flap.

Clinical signs observed include: swelling (often asymmetric) over the frontal and maxillary bones; subcutanous emphysema; uni- or bilateral epistaxis due to hemorrhage from damaged nasal or paranasal sinus mucosa; purulent nasal discharges due to secondary sinusitis; and abnormal respiratory noises due to airflow disturbances caused by engorged nasal mucosae or displaced nasal bones. Severe injuries may cause major skin loss and facial distortion with obstructive dyspnea.

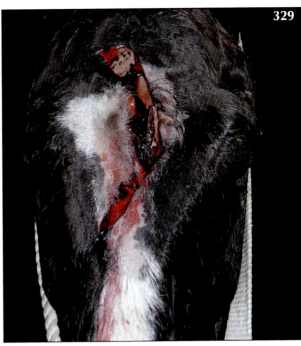

329 This horse has sustained a depressed fracture involving the frontal and nasal bones communicating with the conchofrontal sinus.

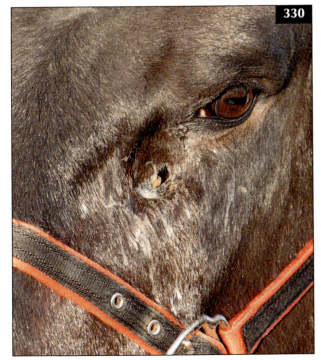

330 This chronic depressed fracture has healed but a sinofacial fistula has remained. Revision surgery can effectively improve such cases if they show drainage of purulent exudates through the facial tract.

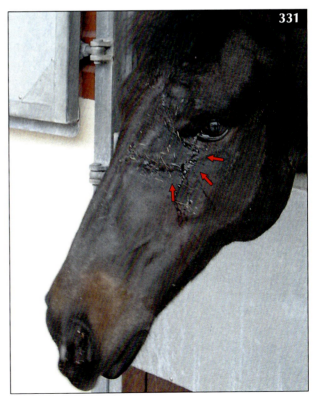

331 The horse from figure **330** has been treated by advancing a skin flap to repair the discharging fistula (arrows).

A careful clinical examination is usually more enlightening than radiology to identify the configuration and margins of a fracture. Figure **332** shows a radiograph of a depressed facial fracture and the difficulty in defining fracture margins.

A neurological examination, including assessment of the cranial nerve reflexes is advisable before sedating the animal. The patient in figure **333** should have a thorough neurological examination.

A detailed inspection of the zygomatic arches for the presence of orbital fractures should be performed. Fracture repair is often delayed by 24 hours to reveal any chronic subdural hemorrhage which may result in delayed-onset neurological signs.

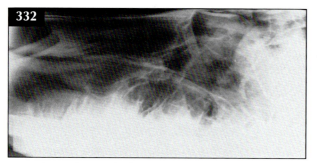

332 This radiograph shows a depressed facial fracture. Such lesions are hard to configure on radiographs due to the complex anatomical superimposition.

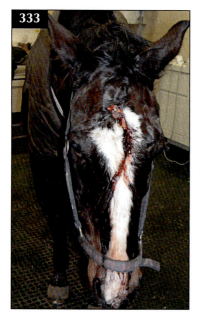

333 Facial injuries may appear very severe and a neurological examination should be performed before embarking on other ancillary tests.

A radiological examination should be performed to detect any latent or nondisplaced fractures and to identify the presence of blood and exudates in the paranasal sinuses. In young horses the suture line between the basi-occipital and basisphenoid bone may be mistaken for a fracture line. Endoscopic examination will identify the presence of hemorrhage from the paranasal nasomaxillary sinus ostia and from the guttural pouches. The latter may indicate avulsion or tearing of the rectus capitis ventralis muscle and could also indicate the presence of a fracture of the base of the skull. Direct sinus endoscopy can be useful to identify the presence of fracture fragments within the sinuses, although the field of view is often impaired by the accompanying hemorrhage. Hemorrhage from the ear should be treated as a suspicious sign of petrous temporal fracture and may be accompanied by neurological defects. Ultrasonography can be particularly useful to image the zygomatic arch and temporomandibular joint and to detect fractures involving the bony orbit caudal to the globe. CT and MRI would be desirable for imaging the skull in three dimensions and to configure fractures more accurately but may be undesirable if general anesthesia is considered a high risk.[9]

After the initial investigation, careful monitoring is advised to detect any deterioration in neurological signs, which may develop up to 24 hours after the initial injury.

Small, or nondisplaced skull fractures may be left to heal conservatively These injuries have a good prognosis and an acceptable cosmetic outcome. Larger or unstable fractures, particularly involving the zygomatic arch, are best treated by removal of devitalized bone fragments and contamination and attempted reduction and stabilization of the fracture. Surgical immobilization of fractures is best achieved under general anesthesia although stabilization of the patient for 24–48 hours post injury is advised. Reconstruction of the zygomatic arch using stainless steel wire or small orthopedic plates can be performed to protect the eye. Contraction of lacerated skin occurs rapidly and can further delay attempts to achieve primary wound closure. Some form of head protection, such as padded stockinette tubular bandage with precut eye-holes may be desirable during induction of anesthesia, and for protection postoperatively (**334**).

The goal of surgical repair is to remove contaminants and devitalized tissue, to stabilize the supporting skull bones, and to restore the facial contour. Extensive skin incisions may be necessary to expose the margins of the fracture. Depressed fragments can be elevated using elevators placed through trephine holes drilled around the fracture or by using bone hooks. Careful elevation of depressed fragments of the zygomatic arch can be assisted using an instrument (e.g. the blunt handle of a small animal dental extraction forceps) placed in the conjunctival fornix. Fractures of the bones adjacent to the medial canthus should be handled carefully to avoid additional trauma to the nasolacrimal duct. Reconstruction of a nasal bridge is important to enable normal airflow, especially in young horses intended for an athletic career. In addition, the facial crest provides strong support for the interposed maxillary bones. Blood clots and debris are lavaged from the nasal passages and paranasal sinuses before closure. The larger fragments are reduced and fixed to stable fragments using 1–1.2 mm diameter stainless steel cerclage wire, which can be placed through small holes drilled with a small drill bit or Steinmann pin. Cuttable bone reconstruction plates[10] and T-plates have also been used for very severe facial fractures.[11] Carbon fiber implants have been used in isolated cases to assist with cosmetic reconstruction.[12] Careful closure of the periosteum, using an absorbable material, including over defects where bone fragments are absent, results in successful healing. The skin can be closed using cyanoacrylate adhesives, sutures, or skin staples. If extensive skin loss is a feature the creation of advancement flaps can assist wound closure. Where there is extensive exudation into the paranasal sinuses, placing an indwelling drain into the frontal or maxillary sinuses before closure will allow lavage of exudates from the sinuses in the ensuing days and prevent the development of sinusitis. A padded stent bandage is advisable to protect the repair during the horse's recovery from general anesthesia and padded halters and assisted recovery techniques can be used. Severely unstable fracture repairs are vulnerable to additional trauma during recovery and assisted recovery in these cases may be desirable.

Postoperatively most repairs need minimal care other than lavage of the sinuses for 3–5 days as described. Implants are not normally removed. Head bandaging may be advisable to prevent wound dehiscense and contamination or self-trauma if the horse rubs its head on stable fittings. If the infraorbital nerve is involved in the injury some abnormal sensations resulting in perceived pruritus can be anticipated. Movement of the skull bones abutting into suture lines at the fracture line or during repair may result in a reactive suture periostitis producing linear exostoses for many months following injury (**335**). Serum discharge from such suture periositis can occur but is usually not indicative of infection.

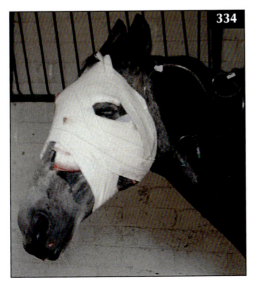

334 Protection should be given to the head after skull fracture repair.

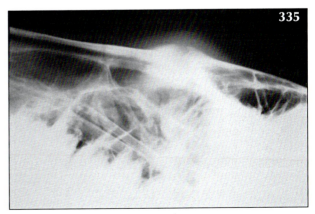

335 Following trauma to the face, a reactive suture periostitis can ensue. These nonpainful lesions are mostly cosmetic and gradually improve with conservative management.

Chronic discharging facial tracts or nasal discharges are usually indicative of fragment sequestration, and removal of devitalized fragments will be necessary for healing to progress.

The prognosis is good with healing of most facial wounds including a satisfactory cosmetic result, even in the presence of defects in the underlying bones. A positive cosmetic result is shown in figure **336**.

Chronic fistula or sinus tract formation can occur following a depression fracture. An example of an oronasal fistula is shown in figure **337**. Its repair is shown in figure **338**. Such injuries lend themselves to cosmetic reconstruction using sliding skin flaps or muscle pedicle graft techniques.[13]

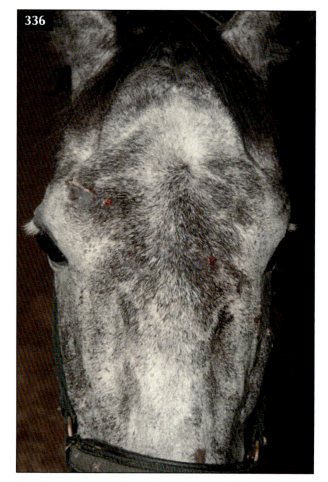

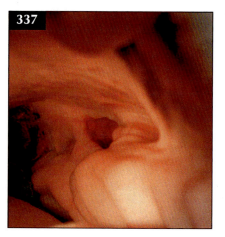

337 Oronasal fistulae are occasional complications of extraction or fracture.

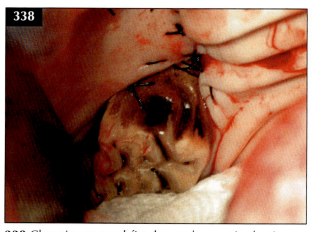

336 A good cosmetic outcome is possible as shown by this horse 3 months after repair of a depressed facial fracture.

338 Chronic oronasal fistula can be repaired using a sliding mucoperiosteal flap.

SKULL BASE FRACTURES

Skull base fractures are most commonly the consequence of a horse rearing over backwards and striking the poll. The fracture occurs while there is tension between the tensed ventral muscles of the neck and the weight of the upsidedown head. Injuries to the base of the skull may also result in tearing of the rectus capitis muscles or avulsion from the occipital bone, avulsion of the insertion of the ligamentum nuchae, fracture of the basihyoid or basisphenoid bones, or fracture of the petrous temporal bone, depending on the position of the head at the time of impact. Injuries to the calvarium and CNS trauma, possibly associated with intracranial hemorrhage or edema, can occur after such traumatic events even in the absence of any fractures.

Clinical signs, which may accompany skull base or cranial injuries, include: hemorrhage from the ear, epistaxis, vestibular defects, and ataxia. Although radiology can confirm the presence of a fracture, movement of the horse to a suitable facility may be impossible until neurological signs have been stabilized or the horse is safe to be moved. Neurological signs can deteriorate after the horse has regained a standing position as a result of intracranial hemorrhage and inflammation. Mannitol, soluble corticosteroids, and diuretics (e.g. furosemide) have been used to prevent CNS edema. Broad-spectrum antibiotics should be administered to prevent transmission of pathogens from the guttural pouches into the meninges, which may communicate in the presence of a fracture.

Skull base fractures are difficult to detect on radiographs and should be interpreted cautiously in light of clinical data.[14] CT or MRI may be more useful to configure the fracture accurately. Endoscopy can identify hemorrhage from the guttural pouches and any pharyngeal or laryngeal motor neurological defects. The treatment of horses with nondisplaced fractures with neurological defects involves symptomatic treatment and anti-inflammatory therapy with glucocorticoids or NSAIDs and mannitol. Dimethyl sulfoxide has also been used although its efficacy is unproven. The prognosis depends on the severity and progression of neurological signs. Complications can include chronic vestibular defects, although horses show a good ability to compensate visually for minor vestibular defects. Blindness has also been reported following lesions involving the optic chiasma and temporohyoid arthropathy. Anesthesia of horses with skull fractures should be delayed until stabilization of any neurological signs and cessation of hemorrhage.

HYOID BONE FRACTURES

Hyoid bone fractures are rare and usually occur as a result of falling over backwards or excessive trauma on the tongue. Stylohyoid bone fractures are most commonly detected secondary to a chronic inflammatory process resulting in ankylosis of the petrous temporal–stylohyoid articulation; they are generally presented with no history of trauma.

Horses with hyoid bone fractures may present with dysphagia with a protruding tongue, which is painful to palapate. In addition, signs of defects associated with cranial nerves VII and VIII (e.g. head tilt) may also be present. Open fractures may present with epistaxis or oral hemorrhage. Lateral and dorsoventral radiographs and nasal endoscopy are useful diagnostic aids. Stylohyoid fractures can be readily identified radiographically. Hyoid bone fractures are treated conservatively, assisted by dietary management involving the feeding of liquidized gruel. The prognosis is fair for unilateral fractures of the stylohyoid bone, which are reported to be able to heal over 2 months. Bilateral fractures carry a poor prognosis and such injuries are usually accompanied by cranial nerve damage. Euthanasia is indicated if oral dysphagia or other severe neurological signs show no improvement after 4 weeks. Ankylosis of the stylohoid petrous articulation may be treated by surgical disarticulation of the hyoid apparatus by removal of the keratohyoid bone.[15,16]

COMPLICATIONS ASSOCIATED WITH SKULL FRACTURES

The prognosis for repair of many skull fractures is good provided that there are no significant neurological deficits. Complications which can occur during their healing include: chronic sinusitis due the presence of sequestra or debris in the paranasal sinuses, discharging facial tracts due to sequestra or infected implants, nasofrontal suture periostitis, and cosmetic deficits due to failure to support depressed fracture fragments. Horses with severe head injuries may also have permanent neurological defects.

SUMMARY

Head trauma in horses is common. The combination of small mechanical loads and good vascularity to bone and soft tissue contributes to good fixation results. Thorough evaluation, including radiographic examination, is necessary to identify and address problems of teeth, sinuses, and other bony and soft tissue structures. Treatment strategies should include those necessary to address the open, contaminated nature of these injuries as well as methods of maintaining normal occlusion and function of the mastication process. Knowledge of materials, experience with them and with traumatic injuries, and imagination in their employment all contribute to successful management of head trauma in equine patients.

REFERENCES

1. Murch KM. Repair of bovine and equine mandibular fractures. *Canadian Veterinary Journal* 1980: **21**; 69–73.
2. Little CB, Hilbert BJ, McGill CA. A retrospective study of head fractures in 21 horses. *Australian Veterinary Journal* 1985: **62**; 89–94.
3. Schneider RK, Mandibular fractures In: White NM, Moore JM (eds) *Current Practice in Equine Surgery*. Philadelphia: Lippincott, 1980; pp. 589–593.
4. Ragle CA. Head trauma. *Veterinary Clinics of North America: Equine Practise* 1993: **9**(1); 171–183.
5. Henninger RW, Beard WL, Schneider RK, *et al.* Fractures of the rostral portion of the mandible and maxilla in horses: 89 cases (1979–1997). *Journal of the American Veterinary Medical Association* 1999: **214**; 1648–1652.
6. Tremaine WH. Mandibular injuries. *Equine Veterinary Education* 1998: **10**; 146–150.
7. Beslsito T, Fisher AT. External skeletal fixation in the management of equine mandibular fractures: 16 cases (1988–1998). *Equine Veterinary Journal* 2001: **33**(2); 176–183.
8. Lischer CJ, Fluri E, Kaser-Hotz B, *et al.* Pinless external fixation of mandible fractures in cattle. *Veterinary Surgery* 1997: **26**(1); 14–19.
9. Ragle CA. Imaging of the equine head: use of CT and MRI. *Proceedings of the North American Veterinary Conference: Large Animal* 2005: **19**; 272–273.
10. Dowling BA, Dart AJ, Trope G. Surgical repair of skull fractures in four horses using cuttable bone plates. *Australian Veterinary Journal* 2001: **79**; 324–327.
11. Burba DJ, Collier MA. T-plate repair of fracture of the nasal bones in a horse. *Journal of the American Veterinary Medical Association* 1991: **199**(7); 909–912.
12. Valdez H, Rook JS. Use of fluorocarbon polymer and carbon fiber for restoration of facial contour in a horse. *Journal of the American Veterinary Medical Association* 1981: **178**; 249–252.
13. Theoret CL. Wound repair in the horse: problems and proposed innovative solutions. (Wound Management Series) *Clinical Techniques in Equine Practice* 2004: **3**(2); 134–140.
14. Ramirez O, Jorgensen JS, Thrall DE. Imaging basilar skull fractures in the horse: a review. *Veterinary Radiology & Ultrasound* 1998: **39**(5); 391–395.
15. Walker AM, Sellon DC, Cornelisse CJ, *et al.* Temporohyoid osteoarthropathy in 33 horses (1993–2000). *Journal of Veterinary Internal Medicine* 2002: **16**; 697–703.
16. Divers TJ, Ducharme NG, Lahunta A, *et al.* Temporohyoid osteoarthropathy. (Special issue. Neurology) *Clinical Techniques in Equine Practice* 2006: **5**(1); 17–23.

PRINCIPLES OF RESTORATION OF DISEASED TEETH

David O Klugh and Randi D Brannan   Chapter 15

The goal of equine dentistry is to maintain oral health and function. This is achieved by relieving pain, correcting abnormal dental conditions, and by prevention of disease. Many fractured and decayed equine teeth can be restored to health with modern materials that are used in human and small animal dentistry. The goals of restorative dentistry are to protect the pulp, arrest decay, restore the tooth to function, and prevent further disease.

Pulp protection should be achieved in all cases. Thorough debridement arrests the disease process. Restoring a tooth to function may not be practical in all cases, but if the pulp is protected and the decay process is arrested, further disease is prevented.

Materials available for use in restorative procedures for equine teeth are:
- Acrylic resins.
- Amalgams.
- Composites.
- Glass ionomers.
- Dentin bonding agents.

Conditions treated with restorative materials in equine dentistry include:
- Infundibular decay.
- Fractures of the crown.
- Enamel hypoplasia.
- Cavities or caries.
- Endodontic access sites.

GV Black classified lesions and cavities for humans in 1908. This system has been modified for use in small animals[1] and it applies to equine dental lesions also. It is based on both the location of the lesion on the tooth and the location of the tooth involved:
- **Class I:** pits, fissures, and developmental grooves on any tooth (**339**). In equine dentistry, this includes infundibular cavities.

- **Class II:** lesions of the proximal surfaces of posterior teeth (**340**). A common manifestation of this lesion in equine dentistry would be a fractured tooth or decay resulting from periodontal disease affecting the interproximal surface.

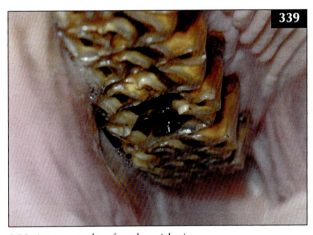

339 An example of a class I lesion.

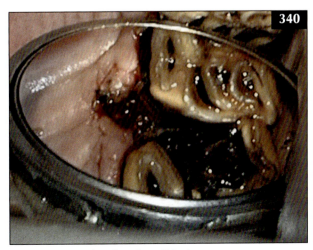

340 An example of a class II lesion.

- **Class III:** lesions of the proximal surfaces of incisors (**341**). This is uncommon in equine dentistry, but would include the same etiologies as class II lesions.
- **Class IV:** lesions at the proximal surface of incisors that involve the incisal or occlusal edge (**342**).
- **Class V:** lesions near the gingiva involving labial, lingual, or palatal surfaces of any tooth (**343**, **344**).
- **Class VI:** lesions involving the incisal or occlusal edge or cusp tips of any tooth (**345**).

The primary usefulness of the classification system is in describing the lesion location and configuration. In

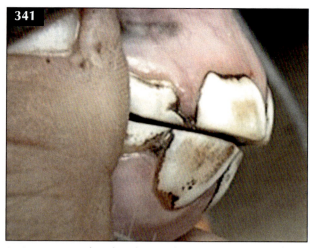

341 An example of a class III lesion.

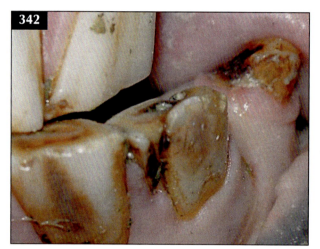

342 An example of a class IV lesion.

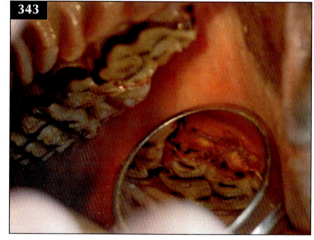

343 An example of a class V lesion: a buccal fracture of a cheek tooth.

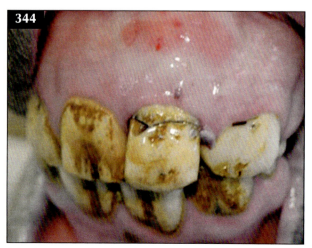

344 An example of a class V lesion: a fractured incisor.

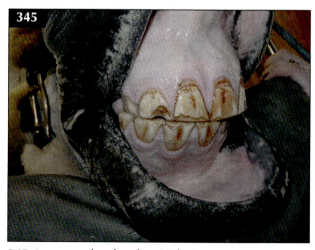

345 An example of a class VI lesion.

brachydont dentistry, this classification system is also used to correlate a dental lesion with a specific type of material most suited for restoration of that lesion. The continually erupting nature of the hypsodont tooth in many cases limits the usefulness of material classification. In class V lesions involving dentin only, in brachydont species, for example, the material choice would include factors such as the chemical nature of the bond and its ability to withstand caries insults. If the class V lesion involved enamel, material flexibility might be a consideration. In equine class V lesions, material strength is a major factor, since the material will ultimately be in occlusal contact. While bond strength is important, the ability of the material to withstand occlusal forces and oral abrasion is also important and would necessitate a material choice different from that used on a brachydont tooth. Appropriate choices of materials are only made with knowledge of their properties and uses. For this reason, in-depth knowledge of dental materials, anatomy, and lesions is necessary for suitable treatment.

MATERIALS

A myriad of materials exists for restoring the structure of a tooth. Each type has specific characteristics that can be advantageous or disadvantageous in specific cases. The ideal restorative material should chemically bond to dentin and enamel, should not break down or become distorted during placement, have the same coefficient of expansion as teeth, low polymerization shrinkage, and should wear at the same rate as the tooth.[1]

Many dental materials are composed of polymers resulting from chemical reactions between basic materials. Polymers are large molecules that are made from smaller monomers. When polymers are created they are smaller in volume than the original components. Consequently they have the potential for leakage around their margins. The coefficient of thermal expansion is the degree to which the material shrinks or expands when heated or cooled. The ideal material shrinks and expands like dentin and enamel.

Acrylic resins are usually methylmethacrylate. Their use in restorative procedures is limited, though they were used for this purpose years ago as the first nonamalgam material. They are composed of a powder polymer and a liquid monomer. They polymerize as the two components are mixed in an exothermic reaction. The heat given off varies with the brand used. Their use in equine dentistry is limited to intraoral splints, patches placed on extraction sites, and in selected cases of periodontal disease as a space-occupying material between teeth. Some veterinary dental practitioners use a glycol methacrylate for patching extraction sites. These products are more exothermic than the methylmethacrylates. The excessive polymerization shrinkage of all acrylics precludes their use in restoration of individual tooth lesions. Some methylmethacrylates shrink up to 21% during the polymerization process.[2]

Amalgams were the first restorative material introduced. Dental amalgams are a mix of a silver alloy and mercury. The silver alloy is composed of silver, tin, and copper. Silver is used to increase the strength and expansion of the material. Tin is used to decrease the expansion and to assist in mixing with the mercury. Recent changes have increased the copper content to give improved strength, hardness, and longevity. Amalgam does not bond to the tooth and requires either an undercut or cement for retention. Additionally, the corrosion of the margin aids in retention. In the high copper amalgams there is less corrosion, thus the need for bonding to prevent marginal leakage.

Composite resins are currently the material of choice for use in areas where there is occlusal contact. They create a smooth surface that wears similarly to enamel. Composites are composed of four components: an organic polymer matrix, inorganic filler particles, silane coupling agents, and the initiator–accelerator system.[3] A dimethacrylate monomer polymerizes during the setting reaction to become the organic polymer resin matrix. *Table 10* lists some resins used in composite materials.

Table 10 Common resins used in composite materials

Common name for simple reference	Chemical name
bis-GMA	bis-phenol-A glycidyl methacrylate
HEMA	Hydroxyethyl methacrylate
TEGDMA	Triethylene glycol dimethacrylate
UDMA	Urethane dimethacrylate

The matrix polymerizes by chemical or light activation. Chemical-cured materials are composed of two pastes that begin reacting when mixed. Light-cured composites begin reaction only when exposed to light of a specific wavelength. The light-cured composites are activated by a blue light that is most intense at 480 nanometers, matching the wavelength needed for the chemical reaction.

The resin matrix alone shrinks volumetrically about 10% during polymerization.[4] Shrinkage is dramatically reduced by the inclusion of filler particles. As filler loading increases shrinkage decreases. Most composites shrink less than 3%.[3]

The filler particles are generally composed of various types of silica glass or quartz. The early composites used quartz particles. The size of the filler particles and percentage content determines the classification of the composite (see *Table 11*).[2] The more filler and the larger the particles, the less the shrinkage, thermal expansion is more like the tooth, and the better the wear resistance. However, they are less esthetic.

Filler particles are covered with a silane coupling agent that bonds the particles to the resin matrix. During setting, the bond between resin matrix and filler particle transfers forces from one particle to another. This represents a major advantage in the physical characteristics of a composite material. However, this bond can be degraded by water during the placement of the material.[3] Therefore, it is important to keep the working field dry when using composite restoratives.

Initiators and accelerators are used in the setting reaction. The setting reaction starts when the initiator is stimulated to begin the polymerization process. Chemical accelerators are used to control the speed of the reaction. Light-cured composites utilize a diketone initiator and an amine accelerator. Chemical-cured composites set by activation of a benzoyl peroxide initiator and a tertiary amine accelerator.

Light-cured composites have less matrix and more filler, making them stronger. Their working time is longer than chemical-cured materials, since polymerization does not begin until it is activated by a curing light.

The first composite introduced in the 1960s was the macrofilled composite, with quartz particles ranging in size from 10–25 μm The finish was rough due to the large size particles, and plaque accumulation was a problem. Their use in equines is limited, though their strength would be valuable in restoration of infundibular cavities.

The need for a smooth finish to prevent plaque accumulation in human dentistry lead to the introduction in the 1970s of microfilled composites. With a particle size of 0.03–0.5 μm and a low fill percent of 40–50%, they have a high coefficient of thermal expansion and less strength. Their modulus of elasticity is low and, therefore, they are more flexible. These are rarely used in equine dentistry due to lack of strength and less demand for a highly polished, esthetic finish.

In the 1980s small particle composites were developed for the purpose of balancing the need for wear resistance and strength and the need for a smooth finish. Particle size ranged from 1–5 μm and the fill percent was 80–85%. The range of particle sizes and higher fill percent produced a material with less shrinkage, good wear and strength, but not the smoothness of the microfills. Their strength allowed use in occlusal locations.

In the late 1980s the hybrid composite was developed. The particle size ranged from 0.5–1 μm with a fill percent of 75–80%. These materials are a balance between the small particle and the microfills. They have better strength and wear resistance than

Table 11 Composite material classification

Classification[2]	Average particle size (μm)[2]	Filler %[2]	Shrinkage %[3]
Macrofilled (traditional)	8–12	70–80	---
Small particle	1–5	80–90	---
Microfilled	0.04–0.4	35–60	2–3
Hybrid	0.6–1.0	75–80	0.7–1.4

microfills with a finish almost as smooth. They are used in equine dentistry for restoration of occlusal lesions, such as those resulting from infundibular disease.

Flowable composites are low-viscosity, light- or chemical-cured composites. They have a very low modulus of elasticity, and thus are flexible. They have high polymerization shrinkage and low filler percent, which gives them low wear resistance. They are used in equine dentistry as liners under other restorative materials.

Packable composites are a recent introduction in the world of restorative materials. They were developed to address shrinkage, wear, and handling. They have high strength, similar to that of amalgam. They have a higher filler content than other composite materials, usually greater than 80%.[4] Filler particles are irregular in size and shape. The amount of resin is reduced, thus shrinkage is reduced.

Glass ionomers are an adhesive material of polyacrylic acid and powdered fluoroalumino-silicate glass. They release fluoride and chemically bond to the tooth. Retention is assisted by micromechanical adhesion to dentinal tubules. They are chemically cured materials. Light-cured glass ionomer materials are those that are resin reinforced.

Setting of a glass ionomer occurs in three phases involving an acid–base chemical reaction. On mixing the two parts, or on light activation of a premixed material, protons (hydrogen ions) are formed in the ionization of polyacrylic acid when it reacts with water. The glass particles are attacked in phase two to release calcium, aluminum, and fluoride ions. As the pH increases, calcium and aluminum ions react with the polyanions remaining from the acid to polymerize the cement as a polycarboxylate chain. Phase three is a slow hydration process that strengthens the cement.[3]

Glass ionomer cement (GIC) chemistry results in an ionic bond between the carboxyl (COO^-) ions in the cement acid and the calcium (Ca^{++}) ions in dentin and enamel.[5] This bond has been shown by x-ray photon spectrophotometry.[6]

Fresh mixtures of GIC create a mild inflammatory reaction in pulp cells when directly exposed. In one study, the reaction was assessed at 3 days,[7] while in another study samples were examined at 8 days.[8] In both studies, inflammation subsided by day 30. There is variation in inflammatory response beteen GICs from different manufacturers. The resin-modified GICs are particularly irritating when the resin is incompletely cured. Components suspected of causing pulp reaction include HEMA and TEGDMA (see *Table 10*).[9] It is important to light cure resin-modified composites thoroughly. Dentin bridge formation is not impaired by the presence of GICs.[7]

The physical properties of glass ionomers have advantages and disadvantages.[2] These materials are brittle, lack wear resistance, are subject to abrasion, and are not resistant to fracture.[10] Their coefficient of thermal expansion is similar to tooth structure and, as such, they have minimal shrinkage when cured. The material bonds to dentin micromechanically and aids in prevention of marginal leakage.[11]

Three types of glass ionomer preparations are used. Type I is used for cementing or 'luting' crowns and bridges. Type II is used as a restorative material. Type III is used as a base or liner to separate a pulp treatment from the final restorative material used in closing the endodontic access site.[2,11]

More recent modifications to the basic GIC have been made.[2,5,11] Metal-modified GICs were introduced in an effort to add strength, wear resistance, and fracture toughness. While improved over conventional GICs, they are not as strong as other materials, such as composites. They are also not esthetic like composites.

Resin-modified GICs were introduced to add strength and prolong working time over conventional glass ionomers. They have the additional benefit of creation of a hybrid bond similar to that of composites. This bond is created by the resin included in the material. This resin is very similar to that used in composites.[2] Additionally, this gives the material improved moisture resistance. These materials are still not strong enough to be used in restoration of occlusal lesions in equine dentistry.

Dentin bonding agents are used with composite materials. They are unfilled dimethacrylate monomers. Bonding agents assist in creation of a complete seal and strong bond between the tooth and the restorative material. Composites by themselves do not bond to tooth material. Dentin bonding agents are used as an intermediate material to which both the tooth and the composite material will adhere. These products include a chemical that etches enamel and dentin, a primer that forms an interlocking micromechanical bond in the dentin, and an adhesive for sealing the margin and creation of a layer to which the restorative material can adhere. Exposure to curing light polymerizes the material and creates a micromechanical bond to the tooth. These materials occlude dentinal tubules and form an interlocking layer with collagen, called a hybrid layer (**346**). Good marginal seal prevents bacterial penetration of the restored tooth.

Dentin bonding agents have evolved through seven 'generations' of products.[12,13] The first four 'generations' were developed in efforts to find materials that actually retain composite materials. Fourth-generation bonding introduced the concept of etching the surface of the tooth to remove completely the smear layer and open the dentinal tubules to improve penetration. The acid used decalcified collagen, allowing the formation of micromechanical infiltration of the collagen matrix with the primer/resin tags. Fourth-generation bonding introduced the concept of maintaining a moist environment so that decalcified collagen does not collapse and prevent impregnation of the collagen matrix with primer/resin.

Fifth-generation bonding materials included simplification of the clinical procedure by combining steps involved. The primer and adhesive are combined in the one bottle. These products are the most commonly used products in equine dentistry today. They are simple to use, not technique sensitive, and result in high bond strength.

Sixth-generation bonding agents were developed in an effort to eliminate the need for a separate etching agent. Sixth-generation type 1 products include the 'self-etching primers'. These products eliminate the need to wash off the etchant, thus reducing the risk of collapse of the collagen matrix when dried. These products are applied separately to the tooth. Self-etching primers produce less bond strength and have higher marginal leakage than fifth-generation products.

The sixth-generation type 2 products are composed of two solutions that are mixed immediately prior to use. They provide good dentin bonding, but less effective enamel bonding than fifth-generation bonding agents.[12]

Seventh-generation products have been developed to further simplify the bonding procedure. These products do not have to be mixed prior to use, as the sixth-generation products require. However, their bond strength to enamel is weak compared to fifth-generation bonding agents.[12]

The acid-base considerations of sixth-generation type 2 and seventh-generation bonding agents preclude proper curing of many self-curing composites, and so are contraindicated in such cases.[13]

DENTAL PRINCIPLES IN THE EQUINE PATIENT

Most research in the development of restorative materials has been performed to benefit brachydont species, i.e. man and small animals. Therefore it is instructive to understand the needs of those species as they relate to materials usage and, when applicable, how the equine patient's needs differ.

All species have the need for materials with strength, wear resistance, and elasticity resembling normal tooth structure. Biocompatibility is also important in all species, though the dynamic equine pulp may be able to respond in some situations where the brachydont pulp may not.

BONDING AND MICROLEAKAGE

Composite restorative materials are micromechanically bonded to tooth structure in brachydont species. The nature of this hybrid bond of resin tags interlocking with collagen fibers and dentinal tubules has been well studied. Its character in equine teeth is not known. It may be that composites are retained in equine teeth primarily or entirely by macro-mechanical means. The uneven surface of the cavity preparation may be sufficient to retain the material. Research is needed in this area.

All dental materials need to be placed, bonded, and cured such that technique does not lead to microleakage. A good marginal seal prevents access by micro-organisms to tooth structure. Invasion of bacteria can result in secondary caries or failure of

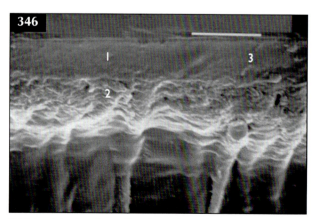

346 In this demineralized section, the arrow indicates the bonding agent extending into the dentinal tubules. The adhesive layer (1) is identified as is the hybrid layer (2), or layer of adhesive intertwined with collagen fibers. **3**: single bond

endodontic therapy. Correct placement, good bonding, appropriate choices of materials, and a final surface sealant all contribute to minimizing marginal leakage.

The problem of marginal leakage in hypsodont teeth is complicated by tooth eruption and attrition. Eruption exposes the deeper part of the original filling. The need for correct placement techniques and correct materials choices becomes important when this part of the original filling is exposed to the oral cavity. The cavity must be completely filled, or occlusal exposure will result in damage to the filling or secondary caries.

The importance of the final surface sealant placed over the filling in brachydont species and its role in preventing marginal leakage is lost quickly in the erupting hypsodont tooth. This thin layer of unfilled resin suffers rapid attrition during mastication within a matter of weeks, thus losing its effectiveness. It should be placed initially, but one must understand that it is short lived.

Further, the role of progression of secondary decay may or may not be greater than the rate of tooth eruption and attrition. The visible presence of a line of secondary decay on follow-up examination of infundibular cavities suggests that the rate of development of secondary decay is faster than the rates of attrition and eruption. However, yearly examination of these fillings (**347**) does not reveal further measurable peripheral extension of decay. Research is needed in this area.

FINISHED RESTORATIVE SURFACE

Surface smoothness of the final restoration is important in brachydont teeth. Plaque adheres best to irregular surfaces, thus leading to decay and periodontal disease. Early composite materials were developed to create a highly polished, very smooth surface to which plaque has difficulty attaching. Periodontal disease in hypsodont teeth is not a result of plaque adhesion. Rather, it results from accumulation of feed materials around and between teeth and the subsequent breakdown of this feed material. Consequently surface smoothness of the finished restoration is less important in hypsodont teeth. A more important principle in equine dentistry is even tooth contact for purposes of efficient and comfortable mastication.

GLASS IONOMER USAGE

GICs and restorative materials were developed as direct bonding materials. Their chemistry assists in both reduction of demineralization of teeth and in remineralization of carious dental structure.[14] These effects are a result of fluoride release from the material into the fluids of the oral cavity.[15] The effects of fluoride release are both chemical and biological.[2]

The chemical effect of fluoride release is to become incorporated into the tooth structure as fluoroapatite. This crystal is more resistant to acid-mediated decalcification than hydroxyapatite.

Fluoride also acts as a catalyst for uptake of calcium and phosphate. Secondary caries is minimized, since the fluoride penetrates carious dental tissue and forms fluoroapatite. The result is resistance of decay and promotion of remineralization. However, a recent evidence-based review of literature demonstrated 'no conclusive evidence for or against a treatment effect of inhibition of secondary caries by the glass ionomer restoratives'.[16]

Glass ionomers bond directly to tooth structure as carboxyl groups of the polyacids react with calcium of the enamel and dentin.[2] Bond strength is higher to enamel than to dentin because of the higher inorganic content of enamel.

Glass ionomers are biocompatible. They cause minimal pulp irritation when placed close to the pulp or directly on the pulp after bleeding stops. These products are used in many cases of pulp capping a

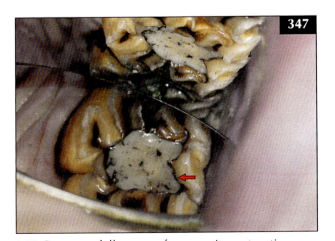

347 One year follow-up of composite restoration demonstrates normal wear with secondary caries of the margin (arrow). This patient exhibited greater than normal staining and adhesion of feed materials to the composite. This condition remains constant on repeated annual examination.

direct pulp exposure and as a liner for indirect pulp capping procedures.

The use of glass ionomers in equine dentistry is limited to locations where pulp protection is needed. This is generally the case in deep cavity preparations and pulp capping procedures. Important considerations include their ability to bond directly to the tooth without any conditioning; their pulp protective character; and possibly their ability to facilitate remineralization. They may be useful in prevention of secondary decay in diseased teeth, and therefore their use as a base or liner should be considered. An example of their use is in figure **348**, where a cavity was in close juxtaposition to the pulp of this tooth. Prevention of indirect pulp exposure and subsequent pulpitis is achieved with the use of a glass ionomer as a liner for this filling.

Lack of strength of glass ionomers precludes their use on the tooth surface, as their low strength will not withstand occlusal forces. Eruption and tooth attrition will eventually result in occlusal exposure of most gingivally oriented placements. Therefore, when used, they should be placed as liners and bases only. Direct placement composites should be used to complete the restoration.

ESTHETICS

In man and small animals, the esthetics of dentistry is of utmost importance. In equine dentistry it is less important. The equine incisor is covered on its labial surface by cementum which takes up pigments from feed due to its porosity and high organic content. This results in significant staining that is highly variable in color. It is usually dark brown and causes a very mottled appearance of the tooth surface (**349**). While it can be readily cleaned, it recurs quickly. This staining is not pathological. Color matching should be compared to exposed enamel. This is done using a template provided by most vendors (**350**).

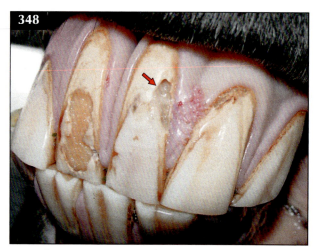

348 Glass ionomer is used as a liner for this filling to protect the pulp (arrow).

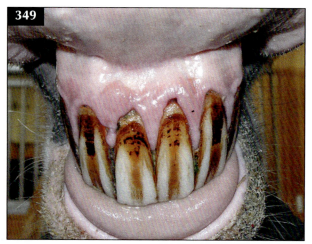

349 The uneven brown staining of the labial surface of these incisors is a result of pigments from feed that are taken up by the porous cementum.

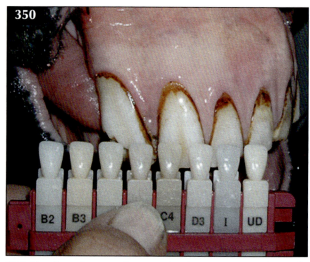

350 Tooth color can be matched using a template of the various shades of composite materials.

AMALGAMS

Amalgam is infrequently used in veterinary dentistry. Use of amalgam requires undercuts or the use of bonding adhesives, because it does not bond directly to the tooth. The corrosive nature of the amalgam results in mechanical retention.

DENTINAL SENSITIVITY

Sensitivity of exposed dentin in cavity or crown preparations, or in recent fractures in brachydont teeth, has lead to significant research into its mechanics and control. The odontoblast process in the dentinal tubule is thought to be a receptor that senses fluid movement within the tubule. This fluid is a normal component of the dentinal tubule. As fluid movement occurs, a signal is sent from the odontoblast process to the nerves of the pulp. This signal is then interpreted as pain.[17]

Sensitivity can be reduced or eliminated with the use of cement bases and dentin bonding agents. Cement bases are used to protect the pulp and exposed odontoblast processes from thermal and chemical irritation in cavity preparations. They are thick materials that provide good insulation.[2]

Dentin bonding agents may be applied to exposed dentin. The unfilled resin fills the first few microns of the exposed dentinal tubules. This creates a protective layer for odontoblast processes.

In equine and small animal dentistry the concept of dentin sensitivity is difficult to evaluate due in part to the stoic nature of the patients. However, it is appropriate to use dentin bonding agents in cavity preparations and on exposed dentin in situations where much crown has been removed during occlusal equilibration. The use of cement bases may be considered in deep cavity preparations. An example is a glass ionomer.

SPECIFIC USES OF RESTORATIVE MATERIALS IN EQUINE DENTISTRY

INFUNDIBULAR DECAY
Anatomy

The gross anatomy of equine teeth has been described in Chapter 3. The occlusal surface of the equine tooth is composed of cementum, dentin, and enamel. The peripheral enamel is coated by cementum. Incisors have a central infundibulum composed of a layer of enamel in the form of a cone filled with cementum. Each upper cheek tooth has a pair of crescent-shaped infundibula variably filled by cementum.

During development, the cementum fills the enamel-lined infundibulum from the occlusal surface apically. A normal infundibulum is shown in figure **351**. It is common for the infundibulum to be incompletely filled with cementum during the process of embryological development. In many cases the apical portion of the infundibulum is void of cementum.

The most important complication of infundibular disease is sagittal fracture and premature tooth loss. It is important to recognize the problem as early as possible in order to maximize the treatment effect. Pulpitis is possible, but uncommon.

In some cases of apical pulpitis in young horses, the route of infection is suspected to be through the infundibulum.[18,19] Other cases of apical pulpitis become infected via anachoresis. This is suspected to be the major route of infection in young horses.[20] To understand better the relationship between apical pulpitis and infundibular disease, it is instructive to consider how mineralization of the crown enamel develops in relation to tooth eruption. This would explain how an anachoretic route of infection of an unmineralized crown might result in both pulpitis and infundibular disease.

Mineralization of the crown has been assumed to be complete prior to its eruption.[21] In an investigation of the timing of enamel mineralization in equine mandibular premolars and molars, Hoppe *et al.* demonstrated that mineralization continues for up to

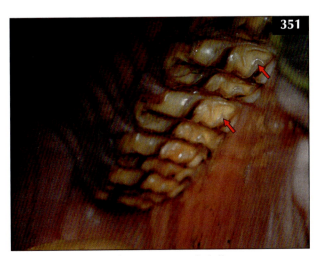

351 The arrows indicate a normal, fully cementum-filled infundibulum.

15 months after eruption.[22] *Table 12* summarizes the findings.

When considering the etiological relationship of apical and infundibular disease, it is instructive to understand that the apical portion of the crown, including the apical infundibulum is not entirely mineralized in young patients. In some cases this portion of the tooth may not be completely developed. This undeveloped or unmineralized soft tissue would likely be subject to inflammatory change and infection when micro-organisms are delivered via anachoresis. Altered vasculature and soft tissue anatomy may result. This may explain some observations of apical communication between the vasculature of the infundibulum and pulp in young horses.

Pathology

Microscopically, the disease begins with cemental hypoplasia. Decay begins within the cementum and progresses peripherally as cemental canaliculi fill with food residue and micro-organisms. Continual decay involves the surrounding enamel and later the dentin.

In stage 1 teeth there may or may not be decay present. If present, the decay process is confined to the cementum and is restricted from expansion by the enamel border. In the vast majority of teeth, the disease remains limited to this stage. Few of these cases progress to stage II.

In some cases the pathology extends to involve the enamel and the dentin surrounding the infundibulum. In such cases, the dentin and enamel separating the two infundibula may be lost either by fracture or further decay. The resulting coalescence of the two infundibula creates a large defect in the occlusal surface. The tooth is then at high risk of fracture and premature loss. An example of sagittal fracture is shown in figures **352**, **353**.

Table 12 Posteruption mineralization of mandibular cheek teeth

Tooth	Age at start of mineralization	Age at end of mineralization	Age at eruption	Months after eruption to end of mineralization
Molar 1	0.5 (± 1)	23 (± 3)	8–12	11–13
Molar 2	7 (± 1.5)	37 (± 3)	20–26	13–15
Premolar 2	13 (± 1)	31 (± 2)	27–32	1–2
Premolar 3	14 (± 1)	36 (± 3)	30–38	1–4
Premolar 4	19 (± 3)	51 (± 2)	42–50	3–6
Molar 3	21 (± 3)	55 (± 2)	39–51	7–13

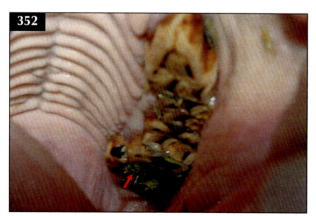

352 A clinical view of a sagittal fracture of 209 (arrow).

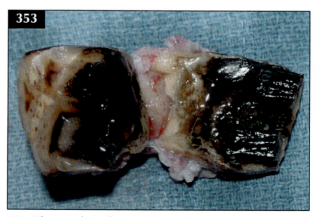

353 The tooth in figure **352** is shown after extraction.

Stages of infundibular decay

Progressive stages of infundibular decay are graded according to the extent of decay of the tissues involved.[20,23,24] On routine examination of the oral cavity, infundibular disease appears as either a darkened spot on the arcade (**354**), or as feed material adherent to the tooth surface (**355**). Further examination with a mirror is necessary to determine the severity of disease. Treatment strategy depends on the stage of the disease:

- Stage I is defined as involving the cementum layer only (**356**).
- Stage II is defined as decay involving the cementum and surrounding enamel (**357**). Dark staining of the enamel indicates decay. The enamel is pitted and subject to fracture.

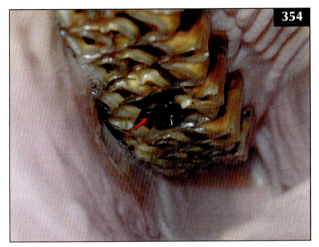

354 The arrow indicates a diseased infundibulum as seen on routine oral examination.

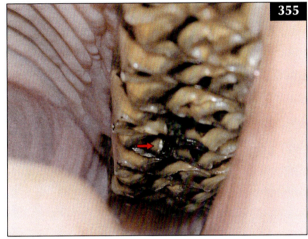

355 The clinical appearance of diseased infundibula may present as feed accumulation in the cavity and adherent to the tooth surface (arrow).

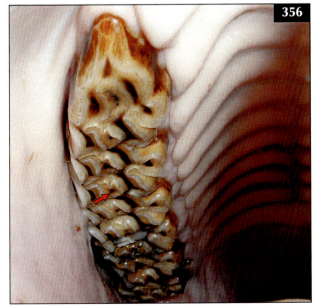

356 Stage I infundibular decay is characterized by cemental hypoplasia, where the cementum does not completely fill the enamel lake (arrow).

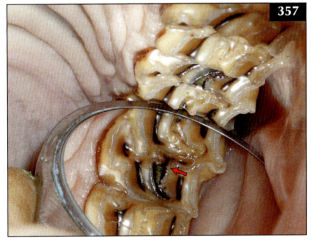

357 Stage II infundibular cavity with decayed enamel (arrow).

- Stage III infundibular decay is defined as extending further and involving the dentin as well as the cementum and enamel (**358**, **359**).

Gradation progresses peripherally. No measurement of the depth of involvement is used in this system of classification. Measurement of depth as a routine step in classification is complicated by the uneven nature of cemental hypoplasia within the infundibulum and the variable depth of the enamel lining. Intraoral radiographs are very helpful in demonstrating the extent of decay (**360**).

Treatment strategies

Studies totaling thousands of horses reveal an overall incidence of cemental hypoplasia of about 70% of all horses over the age of 15. This incidence represents all stages, with stage I predominating.[23–26]

The definition of stage I is involvement of the cementum only. The primary lesion is cemental hypoplasia, with or without cemental decay. In cases examined by the author where a stage I infundibulum was filled and attrition revealed the apical region of the infundibulum, that area of the tooth was found to have suffered further decay. This was evidenced by peripheral extension of decay of both the mesial and distal infundibulum. Filling a stage I lesion does not appear to prevent further decay.

As the disease progresses to involve peripheral tissues, previously described risks to the health of the tooth increase. The most severe consequence of infundibular decay is fracture of the tooth. Intervention for the purpose of prevention of fracture is supported. It is suggested, therefore, that stage II infundibular cavities be filled to prevent fracture.

Stage III involves dentin. Some of the pathological changes previously discussed may have already occurred to stage III teeth prior to presentation to the attending veterinarian. Even after filling, these teeth are at risk of premature loss, though the risks are reduced by restorative procedures. Figure **361** shows attrition of the occlusal surface of a restoration seen at the time of the annual examination. Peripheral decay is seen, though the restorative is intact and functioning normally.

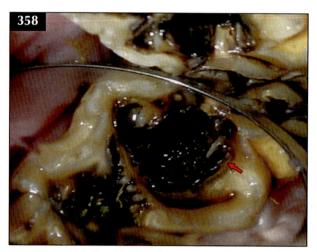

358 Stage III infundibular decay extending into the dentin (arrow).

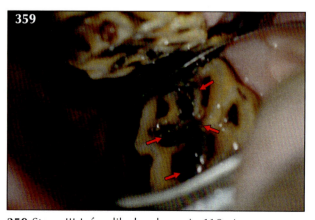

359 Stage III Infundibular decay in 110. Arrows indicate dentin involvement.

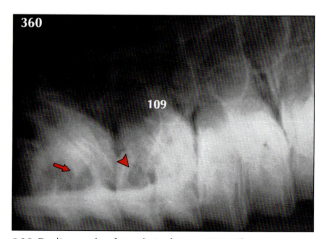

360 Radiograph of tooth in figure **359**. The arrow indicates stage III infundibular decay of 110. 109 also has infundibular disease (arrowhead).

The goal of treatment of infundibular disease is to arrest the decay process, to reduce the risk of sagittal fracture, and to restore the tooth to function. Since infundibular disease is a class I lesion, the use of posterior composite materials would be the appropriate restorative choice. This would correspond to a similar selection of materials used in brachydont teeth.

DECAYED OR FRACTURED TEETH

Fractured and decayed teeth require close examination orally and radiographically to determine the extent of damage to the tooth structure, vitality of the pulp, and health of the root apex. The lesions resulting from fracture or decay result in the gamut of other classes II through VI. In these lesions, the primary consideration is pulp protection.

Immature teeth are those under 7 years old. In such teeth the pulp is large and the apex is wide. The pulp of immature teeth may withstand inflammation without suffering necrosis. Older teeth with limited blood supply may be more likely to suffer necrosis if exposed by fracture. Pulp exposures, both direct and indirect, are addressed according to endodontic principles.

Goals for restoration of fractured or decayed teeth are the same as previously described. Therapeutic procedures are also the same. The important difference is that protection of the pulp is of critical importance in teeth suffering recent fracture. Restoration to mastication function is secondary to preservation and protection of a vital pulp. In many cases it is advisable to delay restoration until pulp exposure is resolved. In other cases the difficulty of exposure and access to the fracture site precludes complete restoration anyway. In such situations treatment procedures for the purpose of pulp protection are sufficient and appropriate.

The decision to pursue restoration to mastication function depends on access and character of the exposed dentin. If diseased dentin can be debrided and substantial tooth remains, full restoration can be performed.

Follow-up evaluation of the restoration should be performed within 4–6 weeks. Radiographic evaluation of the pulp should be done after 3–6 months.

ENAMEL HYPOPLASIA

Defects in enamel formation occur in embryological amelogenesis. They result from either death of ameloblasts or incomplete mineralization of enamel matrix.[27] Exposure of the enamel defect to the oral cavity can result in a decay process that can involve much underlying dental structure. Figure **362** displays a typical appearance of the condition. Radiographs are necessary to determine size of the defect and proximity to the pulp. Complete debridement will frequently result in a large cavity. These class V defects can be restored with composite materials. When the defect is close to the pulp, GICs should be used as a base material to protect the pulp. When the prepared cavity has a markedly uneven surface, a flowable composite can be used as a base preparation. Both materials should be covered with a hybrid composite material.

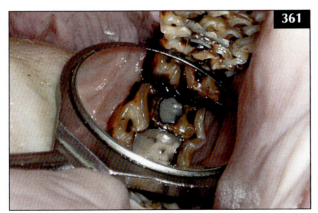

361 Annual follow-up examination reveals normal wear rate of the composite material and normal function of the tooth. Peripheral decay of secondary caries is present.

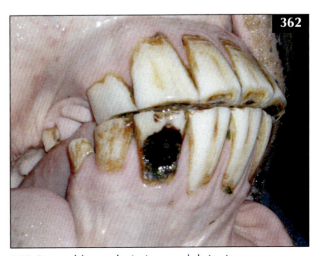

362 Enamel hypoplasia in an adult incisor.

PROCEDURES FOR PLACEMENT OF COMPOSITE RESTORATIVE MATERIALS

Composite resin is the most commonly used material for direct placement restorations. It is bonded to the tooth with dental adhesive. The dental adhesive bonds to both enamel and dentin. Bond strength to cementum is unknown. Support of the restoration is either by chemical or mechanical retention. The technique of application of the resin utilizes the same protocol as in other species. Instrumentation used is shown in figure **363**. A spatula is used to place the material in the debrided cavity. The plugger/condenser is used to tap the composite material into the uneven topography of the cavity. Various sizes are available to fit large and small cavities. The material is spread into approximately 2 mm thick layers. After filling the cavity to the occlusal surface the burnisher is used to smooth the surface before light curing.

There are several steps used in composite placement in restorative procedures. They are described in the following steps and demonstrated in figures **364–372**.

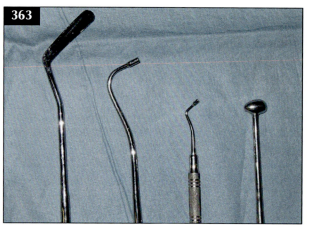

363 Restorative placement and manipulation instruments are shown. The composite material is placed with the spatula on the left. The two plugger/condensers in the center are used to pack the material in place. The burnisher on the right is used to smooth the final surface before light curing.

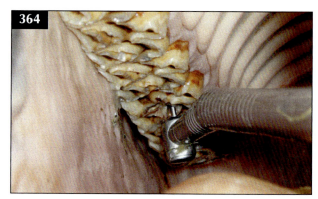

364 The diseased cavity is debrided. The depth of potential debridement is limited by the length of the surgical length No. 8 round bur.

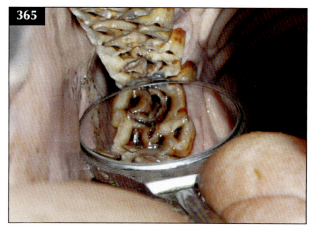

365 The extent of debridement is shown. The bur length limits debridement of the apically oriented infundibulum. In all cases the cavity is debrided as much as possible.

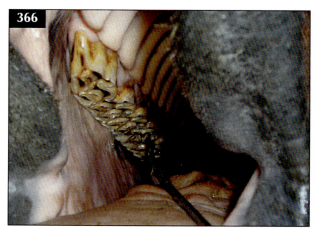

366 The prepared cavity is rinsed and dried with an air water syringe.

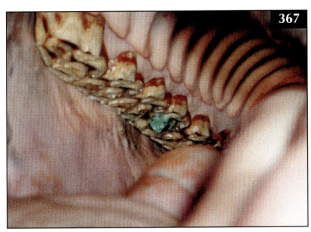

367 Etchant is applied to prepare the cavity surface for bonding.

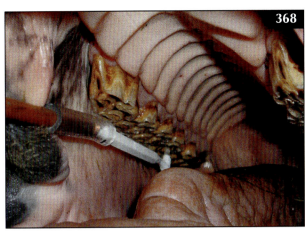

368 After rinsing etchant, the dentin bonding agent is applied.

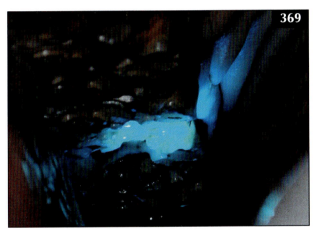

369 The bonding agent is light cured.

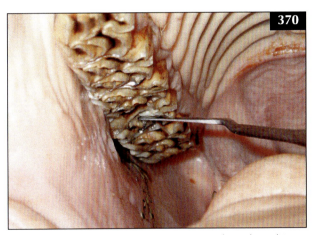

370 The composite restorative material is placed in the cavity with the spatula.

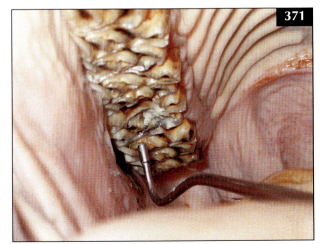

371 The material is 'tapped' into place and spread with the plugger/condenser into layers 2 mm thick.

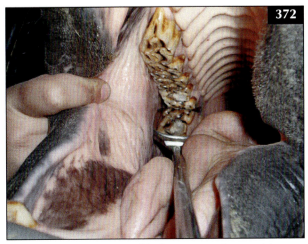

372 After placement and light curing of several layers, the composite material is smoothed and light cured. A final layer of sealant is applied and light cured.

1. Clean debris from infundibulum or disease site with hand instruments or air abrasion.
2. Debride decay with No. 8 round or No. 702 SL bur on high-speed handpiece.
3. Etch with 37% phosphoric acid according to manufacturer's directions.
4. Rinse the cavity for 30 s and air dry to a 'frosty' appearance. Do not dessicate.
5. Apply a layer of dentin bonding agent/adhesive to cover the walls of the cavity. Air dry.
6. Light cure according to manufacturer's specifications.
7. Fill cavity with composite material in layers as in manufacturer's directions. Some allow up to 40 mm per layer.
8. Pack or 'tap' the composite material into the uneven depressions of the cavity with a plugger/condenser.
9. Light cure each layer.
10. In some cases a flowable composite material can be used to fill the small crevices of the cavity, or a glass ionomer can be used as a base or liner.
11. Smooth the final layer with a burnisher.
12. Apply a sealing layer of bonding agent.
13. Light cure the final layer.
14. Check the occlusal surface for marginal seal with dental explorer.

In treatment of diseased infundibula, thorough debridement of the affected area is important. In many cases the volume of decayed tooth material is much greater than clinically evident on initial examination. Thorough debridement assists in creation of a strong bond between the tooth and restorative material. The result is maximum strength and ability of the restored tooth to withstand mastication forces.

An additional procedure that assists in retention of the composite material is the use of an undercut in the margin of the cavity. Use of an inverted cone-shaped bur such as a No. 35 or No. 37 creates a groove under the border of the cavity preparation. The material placed in this groove results in a strong mechanical bond.

In treatment of all diseased teeth it is important to evaluate radiographically the proximity of the pulp to the tooth preparation. While it is unusual to be in close proximity, protection of the pulp with a glass ionomer may be indicated.

SUMMARY

Indications for restoring equine teeth are:
- Protection of vital pulp.
- Restoring mastication function.
- Arresting decay.
- Prevention of further disease, such as sagittal fracture of cheek teeth.

Infundibular disease should be assessed for the stage of the decay process and treated accordingly. Restoration is not indicated for all infundibular disease.

Filling stage I disease does not prevent progression to stage II. It is recommended for stage II and stage III infundibular decay, but not for stage I.

Fractured teeth require close oral examination, including radiographs. Pulp health should be monitored. Complete debridement and pulp protection should be achieved in all cases for elimination of pain and prevention of further disease.

REFERENCES

1. Wiggs RB, Lobprise HB. *Veterinary Dentistry: Principles and Practice*. Philadelphia: Lippincott-Raven, 1997; p. 353.
2. Soderholm KJ. Chemistry of synthetic resins. In: Anusavice KJ (ed) *Phillip's Science of Dental Materials*, 10th edition. Philadelphia: WB Saunders, 1996; p. 232.
3. Powers JM. Composite restorative materials. In: Craig RG, Powers JM (eds) *Restorative Dental Materials*, 11th edition. St. Louis: Mosby, 2002; pp. 232–257.
4. Fortin D, Vargas MA. The spectrum of composites: new techniques and materials. *Journal of the American Dental Association* 2000: **131**; 26S–30S.
5. Tyas MJ, Burrow MF. Adhesive restorative materials: a review. *Australian Dental Journal* 2004: **49**(3); 112–121.
6. Yoshida Y, Van Meerbank B, Nakayama Y. Evidence of chemical bonding at biomaterial-hard tissue interfaces. *Journal of Dental Research* 2000: **79**; 709–714.
7. Six N, Lasfargues JJ, Goldberg M. *In vivo* study of the pulp reaction to Fuji IX, a glass ionomer cement. *Journal of Dentistry* 2000: **28**(6); 413–422.

8. Shimada Y, Sasafuchi Y, Arakawa M, *et al.* Biocompatibility of a flowable composite bonded with a self-etching adhesive compared with a glass ionomer cement and a high copper amalgam. *Operative Dentistry* 2004: **29**(1); 23–28.

9. Stanislawski L, Daniau X, Lautie A, Goldberg M. Factors responsible for pulp cell cytotoxicity induced by resin-modified glass ionomer cements. *Journal of Biomedical Materials Research: Applied Biomaterials* 1999: **48**(3); 277–288.

10. DuPont G. The bonded composite restoration. *Proceedings 15th Annual Veterinary Dental Forum* 2001; pp. 57–60.

11. Brannan RD. Dental materials in veterinary dentistry. In: Baker GJ, Easley J (eds) *Equine Dentistry.* London: Elsevier Saunders, 2005; 303–312.

12. Kugel G, Ferrari M. The science of bonding: From first to sixth generation. *Journal of the American Dental Association* 2000: **131**; 20S–25S.

13. Farah JW, Powers JM. Self-etching bonding agents. *The Dental Advisor* 2003: **20**(8); 1–2.

14. Ten Cate JM, van Duinen RN. Hypermineralization of dentinal lesions adjacent to glass-ionomer cement restorations. *Journal of Dental Research* 1995: **74**; 1266–1271.

15. Swartz ML, Phillips W, Clark HE. Long-term F release from glass ionomer cements. *Journal of Dental Research* 1984: **63**(2); 158–160.

16. Randall RC, Wilson NH. Glass-ionomer restoratives: a systematic review of a secondary caries treatment effect. *Journal of Dental Research* 1999: **78**; 628–637.

17. Torneck CD. Dentin-pulp complex. In: Ten Cate AR (ed) *Oral Histology: Development, Structure and Function.* St. Louis: Mosby, 1998; 169–217.

18. Pascoe J. Oral cavity and salivary glands. In: Auer JA and Stick JA (eds) *Equine Surgery* 2nd edition. Philadelphia: WB Saunders, 1999; p. 191.

19. Dixon PM, Tremaine WH, Pickles K, *et al.* Equine dental disease. Part 4 A long-term study of 400 cases: apical infections of cheek teeth. *Equine Veterinary Journal* 2000: **32**(3); 182–194.

20. Dacre IT. Equine dental pathology. In: Baker GJ, Easley J (eds) *Equine Dentistry.* London: Elsevier Saunders, 2005; 91–110.

21. Bryant JD, Froelich PN, Showers WJ, Genna BJ. A tale of the quarries: biologic and taphonomic signatures in the oxygen isotope composition of tooth enamel phosphate from modern and Miocene equids. *Palios* 1996: **11**; 397–408.

22. Hoppe KA, Stover SM, Pascoe JR, Amundson R. Tooth enamel biomineralization in extant horses: implications for isotopic microsampling. *Paleogeography, Paleoclimatology, Paleoecology* 2004: **206**; 355–365.

23. Honma K, Yamakawa M, Yamauchi S, Hosoya S. Statistical study on the occurrence of dental caries of domestic animals. *Japanese Journal of Veterinary Research* 1962: **10**(31); 31–37.

24. Baker GJ. Some aspects of equine dental disease. *Equine Veterinary Journal* 1970: **2**; 105–110.

25. Colyer F. Abnormal conditions of the teeth of animals in their relationship to similar conditions in man. *The Dental Board of the United Kingdom* 1931; 36–38.

26. Merrillat LA. *Veterinary Surgery,* Volume 1. Chicago: Alexander Eger, 1906; p. 32.

27. Eisenmamm DR. Amelogenesis. In: Ten Cate AR (ed) *Oral Histology: Development, Structure and Function.* St. Louis: Mosby, 1998; 239–256.

PRINCIPLES OF PERIODONTAL DISEASE

David O Klugh   Chapter 16

Periodontal disease is pathology of the attachment apparatus which holds the tooth in the alveolar socket. When left undiagnosed and untreated, destruction of the periodontium results in tooth mobility and premature exfoliation. The disease most commonly affects aging patients. When affecting younger patients, the disease is usually concurrent with the processes of eruption of a permanent tooth and exfoliation of a deciduous tooth. Pain is significant whether one or several teeth are affected. Mastication is inefficient in patients with loose, painful teeth due to both the instability of the affected tooth or teeth and the pain caused by the destruction of attachment. Many patients with periodontal disease have bitting or behavioral problems. Periodontal disease has detrimental effects on the overall health, condition, and performance of the horse. *Table 13* summarizes the incidence of periodontal disease.

Multiple factors influence the etiology and pathogenesis of periodontal disease including eruption physiology, mastication biomechanics, orthodontic forces, bacterial involvement, and host defense mechanisms. Consideration of the principles of anatomy, physiology, etiology, pathogenesis, clinical examination, and treatment of periodontal disease in horses leads to proper recognition of disease and early intervention. The gold standard of all medicine, including periodontal disease, is prevention.

TERMINOLOGY, ANATOMY, AND UNIQUE CHARACTERISTICS OF THE EQUINE PERIODONTIUM

The periodontium consists of gingiva, PDL, cementum, and alveolar bone. *Periodontal disease* is a general term referring to the altered state of the periodontium. It includes both the active and resting states of the disease process. *Periodontitis* refers to the active state of disease with inflammation of the periodontium. *Gingivitis* refers to inflammation of the gingiva only.

Gingiva is that part of the oral soft tissue that is tightly adherent to the crowns of unerupted teeth and encircling those that have erupted.[4] *Mucosa* is the

Table 13 The incidence of periodontal disease

Date	Author	Age of subjects	Number affected	Total (%)
1905	Colyer[1]	All ages	166 of 484	34
1937	Voss[2]	All ages	213 of 647	34
1937	Voss[2]	13 and older	87 of 142	61
1970	Baker[3]	15 and older	218 heads of all ages were evaluated	60

thin, slightly mobile, fragile part of the oral soft tissue that is continuous with the mucous membranes of the cheek, lips, and floor of the mouth.[5] The two tissues meet at the *mucogingival junction.* These structures are demonstrated in figure **373**.

The anatomy of the gingiva can be further divided by location. *Marginal gingiva* is the unattached terminal edge of the gingiva that surrounds the tooth in a collar-like fashion. The *gingival sulcus* is the shallow space around the tooth bounded by the tooth on one side and the gingiva on the other. *Attached gingiva* is continuous with marginal gingiva. It is tightly bound to the underlying periosteum and alveolar bone and extends to the loose alveolar mucosa at the mucogingival junction. The interproximal space is occupied by the *interdental gingiva* or *interdental papilla.* Figure **374** demonstrates the relationship between the tooth and the gingiva.

Equine periodontal anatomy exhibits unique characteristics. The interproximal space is very large, making the interdental papilla significantly wider bucco-lingually than in brachydont teeth of man and small animals. The close contact between adjacent teeth makes this tissue very thin, and easily damaged by periodontal inflammation.

Equine teeth are known as radicular hypsodont teeth. This means that they are continuously erupting teeth with roots that elongate as the tooth erupts. Brachydont teeth erupt to the point of occlusion and stop.

Hypsodont equine teeth have no cementoenamel junction. In brachydont teeth, the cementoenamel junction is the general area of attachment of the gingiva. Gingival recession is measured from that point. Since this anatomical landmark does not exist in horses, gingival recession is estimated by comparison with the gingival height of adjacent teeth.

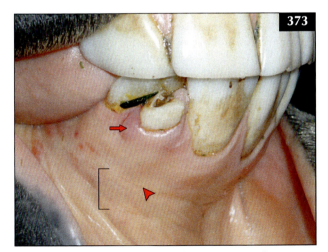

373 The gingiva, mucosa, and mucogingival junction are identified. The arrow indicates inflamed gingiva surrounding retained deciduous 803. Bracket indicates mucosa. The arrowhead indicates the fold marking the mucogingival junction.

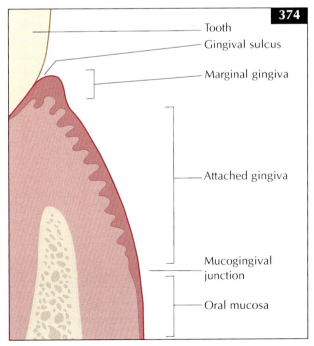

374 The various divisions of the gingiva are identified. (Copyright © 2002. WB Saunders Company[16].)

The hypsodont equine tooth is completely enveloped by cementum at eruption. The occlusal surface is covered by cementum until occlusal attrition exposes a normal mastication surface of enamel, dentin, and cementum. Brachydont teeth have no cementum on the crown. In these teeth, cementum is present only as part of the attachment apparatus of the root. Equine teeth also have cementum as part of the attachment apparatus.

Histologically, the gingival epithelium is divided by anatomical location (**375**). The outer epithelium covers the crest of the gingival margin and the oral surface of the marginal and attached gingiva. Sulcular epithelium lines the gingival sulcus. Junctional epithelium consists of a band of cells that surround the tooth at the bottom of the gingival sulcus. These cells are closely adherent to the tooth. Regeneration of cells from basal layers of the junctional epithelium proceeds coronally and centrifugally.[6] As dividing cells migrate, continuous attachment to the tooth is maintained by attachment to a basal lamina.[7] Aging cells are shed into the sulcus or directly into the oral cavity.

Equine gingival connective tissue consists of collagen fibers and ground substance, consisting of water, hyaluronic acid, chondroitin sulfate, and glycoproteins. Connective tissue fibers include collagen and oxytalan.

Cells of the gingival connective tissue consist primarily of fibroblasts. A few leukocytes are present even in the absence of inflammation.[8] They reside in connective tissue surrounding the vasculature. The blood supply to the gingiva comes from arterioles that emerge from the alveolar crest in the interdental papilla, along with subperiosteal vessels[9] and some from the PDL.[10] Innervation of the gingiva is from branches of the greater palatine and infraorbital branches of the maxillary nerve for the upper arcades and mandibular nerve for the lower arcades. These are segments of the trigeminal nerve.[11]

The connective tissue of the PDL is continuous with that of the gingiva. The major fibers are called principal fibers.[12] Principal fiber bundles consist of a network of interconnected individual fibers that attach the tooth to the bone. These fibers terminate in the cementum as Sharpey's fibers. They are made of type 1 collagen which is synthesized by PDL fibroblasts. Principal fiber arrangement consists of large fascicles with multiple fiber bundles comprised of individual fibers.[13] Fascicles vary from less than 100 μm to greater than 200 μm in diameter.[13]

Mandibular principal fibers had a unique arrangement as compared to those of brachydont teeth in a study by Mitchell.[14] The buccal fiber arrangement is similar to that of brachydont teeth, with horizontal and oblique fibers extending from the cementum to the alveolar bone. The lingual fibers are arranged in a crosshatched or basketweave formation. The PDL is much thicker lingually than buccally. There are many more elastic fibers in the equine PDL than in the brachydont PDL. Trans-septal fibers connect cementum of proximal teeth. Figure **376a,b** demonstrates the arrangement of periodontal fibers.

Staszyk[13] looked at the structure and orientation of PDL principal fibers. The arrangement of fibers closely resembled the gingival and principal fiber array of brachydont teeth. Corresponding terminology is described in *Table 14*. Gingival fibers and

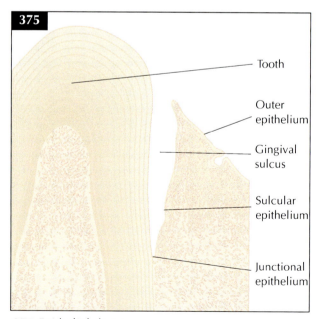

Tooth

Outer epithelium

Gingival sulcus

Sulcular epithelium

Junctional epithelium

375 Epithelial divisions.

376 The pattern of periodontal ligament fiber attachment in the equine mandibular tooth as described by Mitchell *et el.*[14]

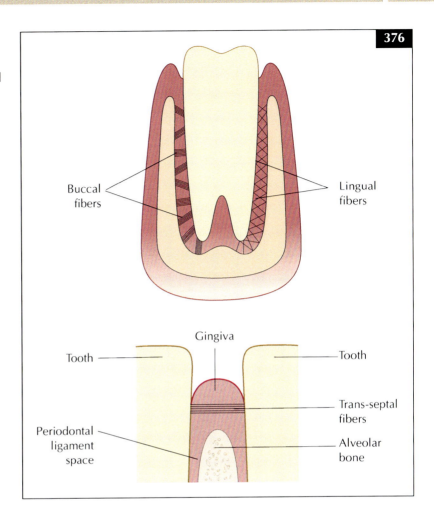

Buccal fibers

Lingual fibers

Gingiva

Tooth

Tooth

Trans-septal fibers

Periodontal ligament space

Alveolar bone

Table 14 Comparison of terminology of gingival fibers

Staszyk description[13]	Brachydont term
Cementogingival	Gingivodental group: cementum to gingiva
Cementogingival	Gingivodental group: cementum to outer surface of gingiva
Periostealgingival	None
Cementoperiosteal	Gingivodental group: cementum to periosteum
Alveolocemental	Principal fiber group: alveolar crest group
Cementoperiodontal	Circular group
Cementocemental	Circular group
Alveoloalveolar	Circular group
Periodontoperiodontal	Circular group
Gingivogingival	Circular group

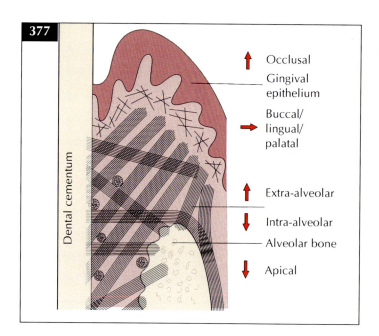

377 Fiber arrangement of gingival fibers. (From Staszyk *et el.*[13])

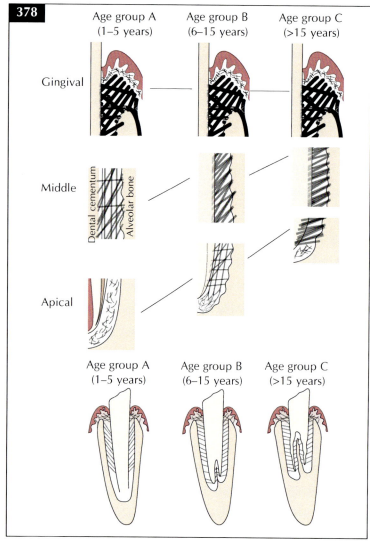

378 Principal fibers, showing age-related changes. Apical fibers are not organized in young horses 1–5 years of age. In horses over 15 years of age, fiber attachment includes the entire tooth, including the roots. (From Staszyk *et el.*[13])

principal fibers are shown in figures **377** and **378** respectively. The continuous eruption and multicingular suface anatomy of the hypsodont tooth creates the need for a more complex arrangement of principal fibers of the PDL. Brachydont principal groups of trans-septal, alveolar crest, horizontal, oblique, and apical fibers are present in hypsodont teeth, though their arrangement is generally more complex. Inter-radicular fibers were not described by Staszyk.[13]

The PDL contains numerous types of cells. The fibroblast is the predominant cell type. Other connective tissue cells include cementoblasts, cementocytes, and osteoblasts. The epithelial cell rests of Malassez are located close to the cementum. These epithelial cell rests are considered to be important in the differentiation of cementoblasts.[15] They are found throughout the length of the PDL, and are located near the cementum. Immune system cells are also present. The ground substance of the PDL has three main constituents: glycosaminoglycans, glycoproteins, and water.

Equine cementum has many unique features.[14] It covers the entire tooth at eruption. The cementum of maxillary cheek teeth is thicker buccally than palatally whereas the cementum of mandibular cheek teeth is thicker lingually than buccally. This difference in thickness coincides with thinner enamel in the same areas.

The matrix of equine cementum is composed of mineralized collagen fibers termed intrinsic and extrinsic fibers, together with living cells, viable blood vessels, and functional nerves. Classification of cementum can be based on the timing of its production. Primary cementum is produced first, with secondary next, and tertiary last. Primary cementum is the oldest cementum and is the most highly mineralized. Secondary cementum is somewhat less mineralized and tertiary cementum is least mineralized of all. Cementum can also be classified as peripheral or infundibular, based on its anatomical location.

A collagen fiber framework provides the foundation for mineralization of the cementum. Intrinsic fibers produced by cementoblasts are collagen fibers that provide an attachment framework for extrinsic fibers. Extrinsic fibers produced by fibroblasts are thicker collagen fibers that attach the cementum to the alveolar bone. They terminate as Sharpey's fibers.

Cells of the cementum include cementoblasts and cementocytes. Cementoblasts produce the collagen

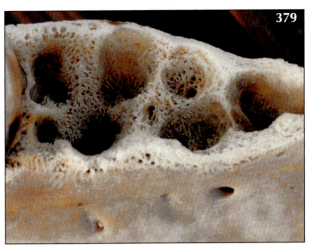

379 Alveolar bone of the mandible in an aged horse.

matrix of intrinsic fibers. As these cells transition to cementocytes, their function is to mineralize the matrix. Cementocytes are active cells when incorporated into the mineralized cementum. Viable blood vessels and functional nerves are also present within the mineralized cementum, making it a living tissue.

Primary cementum is thin and well mineralized. It completely envelopes the tooth and attaches to the enamel. Overlying primary cementum is a thicker layer of secondary cementum that is also cellular, and contains intrinsic and extrinsic fibers. Secondary cementum provides the attachment for the PDL to the alveolar crown. Tertiary cementum covers the gingival and clinical crown.[14] It is very thick and fills in the folds of the enamel. It attaches the gingival crown to the PDL.

The alveolar process is the portion of the mandible or maxilla that houses the tooth. It consists of: an external plate of cortical bone; an inner socket wall sometimes referred to as alveolar bone proper; and trabecular bone between the two. The alveolar bone proper is seen radiographically as the lamina dura and is sometimes also called the cribriform plate. It has many openings through which neurovascular bundles supply the PDL. Figure **379** shows alveolar bone of an aged patient's mandible.

PHYSIOLOGY OF THE PERIODONTIUM

The gingiva protects the tooth and underlying structures. Gingival fibers mechanically support the gingiva and hold it tightly against the tooth, deflecting food and debris away from the tooth and gingival sulcus. Gingiva is lined by epithelium, with the oral surface covered by the outer epithelium and the sulcular epithelium lining the gingival sulcus. Sulcular epithelium acts as a semi-permeable membrane through which fluids, inflammatory cells, and cell by-products can pass. The character of cells, fluids, and cell by-products varies in response to external stimulus. Bacteria and their by-products pass through the epithelium into the gingiva to cause an inflammatory reaction.

One of the protective mechanisms of the gingival epithelium is a rapid turnover rate. Regeneration of the thin lining of the gingiva maintains a mechanical barrier to outside insult.

Cementum is added to the gingival crown (that portion above the alveolar bone and surrounded by gingiva) during eruption in the form of tertiary cementum. It provides a smooth surface for oral soft tissue contact. It supports the enamel folds during mastication and fills around the teeth creating tight contact between cheek teeth.

Alveolar bone is a mixture of fibrous connective tissue, less dense bone, and bundle bone. Alveolar bone adapts to occlusal forces. Radiographically, the lamina dura becomes more dense as a result of these forces. An example is seen on the lower cheek teeth in figure **380**. These teeth are angled mesially. Compression or crushing forces of mastication tip these teeth mesially. Increased density of the lamina dura is observed on the mesial aspect of the alveolus. This increased density is a result of prolonged heavy forces delivered to that area causing the lamina dura to undergo sclerosis.

Table 15 Common oral flora (From Baker.[17])

High counts of:
- Streptococci
- Micrococci
- Starch hydrolyzers

Intermediate counts of:
- Anaerobes
- *Veillonella* spp.
- H_2S producers

Low counts of:
- *Lactobacillus* spp.
- *Fusobacterium* spp.
- Coliforms

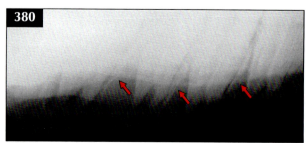

380 Arrows indicate sclerotic mesial alveolar bone.

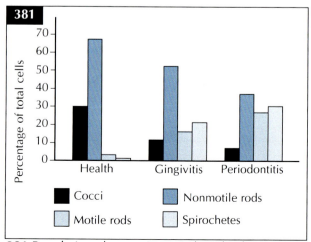

381 Population changes in periodontal infection.

PATHOPHYSIOLOGY OF THE PERIODONTIUM

The normal oral flora consists of populations of different bacteria. A shift in the populations of bacteria can start the pathological process leading to gingivitis and periodontitis.[16]

In the brachydont, the normal flora of Gram-positive cocci and rods colonize the surface of the tooth. Their populations are significantly higher than other bacteria such as Gram-negative anaerobic rods and spirochetes. In 1979 Baker characterized the species cultured from normal equine tooth surfaces (*Table 15*).[17]

The populations of bacteria shift as gingival inflammation progresses. The number of Gram-positive cocci and rods decreases and the population of Gram-negative aerobes and anaerobes increases (**381**). The increase in Gram-negative aerobes, anaerobes, and spirochetes occurs as attachment loss develops in the deeper tissues of the PDL.

All stages of periodontal disease are accompanied by mixed infections and most of the same bacteria are present in all stages. The pathological process is one of population change. The result is a sufficient number of pathogenic organisms to produce an inflammatory response and subsequent degradation of host tissues. The culture results in *Table 16* exemplify a clinical case of periodontal disease.

A pathophysiological response by the host occurs as a result of interactions between the host and invader. The host maintains significant defense mechanisms. The inflammatory exudate produced in the gingival sulcus or crevice is called gingival crevicular fluid (GCF). It contains leukocytes, antibodies, enzymes, and electrolytes. The volume of fluid produced increases with inflammation and mastication. The GCF functions to provide a medium for the immune system to respond to bacterial invasion, while flushing bacteria and desquamated epithelial cells.

Saliva provides significant assistance in the defense of the periodontium.[18] The glycoprotein content of saliva is both lubricating and protective. The salivary pellicle forms a barrier which protects against minor trauma and prevents adherence of bacteria to the tooth surface. The fluid consistency of saliva helps cleanse nonadherent bacteria and debris from the tooth surface.

Saliva's buffering action is beneficial in a number of ways. Secreted saliva maintains a specific pH in the oral cavity in which certain pathogenic bacteria cannot flourish. Acids produced by oral micro-organisms can damage oral tissues. Salivary bicarbonate, phosphate ions, and other chemicals prevent tissue damage by buffering these acids.

Saliva has a direct antibacterial effect. Lysozyme is a salivary enzyme that hydrolyzes bacterial cell walls. Lactoferrin in saliva binds free iron which is an essential element for many pathogenic bacteria. Antibodies, such as IgA, agglutinate bacteria which can then be flushed out of the oral cavity.

The host's immune system acts further to arrest the infectious process. Initially, the focus of the immune system is to overcome the infection. As the disease process progresses the immune response includes isolation of the infection to local tissues and protection of the rest of the body from spread of disease. The progression of response leads to rejection of the tooth. The progression from protection of the body to rejection of the tooth is an important part of the pathophysiology of periodontal disease that involves dynamics of the immune system as it responds to invasion. Understanding the dynamics of the immune response assists in diagnosis, implementation of treatment measures, and emphasizes the importance of prevention.

Table 16 Culture results from incisor periodontal disease

Bacillus spp.

Streptococcus spp.

Corynebacterium spp.

Bacteroides spp.

Fusobacterium spp.

Bacteria can have a number of effects on the host. Some act directly by causing tissue destruction, while others act indirectly by chemical stimulation of host defenses. Pathogenic bacteria cause direct tissue destruction by proteolytic enzymes and endotoxins.[19] Leucotoxins destroy host leukocytes. Some bacteria directly inhibit host tissue metabolism and cellular growth, further inhibiting host response.

Host polymorphonuclear cells are sensitized by bacterial exposure to produce proteinase enzymes such as collagenase, resulting in breakdown of the attachment apparatus and gingival support structure. Collagenase is also produced by macrophages and fibroblasts as inflammation progresses.

Further inflammation results from white blood cell production of interleukins and tumor necrosis factor. These cytokines act to induce production of more proteinases and stimulate osteoclastic bone loss.[20] White blood cell production of prostaglandins (PGs) (specifically PGE_2) also directly stimulates osteoclastic bone loss. PGE_2 is a major mediator of the immune system response. As the rejection process continues, fibroblastic phagocytosis of collagen further destroys tooth attachment.[21]

The initial clinical sign of the pathological process is gingivitis. This is recognized as edematous and reddened gingiva. Sulcular epithelium is inflamed and gingival collagen support is lost as inflammation progresses.

Periodontal pocket formation occurs as junctional epithelium proliferates apically in an attempt to maintain tooth contact while detachment occurs at the coronal margin.[22] Invasion of bacteria results in inflammation and thickening of sulcular epithelium. This tissue eventually becomes necrotic. If uninterrupted, the vicious cycle continues until the tooth is exfoliated.

Equine dental anatomy is unique in that the cementum of the clinical and reserve crown is involved in the periodontal disease. Supragingival and subgingival cementum become necrotic and destroyed. Cemental disease can extend interproximally or apically.

In animals with brachydont teeth, change in oral flora is coincident with the accumulation of plaque and calculus. While plaque and calculus are seen in equine teeth they rarely lead to attachment loss. In most cases of equine periodontal disease no calculus or plaque is present. The triggering event in horses is stasis of feed material and its resulting decomposition.[1,23,24] Feed stasis and putrefaction result from several factors.

These include alteration of normal range of motion of mastication, direct gingival abrasion, and orthodontic tooth movement by malocclusion.

Protuberant crowns alter the normal range of motion of mastication by causing dental interlock (occlusal interference). The normal diagonal movement of the mandible is blocked by overlong teeth. The mandible is forced to move directly medially and crushing forces are increased. The result is packing of feed into gingival depressions in the normal topography of the periodontium.

An important concept associated with decreased range of motion of mastication is that of orthodontic tooth movement. There are two aspects to this principle. The first is the creation of abnormal forces. For example, it is well recognized that rostral hooks on upper second premolars (106 and 206 in the Triadan system) cause these teeth to move in a mesial direction by forces of mastication. This movement results in widened interproximal spaces where feed material can accumulate and decompose. Reduction of this malocclusion often results in closure of the interproximal space. This type of orthodontic movement can be seen in other teeth as well.

The second orthodontic principle related to decreased range of motion of mastication is reduction of normal forces. As a horse ages, the teeth drift mesially in the arcade. The mechanism may involve elastic trans-septal fibers keeping the teeth in close contact. The eruptive process and compressive angulation of the teeth also help maintain a tight-fitting dental battery which drifts mesially over time.

The same forces that result in abnormal orthodontic movement can also limit normal mesial drift of the teeth as the patient ages. Interproximal spaces are created as elongated crowns limit mesial drift in some teeth and not in others. The resulting increased interproximal space involves a recession of the interdental papilla which compromises the elastic trans-septal fibers. Older teeth have less reserve crown and less eruptive potential because eruption rates slow with age. Since the periodontal mechanism for resolving the increased interproximal space is compromised by reduction in function, the abnormally positioned geriatric tooth has very limited ability to correct itself.

Moisture content plays an important role in limiting stasis and putrefaction as a result of alteration of mandibular motion in mastication. When feedstuffs are moist and soft, such as in lush pasture, a wider range of mandibular motion is employed.[25] This wide range of motion creates a large amount of soft tissue contact, and increases GCF flow and salivary production. The soft tissue contact, coupled with saliva, mechanically cleanses the teeth and prevents feed stasis.

Horses secrete up to 50 mL/min of saliva from the parotid salivary gland. Salivary flow is stimulated by mastication. Without mastication, salivary flow is limited to that amount needed to maintain a moist intraoral environment. Horses in free-range situations have been shown to feed for about 14 hours per day. By calculation only, not by direct measurement, that would mean horses could create over 40 L of saliva per day when feeding on grass from one gland alone. The benefits of saliva are lubrication, barrier formation, mechanical cleansing, acid buffering, delivery of antibodies, and direct antibacterial activity. The benefits of GCF are leukocyte and antibody delivery. They are important in prevention of gingivitis and periodontal disease.

When horses consume drier and harder feeds such as hay and grain, all the above parameters change in favor of the development of periodontal disease. Range of motion is reduced; teeth become protuberant; feed stasis occurs followed by decomposition, and the cascade is set in motion. The saliva that is produced is absorbed by the dry feed to some degree, thus reducing its effectiveness. Since the time of feeding is reduced, the total daily saliva and GCF production is dramatically reduced. The net result is a much greater time for static feed material to break down. Reduced soft tissue contact and reduced range of motion leads to, putrefaction of feed material, thus creating the environment in which periodontal disease can flourish.

EXAMINATION

All parts of the periodontium must be examined for accurate determination of attachment loss. This includes characterization and measurement of the gingiva, cementum, alveolar bone, and PDL.

Oral examination begins with removal of feed debris. The tooth and periodontium are examined for gingival inflammation, ulceration, and recession, condition of sulcular epithelium, pocket depth and mesial/distal length, condition of the cementum, and tooth mobility. Pocket depth and length are measured with a periodontal probe. Decayed cementum is black and pitted. When decay is severe, cementum may be destroyed leaving enamel on the tooth surface. These measurements are charted. The conclusion of the examination is determination of attachment loss and staging of disease.

Since periodontal disease is defined by attachment loss, determination of the degree of advancement of the disease is critical in treatment and prognosis. When attachment loss cannot be fully characterized clinically, it must be determined radiographically. Radiographic evaluation of periodontal disease is adapted from techniques for intraoral radiography used in brachydont species. A technique for intraoral radiography in equine patients has been developed.[26] Follow-up radiographic evaluation of ongoing disease provides valuable information about treatment strategies.

Guidelines for assessment of percentage of attachment loss have been determined for use in small animals. The author uses the Veterinary Periodontal Disease Index adapted for equine anatomy (*Table 17*).[27]

Table 17 Stages of periodontal disease

0	**Normal:** No attachment loss. Probing depth <5 mm
1	**Gingivitis:** No attachment loss. Probing depth <5 mm
2	**Early periodontal disease:** <25% attachment loss and/or crestal bone loss around teeth
3	**Moderate periodontal disease:** 25–50% attachment loss or bone loss <50% around tooth root(s)
4	**Advanced periodontal disease:** >50% attachment loss or bone loss >50% around tooth root(s)

The pathological endpoint of periodontal disease is exfoliation. The reason for intervention is prevention of this eventuality. Affected teeth gradually become loose when the degree of attachment loss can no longer withstand mastication forces. Grades of mobility of teeth can be measured. *Table 18* is adapted from the Tooth Mobility Index[27] used in small animals, and is used in reference to cheek teeth. Tooth movement is measured at the occlusal surface.

The chart in figure **382** can be used to record findings related to periodontal disease.

STAGING PERIODONTAL DISEASE
Normal periodontium: stage 0
The normal status of the periodontium is characterized clinically by pink gingiva which adheres tightly to the tooth and conforms closely to the topography of the dental arcade. The gingiva has a moist, smooth surface as in figure **383**. The depth of the gingival sulcus is 5 mm or less.

Gingivitis: stage 1
Stage 1 periodontal disease is characterized by gingivitis. On examination the gingiva in figure **384** is swollen and reddened. The gingival sulcus is normal depth, but may bleed on probing. No attachment loss is present. In this stage, the cementum may be normal or may be decayed. Any cemental disease remains supragingival.

Early periodontal disease: stage 2
Periodontal disease is recognized by the presence of feed material in depressions of the periodontal topography as shown in figure **385**. All further progression of disease presents with feed debris packed in a pocket. Characterization of the stage of disease requires removal of debris and close examination with a mirror and periodontal probe.

Stage 2 periodontal disease is characterized by the presence of attachment loss involving up to 25% of the periodontium. The supragingival cementum and gingiva are examined. Subgingival cementum and sulcular epithelium are evaluated. The pocket is measured.

Table 18 Tooth Mobility Index modified for equine dentistry

0	None	Normal
1	Slight	Represents the first distinguishable sign of movement greater than normal
2	Moderate	Movement of up to approximately 3 mm (1 mm in man)
3	Severe	Movement >3 mm in any direction and/or is depressible

---

382

Patient _____ Age _____ Sex _____ Breed _____ Owner _____

Previous history of dental care: _____

Location of peridontal disease: _____

Tooth Mobility:

    M:0 No movement

    M:1 First signs of movement

    M:2 Movement of up to 3 mm at the occlusal surface

    M:3 Movement of 3 mm or more at the occlusal surface

Cementum:

Supragingival:	Normal	Stained	Decayed
Subgingival:	Normal	Stained	Decayed
Gingiva:	Normal	Recessed	Inflamed Ulcerated
Sulcular epithelium:	Normal	Inflamed	Necrotic

Pocket length: _____ mm

Pocket depth: _____ mm

Radiographs: Yes/No

Findings:

_____

_____

_____

Stage of disease related to percentage of attachment loss:

Stage 0: 0%

Stage 1: 0%

Stage 2: Up to 25%

Stage 3: 25%–50%

Stage 4: Over 50%

382 Examination chart for periodontal disease.

Probing depth is greater than 5 mm. The gingiva has receded and is ulcerated (**386**). Supragingival cementum is decayed. Sulcular epithelium suffers disease varying from mild inflammation to necrosis. Subgingival cementum is decayed. Tooth mobility is slight when present, or stage 0 or 1.

When determining percentage of attachment loss, the age of the patient is considered. A 5–10 mm deep pocket in a young horse with several centimeters of reserve crown translates to attachment loss of less than 25%. A pocket of the same depth in a 28-year-old patient with less than 2 cm of reserve crown has a higher percentage of attachment loss. In such cases, radiographic evaluation of the periodontium is the only method of determining percentage of attachment loss. Figure **387** shows a young patient with no bone loss.

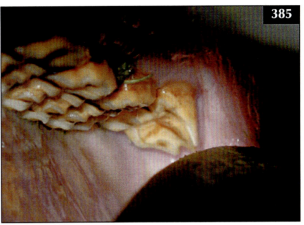

385 Typical periodontal pocket with debris.

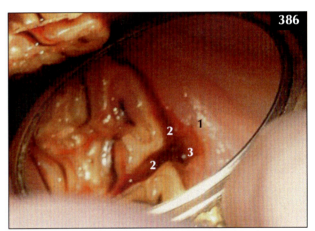

386 Ulcerated, recessed gingiva (1), decayed supragingival and subgingival cementum (2), and inflamed sulcular epithelium (3). Probing depth is 5–10 mm. Tooth mobility is 0.

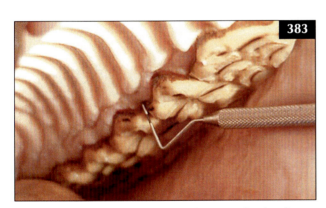

383 Normal gingiva with normal 5 mm depth of gingival sulcus.

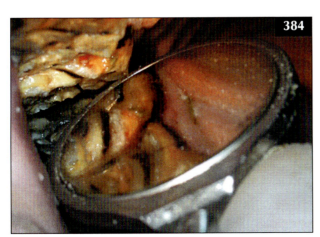

384 Swollen and reddened gingiva of stage 1 periodontal disease.

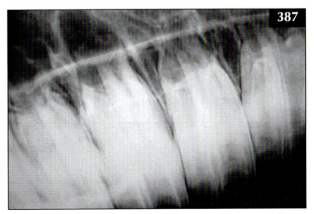

387 Radiograph of patient in figure **386**. Crestal bone height, lamina dura, and PDL space are normal. Conclusion is <25% attachment loss and stage 2 periodontal disease.

Radiographs must be interpreted together with clinical findings, since radiographs provide a two-dimensional view of the tooth and periodontium. The clinical examination determines the three-dimensional shape of the pocket and aids in interpretation of radiographic findings.

Moderate periodontal disease: stage 3

Further attachment loss requires more detailed examination. The importance of detailed clinical evaluation is in implementation of correct treatment measures, accurate prognosis of the disease, and for the purpose of monitoring disease on follow-up examination. On initial presentation, the pockets in stage 3 periodontal disease appear similar to those in stage 2. The clinical examination findings of the gingiva, cementum, and sulcular epithelium are also similar to those of stage 2 (**388**). The probing depth is deeper, and sometimes exceeds the length of the probe. These cases require radiographic characterization of attachment loss (**389**).

Severe periodontal disease: stage 4

Immediately prior to the end stage of periodontal disease, or exfoliation, the extent of disease is widespread and severe. Clinical examination reveals severe gingival disease including recession, ulceration, and edema (**390**). Cementum is decayed supragingivally and subgingivally. Sulcular epithelium is necrotic and a purulent discharge may be present.

Tooth mobility is stage 2 or 3. Radiographic changes demonstrate of loss of alveolar bone, blunting of apices, and lytic changes in subgingival crown and roots (**391**).

TREATMENT STRATEGIES

In order of importance, treatment strategies for stages 0 to 3 include:
1. Occlusal equilibration.
2. Pocket debridement.
3. Perioceutic therapy.

Occlusal equilibration is the first step in treatment of mild to moderate periodontal disease. When disease is identified, the opposite arcade is examined for an overlong tooth located in a position opposite the periodontal disease, causing accumulation of debris or orthodontic movement of the affected tooth. Reduction of the overlong tooth is necessary in all cases of periodontal disease. Many cases of stage 1 and stage 2 periodontal disease are quickly resolved by reducing overlong occlusal surfaces.

After correcting abnormal occlusal surfaces, removing debris from the periodontal pocket, and characterizing the periodontium clinically and radiographically, further treatment measures are instituted. In management of any infected wound, debridement is one of the most important parts

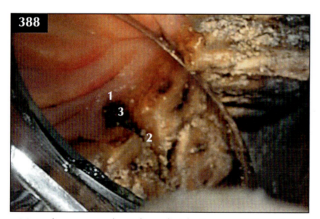

388 A deep periodontal pocket between 208 and 209 with gingival inflammation (1), edema, and recession. Cementum (2) is decayed supragingivally and subgingivally. Sulcular epithelium (3) is necrotic. Tooth mobility is 0 for 208 and stage 2 (<3 mm of movement at the occlusal surface) for 209.

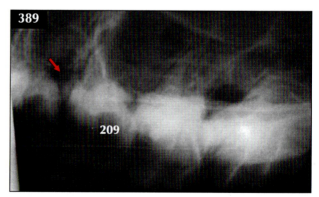

389 Radiograph of the patient in figure **388**. The arrow indicates location of pocket. The radiograph indicates loss of crestal bone, sclerosis of alveolus of mesial 209, and roughened surfaces of lamina dura and tooth reserve crown. All findings are consistent with 25–50% attachment loss and stage 3 periodontal disease affecting 209.

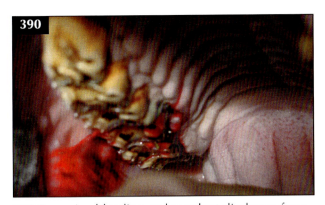

390 Excessive bleeding and purulent discharge from severe periodontal disease affecting 109. Bleeding and purulent discharge resulted from tooth manipulation by molar forceps in determination of tooth mobility. This tooth is stage 3 in the Tooth Mobility Index.

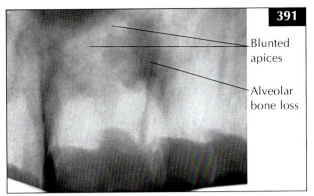

391 Radiograph of the patient in figure **390** with severe loss of alveolar bone, blunted apices, lytic areas of reserve crown and roots, and loss of PDL space. There is >50% attachment loss, or stage 4 periodontal disease.

of treatment. The same is true of treatment of periodontal disease. Diseased epithelium and underlying connective tissue of the periodontal pocket are removed by scraping the lining of the pocket to remove all purple and black necrotic debris. When sufficient diseased tissue has been removed, the remaining healthy gingiva and PDL will bleed. Instruments used for debridement include a sickle scaler (or excavator) or a high-speed handpiece and a bur. High-pressure hydrotherapy and air abrasion can be used for cleaning and debriding the pocket.

Debridement of necrotic cementum prevents extension of the decay process in an apical and peripheral direction, thus arresting the condition. A high-speed handpiece and bur are used for cemental debridement.

Stage 1 mobile teeth are commonly encountered in geriatric patients. Aging causes reduced PDL fiber collagen and ground substance and results in reduced reserve crown length. These factors combine to result in slight mobility of most geriatric teeth. These teeth are stage 1 in the Tooth Mobility Index. They usually require only removal of sharp enamel points that may abrade oral soft tissues. The use of rotary instrumentation minimizes trauma to the remaining crown and PDL. Care should be taken not to further loosen or extract those teeth with high-impact hand or power dental instruments.

Stage 2 mobile teeth are treated by reducing the opposing tooth such that the pair is not in occlusion. By resting the mobile tooth from the forces of mastication, the inflammation of the damaged PDL resolves. Teeth treated in such a manner are rechecked at 6–12 month intervals, and are found to be less mobile. Most are stage 1 and a few are stage 0 at re-examination.

Stage 3 mobile teeth are extracted. By definition these teeth have at least 3 mm of mobility at the occlusal surface. As the degree of tooth mobility increases, more periodontal attachment is lost. Most of these teeth fall into grade 4 in the Periodontal Disease Index, representing at least 50% loss of attachment. These teeth will not re-establish attachment if treated like stage 2 mobile teeth, and will remain painful if left in place.

Many of these teeth can be extracted digitally. However, since there is pain associated with manipulation of these teeth, regional anesthesia is indicated. After the affected tooth is anesthetized, the remaining gingiva is separated from the cementum with a periosteal or gingival elevator. Molar spreaders are used to break down further the mesial and distal PDL. Molar forceps are used to rock the tooth and break down the PDL in the bucco-lingual direction. When sufficiently loose, the tooth is removed from the alveolar socket with molar forceps and a fulcrum. Postoperative radiographs help determine the presence of any root fragments and characterize the alveolar bone. The alveolus is debrided of necrotic PDL and bone. Care must be taken in debriding maxillary alveoli. The maxillary plate is very thin in areas subjacent to the maxillary sinus and can be easily penetrated by forceps or debriding instruments.

The debrided alveolar socket may be patched if necessary. Patching materials include vinyl polysiloxane impression materials and acrylics. The patch must be removed approximately 2–4 weeks postoperatively. Many of these patches will fall out as a result of normal mastication forces. Some alveoli are too shallow for retention of a patch. This is especially true of geriatric patients. Acrylic patches can become a foreign body and cause signs similar to those of the original abscessed tooth if improperly applied or left in place too long. It is important to make an appointment to remove any material used to patch the socket.

The use of perioceutic agents should also be considered. They are secondary in importance to occlusal equilibration and wound debridement. Many perioceutic agents have benefits in addition to antibacterial therapy. Products with citric acid demineralize cementum, thereby exposing cementum collagen and promoting formation of new attachment. Doxycycline inhibits collagen breakdown by the enzyme collagenase which is elaborated from bacteria and polymorphoneuclear cells during the inflammatory process.[28] Ascorbic acid aids in collagen formation. Zinc has antibacterial effects.[29] Chlorhexidine has antimicrobial effects that continue for several hours after oral rinse due to its absorption by oral epithelial cells. Products that contain this disinfectant are very effective in treating periodontal disease. A product containing doxycycline is available

in a soft gel form that is placed in the periodontal pocket. The antibiotic is released over time for continuous treatment of the infected tissue for up to 2 weeks. Shallow pockets frequently fail to retain the product, thus deeper pockets are more amenable to this treatment.

Treatment by enlargement of interproximal spaces is useful in specific cases. In aging patients with triangular-shaped interproximal spaces or the so-called 'valve diastema', removal of a small part of the crown assists in improved flow of feed and reduces decay.[30] Caution must be exercised in all patients with this condition. Young patients have a pulp in close proximity to the occlusal or interproximal surface, while aging patients have pulps that have reduced capability of response to insult. In cases with enlarged interproximal spaces ('diastema' not of the 'valve' type) the procedure of enlargement or increasing the width of the interproximal space may result in further feed accumulation which will prevent physiological closure of the enlarged space. The use of this procedure must be carefully evaluated in all cases.

An alternative treatment for enlarged interproximal spaces in patients of all ages involves the use of polymethylmethacrylate. The spaces are debrided of necrotic material including the cementum. Hand instruments and high-speed burs are used. The 'diastema bur' can effectively debride cementum. The goal is to debride as much necrotic tissue as possible.

After debridement, the space is filled with polymethylmethacrylate (**392**). The material is mixed

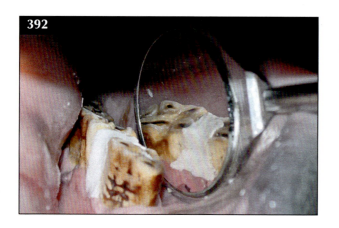

392

392 Interproximal placement of polymethylmethacrylate prevents feed accumulation while protecting underlying tissue, thereby assisting in healing of the periodontium.

according to manufacturer's directions. When it begins to react, it forms a surface layer or 'skin'. With moistened gloved hands, this material can easily be placed and manipulated into proper position. Digital pressure forces the material between teeth and into the periodontal pocket. Further manipulation of the material to extend lingually and buccally around a portion of each tooth assists in retention of the patch. Moisture does not inhibit curing of the material. The elevated temperature of exothermic curing is safe for the oral environment.

The polymethylmethacrylate is placed for the purpose of occupying space. In young horses, growth and normal mesial drift help close the space. In aging patients, the space may never close. When these problems are encountered, the condition must be characterized as previously described. If polymethylmethacrylate is used, it can be replaced as needed.

Limitations include inability to debride the periodontium completely due to limited instrument length and difficult access. In such cases, the patch prevents further accumulation of feed material and the pocket undergoes physiological debridement. Granulation tissue and epithelialization follow as underlying occlusal abnormalities are addressed.

INCISOR PERIODONTAL DISEASE

In the late teenage and older patient, periodontal disease may affect incisors. Though uncommon, the disease can be devastating to the patient. An individual may have severe pain manifest as mastication or bitting difficulties, and halitosis. Varying degrees of severity are presented.

Gingival recession is a common finding in equine incisors. This condition increases with age. Calculus is found on teeth with normal and receding gingiva. Receding gingiva may or may not have calculus. Therefore, while it is possible that calculus plays a role in some cases, it is not a consistent etiological agent, and its removal from all patients will not prevent this condition. In cases of incisor gingivitis caused by calculus, its removal, along with general cleaning and polishing, is temporarily palliative. Calculus tends to recur quickly on those horses that are susceptible to its development initially.

In the equine patient two variations of incisor periodontal disease exist, sometimes together. The first is cemental hyperplasia. This is presented as subgingival nodular enlargements of the reserve crown (**393**). Radiographically, these are dense thickenings of the subgingival tooth. The hyperplastic condition is rarely treated.

The second and more severe condition is characterized by cemental lysis. When gingiva are recessed, cemental lysis is evident clinically on the reserve crown. Changes in sulcular epithelium vary from mild to necrotic. Invasion of bacteria results in osteomyelitis and attachment breakdown with increased tooth mobility. Pulpitis and pulp necrosis may result from apical extension of the disease process. Radiographically, the lytic process progresses to include alveolar bone. Culture and biopsy results indicate mixed infection and inflammatory changes of cementum and surrounding structures, including local osteomyelitis.

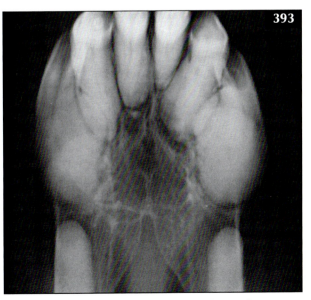

393 A radiograph of the hyperplastic form of incisor periodontal disease.

Examination reveals hyperemic gingiva that are frequently edematous and may be recessed. Examples are seen in figures **394–398**. Some patients have apical fistula formation. Many have teeth with varying degrees of mobility (see *Table 18*). Gingival recession may reveal lytic and hypertrophic changes in the cementum. The condition should be radiographed. Radiographic changes include lysis of cementum and bone, interproximal bone loss, widened PDL space, and cemental hyperplasia. An example of an extracted tooth with cemenal lysis and hyperplasia is shown in figure **399**.

Complications of this condition can include pulp death if the disease process extends apically, and tooth shifting or loss. Painful patients resist application of a speculum for routine dental care.

The underlying pathology is thought to involve stimulation of the epithelial cell rests of Malassez. These cell rests are remnants of Hertwig's epithelial root sheath, which is responsible for root growth and cementum development. In brachydont teeth, the cell rests are responsible for two events. When a tooth has an apical abscess, the cell rests play a role in detruction of tissue[31] seen radiographically as a lytic

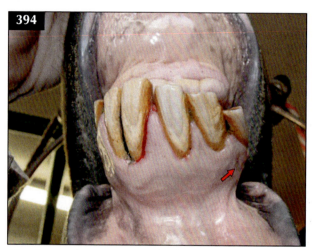

394 Gingival recession and edema, with tooth shifting, and draining tract formation (arrow) indicate severe incisor periodontal disease.

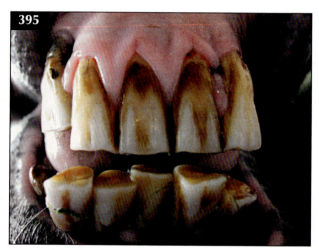

395 Gingival redness, edema, recession, tooth shifting, and pain on examination indicate severe lytic periodontal disease.

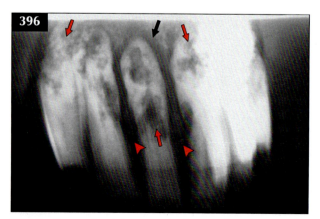

396 Radiograph of the case in figure **395**. Cemental lysis (red arrows) with interproximal bone loss (arrowheads), widened PDL space (black arrow), and tooth shifting seen on clinical examination indicate severe lytic periodontal disease.

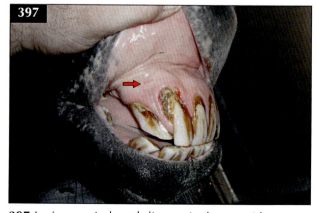

397 Incisor periodontal disease is shown with severe gingival recession, redness, and edema. Teeth are mobile and very painful. The arrow indicates areas of apical fistula formation.

area around the root tip. They also play a role in stimulating cementoblasts to create additional cementum when necessary.[32] An example from brachydont dentistry would be the cemental repair of an endodontically treated tooth where the open pulp at the apex of the tooth is filled physiologically. It is thought that cementum production is regulated by the cell rests in the hypsodont tooth.[33]

The disease usually begins in the Triadan 3s and extends mesially. A possible explanation for the onset of this condition lies in analysis of occlusal forces on aging teeth. As incisors age they normally undergo a rostrally directed tipping movement. The 3s are the most dramatically tipped teeth, and the biomechanical forces are exacerbated by mastication. These forces may be sensed by the cell rests and set off a cascade of events that lead to disease. Occlusal forces directed to a tipping tooth may be misinterpreted or misdirected in some individuals by the cell rests and result in disease. Extension to involve other teeth may be a result of occlusal forces or of chemical communication via cytokine recruitment of inflammation.[34]

Treatment for the lytic condition may invlove extraction. When the third incisors (Triadan 3) are stage 3 in the Mobility Index, they are extracted. If these are the only teeth involved, the disease process is frequently slowed dramatically or arrested. Ideally only 3s are removed. When additional teeth are involved, an intraoral splint (**400**) is used to stabilize all teeth, reducing mobility and pain.

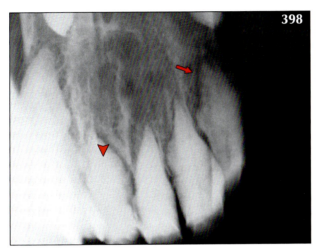

398 Radiographic examination of the patient in figure **397** shows a combination of lysis (arrow) and hyperplasia (arrowhead) of the cementum.

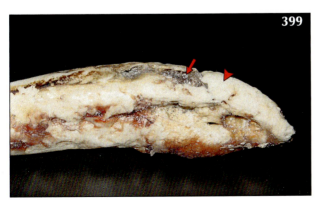

399 An extracted tooth demonstrates cemental lysis (arrow) and mild hyperplasia (arrowhead).

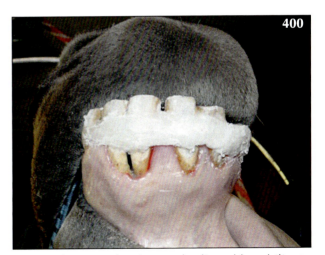

400 Application of an intraoral splint adds stability to all teeth.

In applying interdental splints, the labial surface of teeth must have all cementum removed (**401**). This may be a painful procedure requiring the use of local or regional anesthesia. Diamond burs are used to remove cementum. The enamel is etched with 37% phosphoric acid and dentin bonding agent is applied and light cured. Composite restorative material is placed on the surface. A strip of splint material is pressed into the composite dot on each tooth, thus connecting all the teeth (**402**). The composite is light cured. Additional composite is placed on top of the strip and light cured. The splint is reinforced with polymethylmethacrylate for further stability.

Since the suggested underlying cause is an inflammatory event involving the epithelial cell rests, treatment directed at these cells is indicated. The author uses a regimen of trimcinolone administered at up to 1 mg per site with no more than 6 mg used at a time. If additional treatments are needed they are performed on a monthly basis. Injection is submucosally near the apex of the tooth.[35] Early cases of this condition respond readily to this as the primary treatment. Broad-spectrum antibiotics may be helpful in some cases. A suggested regimen is a combination of sulfa/trimethoprim given orally at 24 mg/kg twice daily and metronidazole given at 10–15 mg/kg orally twice daily.[36]

Incisor periodontal disease can be devastating to the patient and frustrating to the dental practitioner. Early recognition and conservative treatment should be the goal. All cases should be examined radiographically.

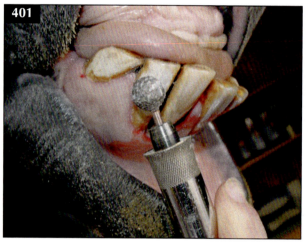

401 Cementum is removed from the labial surface of the tooth with a diamond bur.

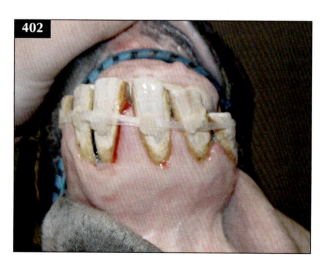

402 After etching and bonding, dots of composite restorative are placed on each tooth and connected by a fiberglass strip. The dots are covered by additional composite.

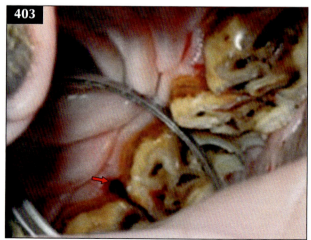

403 A periodontal pocket between 206 and 207 before treatment (arrow).

RESULTS

Treatment of periodontal disease can yield successful results. Pockets can be reduced and gingival attachment to teeth can be established. Reattachment may occur, though the true character of the adherent tissue is unknown. Figure **403** shows the periodontal pocket before treatment. The radiograph in figure **404** indicates widened PDL space. Figure **405** demonstrates a follow-up photograph of the same patient 6 months after treatment, indicating resolution of the periodontal disease.

In the case in figures **403–405**, detailed examination revealed necrotic supragingival and subgingival cementum, recessed and swollen gingiva, and necrotic sulcular epithelium. The tooth was stage 1 in the Tooth Mobility Index. The conclusion is 25–50% attachment loss, or stage 3 periodontal disease.

Treatment included reduction of overlong 306 and 307, debridement of necrotic cementum and sulcular epithelium, and flushing the pocket with 0.12% chlorhexidine gluconate oral rinse.

Since equine teeth undergo continual eruption, reattachment may occur, as there is a normal process of breakdown and re-establishment of collagen fiber connections. This is one of many areas of equine dentistry that need further research.

SUMMARY

Treatment of equine periodontal disease requires thorough evaluation and characterization of the affected tissues. Accurate staging of the disease process leads to appropriate treatment and favorable prognosis.

Strategies for treatment begin with removal of the underlying causes. Occlusal equilibration is critical in reducing the overlong teeth responsible for packing feed in periodontal depressions. Complete debridement of necrotic tissue facilitates healing and prevents the apical and peripheral spread of the disease. Stage 3 mobile teeth are extracted. Antimicrobials and other adjunctive medications further reduce the abnormal bacterial populations and have other effects beneficial to the healing process.

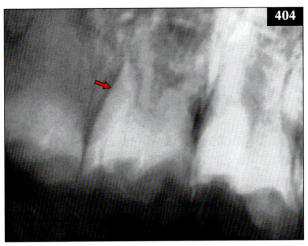

404 Widened PDL space between 206 and 207 (arrow). This is suggestive of attachment loss in this area. On the distal aspect of the tooth there is reduced crestal bone height.

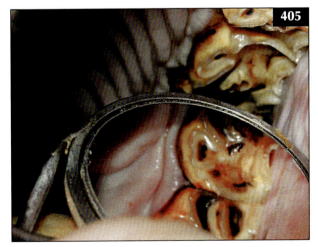

405 Periodontal pocket from patient in figures **403** and **404** 6 months after treatment with gingiva adherent to tooth.

REFERENCES

1. Colyer JF. Variations and diseases of the teeth of horses. *Transactions of the Odontological Society of Great Britain, New Series* 1906: **38**; 42–47.

2. Voss HJ. *Die Zahnfachentzundung des Pferdes.* Stuttgart: Ferdinand Enke, 1937.

3. Baker GJ. Some aspects of equine dental disease. *Equine Veterinary Journal* 1970: **2**; 105–110.

4. Jablonsky S. *Jablonsky's Dictionary of Dentistry.* Kreiger Pub Co., 1992; p. 351.

5. Jablonsky S. *Jablonsky's Dictionary of Dentistry.* Kreiger Pub Co., 1992; p. 515.

6. Listgarten MA. Changing concepts about the dentogingival junction. *Journal of the Canadian Dental Association* 1970: **36**; 70.

7. Loe H, Karring T. A quantitative analysis of the epithelium-connective tissue interface in relation to assessments of the mitotic index. *Journal of Dental Research* 1969: **48**; 634.

8. Laurell L, Rylander H, Sundin Y. Histologic characteristics of clinically healthy gingiva in adolescents. *Scandinavian Journal of Dental Research* 1987: **95**; 456.

9. Egelberg J. The topography and permeability of blood vessels at the dentogingival junction in dogs. *Journal of Periodontal Research* 1967: **2** (Suppl. 1).

10. Carranza FA, Itoiz ME, Cabrini RL. A study of periodontal vascularization in different laboratory animals. *Journal of Periodontal Research* 1966: **1**; 120.

11. Godinho HP, Getty R. Peripheral nervous system. In: Getty R (ed) *Sisson and Grossman's The Anatomy of Domestic Animals*, 5th edition. Philadelphia: WB Saunders, 1975; p. 655.

12. Berkovitz BKB. The structure of the periodontal ligament: an update. *European Journal of Orthodontics* 1990: **12**; 51.

13. Staszyk C, Wulff W, Jacob HG, Gasse H. Collagen fiber architecture of the periodontal ligament in equine cheek teeth. *Journal of Veterinary Dentistry* 2006: **23**(3); 143–147.

14. Mitchell SR, Kempson SA, Dixon PM. Structure of peripheral cementum of normal equine cheek teeth. *Journal of Veterinary Dentistry* 2003: **20**(4); 199–208.

15. Kempson SA. The periodontium of the mandibular teeth of the horse. *17th Annual Veterinary Dental Forum* 2003; p. 204.

16. Haake SK, Newman MG, Nisengaard RJ, Sanz M. Periodontal microbiology. In: Newman MG, Takei HH, Carracza FA (eds) *Carranza's Clinical Periodontology*, 4th editon. Philadelphia: WB Saunders, 2002; pp. 96–112.

17. Baker GJ. *A Study of Dental Disease of the Horse.* PhD thesis, University of Glasgow, 1979; p. 61.

18. Dale AC. Salivary glands. In: Ten Cate AR (ed) *Oral Histology: Development, Structure and Function.* St. Louis: Mosby, 1998; pp. 315–385.

19. Socransky SS, Haffajee AD. Microbial mechanisms in the pathogenesis of destructive periodontal diseases: a critical assessment. *Journal of Periodontal Research* 1991: **26**; 195.

20. Page RC. The role of inflammatory mediators in the pathogenesis of periodontal disease. *Journal of Periodontal Research* 1991: **26**; 230.

21. Deporter DA, Brown DJ. Fine structural observations on the mechanisms of loss of attachment during experimental periodontal disease in the rat. *Journal of Periodontal Research* 1980: **15**; 304.

22. Schroeder HE, Attstrom R. *The Borderland between Caries and Periodontal Disease*, Volume 2. London: Grune & Stratton, 1980.

23. Harvey FT. Some points in the natural history of alveolar or periodontal disease in the horse, ox, and sheep. *Veterinary Record* 1920: **32**; 457–463.

24. Little WM. Periodontal disease in the horse. *Journal of Comparative Pathology and Therapeutics* 1913: **24**; 240–249.

25. Easley J. Equine dental development and anatomy. *Proceedings 42nd Annual Convention of the American Association of Equine Practitioners* 1996; pp. 1–10.

26. Klugh DO. Intraoral radiography of equine premolars and molars. *Proceedings 49th Annual Convention of the American Association of Equine Practitioners* 2003; pp. 280–286.

27. Wiggs RB, Lobprise HB. Dental and oral radiology. In: Wiggs RB and Lobprise HB (eds) *Veterinary Dentistry: Principles and Practice.* Philadelphia: Lippincott-Raven, 1997; p. 197.

28. Jolkovsky DL, Cianco SG. Chemotherapeutic agents in the treatment of periodontal diseases. In: Newman MG, Takei HH, Carranza FA (eds) *Carranza's Clinical Periodontology*, 9th edition. Philadelphia: WB Saunders, 2002; p. 679.

29. Clarke DE. Clinical and microbiological effects of oral zinc ascorbate gel in cats. *Journal of Veterinary Dentistry* 2001: **18**(4); 177–183.

30. Collins NM, Dixon PM. Diagnosis and management of equine distemata. *Clinical Techniques in Equine Practice* 2005: **4**; 148–154.

31. Bykov VL. Epithelial cell rests of Malassez: tissue, cell, and molecular biology. *Morfologia* 2003: **124**(4); 95–103.

32. Hasegawa N, Kawaguchi H, Ogawa T, *et al.* Immunohistochemical characteristics of epithelial cell rests of Malassez during cementum repair. *Journal of Periodontal Research* 2003: **38**; 51–56.

33. Mitchell SR, Kempson SA, Dixon PM. Structure of peripheral cementum of normal equine cheek teeth. *Journal of Veterinary Dentistry* 2003: **20**(4); 199–208.

34. Tadoko O, Maeda T, Heyraas KJ, *et al.* Merkel-like cells in Malassez epithelium in the periodontal ligament of cats: an immunohistochemical, confocal-laser scanning and immuno electron-microscopic investigation. *Journal of Periodontal Research* 2002: **37**; 456–463.

35. Klugh DO. Infiltration anesthesia in equine dentistry. *Compendium on Continuing Education* 2004: **26**; 631–633.

36. Britt B, Byars TD. Hagyard-Davidson-McGee Formulary. *Proceedings 43rd Annual Convention of the American Association of Equine Practitioners* 1997; pp. 170–177.

PRINCIPLES OF ENDODONTICS
David O Klugh and Peter Emily   Chapter 17

Endodontics is the branch of dentistry that addresses the diseases and conditions of the dental pulp. Endodontic treatment of diseased pulp is a standard treatment in man and small animals. Conventional endodontic treatment is performed via access from the exposed crown. Surgical endodontics is performed via bone flap and access to the tooth root. In equine dentistry, only the incisors and canines are routinely amenable to conventional therapy, while premolar and molar pulp disease is treated by surgical access.

Indications commonly found in equine dentistry for endodontic treatment include nonvital pulp exposure (NVPE), tooth discoloration, traumatic injury, selected problems secondary to periodontal disease, radiographic evidence of apical disease, and iatrogenic vital pulp exposure.

Much of the histology, development, and anatomy of equine dentistry are based on understanding of research of brachydont teeth.

PULP DEVELOPMENT AND ANATOMY

Embryological development of the pulp involves the condensation of ectomesenchymal tissue under the inner enamel epithelium of the bell stage. The multicellular character of the pulp develops from undifferentiated mesenchymal cells.

Pulp consists of connective tissue, nerves that provide sensation, blood vessels that provide nutrition to the pulp, immune cells for defense against infection, and formation of dentin by odontoblasts.[1] A layer of odontoblasts lies next to the dentin at the periphery of the pulp. Beneath this layer is the remainder of the pulp. Fibroblasts are the most common cell type.[2] Other cell types include undifferentiated mesenchymal cells and immune cells. Undifferentiated mesenchymal cells are precursors of odontoblasts and fibroblasts. Differentiation varies with the type of stimulus received by the cells and the needs of the pulp. Pulp matrix contents include collagen fibers and ground substance, which is composed of glycoproteins, glycosaminoglycans, and water. Ground substance functions as a transport medium between blood vessels and cells.[2]

The pulp also contains a rich network of blood vessels and nerves. These structures enter the pulp via the apical foramen. Blood vessels entering the pulp are arterioles, with smooth muscle walls. Some vessels anastomose to provide collateral circulation within the pulp.[2] Nerves are primarily sensory from the trigeminal nerve.[2] In brachydont teeth most nerve endings are myelinated A-gamma fibers sensing sharp pain.[2] A-beta fibers sense mechanical tactile input.[2] C fibers are nonmyelinated fibers sensing dull pain and temperature.[3] Some dentinal tubules contain unmyelinated nerve endings. These nerve endings may be more related to mechanical sensation and not pain.

ANATOMY OF THE PULP CAVITY

In all teeth, the pulp cavity begins as a large space within the shell of enamel and dentin. Anatomical terminology is adapted from brachydont dentistry.[4] Maturation results in formation of divisions of the pulp cavity as additional dentin is deposited. At the base of the crown is the pulp chamber. Coronally the pulp cavity continues as the pulp horn(s). Apically from the pulp chamber, the root canal extends toward the apex of the tooth. Figures **406** and **407** illustrate the divisions of the pulp cavity of an incisor and a cheek tooth.

INCISORS

The pulp cavity of incisors begins as a large, cone-shaped cavity that changes conformation as secondary dentin is deposited. Figure **408** shows the pulp cavities of young incisors radiographically. Labio-lingual narrowing of the pulp cavity due to the presence of the infundibulum is evident by the shape of the dental star (**409**).

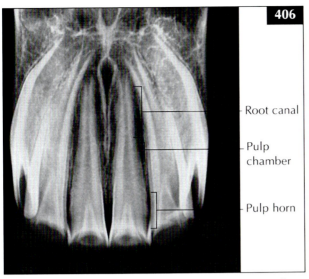

Root canal

Pulp chamber

Pulp horn

406 Divisions of the pulp cavity are demonstrated in an incisor.

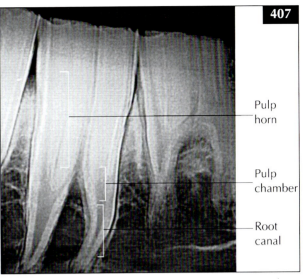

Pulp horn

Pulp chamber

Root canal

407 Divisions of the pulp cavity are demonstrated in a cheek tooth.

408 Radiograph of young incisors showing large pulp cavities of incisors immediately post eruption in this 3-year-old patient.

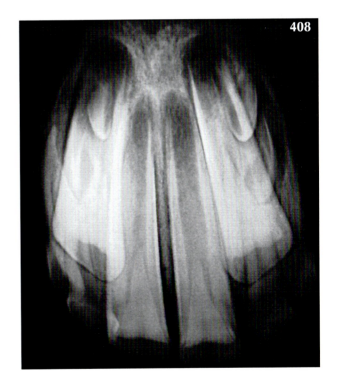

409 The dental star and therefore the pulp canal are compressed labio-lingually by the infundibulum. (arrows)

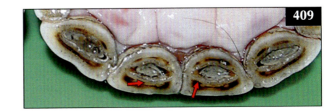

Beyond the infundibulum the middle third of the pulp cavity becomes tube-shaped, as dentin is deposited. The parallel walls are evident radiographically in most cases (**410**).

Further apically, the pulp cavity is unevenly narrowed. Lateral compression of roots results in dentinal deposition such that the root canal inconsistently diverges into two parts. One is labial to the other. Apical openings are variably positioned mesially, distally, or apically. For further discussion of age-related incisor pulp cavity changes, please refer to Chapter 3: Anatomical characteristics of equine dentition.

The divisions of the pulp cavity, i.e. horns, chamber, and root canal are not easily identified radiographically, though their definition and presence remain the same.

PREMOLARS AND MOLARS

The pulp cavities of premolars and molars have similar characteristics. Separation of mesial from distal pulp chamber usually occurs by year 3 or 4 of tooth life.[5] Each root canal is continuous with one pulp chamber. Separation between lingual and buccal pulp chambers may not occur. The mature pulp chamber remains large for many years.[6] The bulbous shape of the pulp chamber (**411**) makes instrumentation difficult when performing root canal therapy on cheek teeth. The large size of the pulp chamber also makes complete sealing of the pulp cavity difficult, as many of the materials used for this purpose are not designed to seal such a large space.

Pulp horns separate as dentinal deposition fills the pulp cavity in the crown. Separation is complete by 6–8 years of tooth age.[6] There are at least five pulp horns in each cheek tooth. Some teeth have six (6s in Triadan system) and others have up to 11 (11s in Triadan system). In the mature tooth, each pulp chamber is contiguous with one or two pulp horns. The horns taper towards the coronal tip. Their length varies, and may be asymmetrical within the same tooth, depending on the occlusal angle.[6] In the geriatric horse, the pulp horns are inconsistently present, and may be filled with dentin.[6] The rate of filling of pulp horns is slower in maxillary cheek teeth than in mandibular cheek teeth.[6]

Within 2 years after eruption, roots are formed. The pulp canals in the roots begin development as roots form in the young tooth. As the root extends in length, the root canal follows. The normal root canal fills with secondary dentin as it ages. The age of the patient that coincides with apical closure is highly variable. Some close in the mid teenage years, while others remain open until the 20s.[6] In equine teeth, there are one or a few apical openings. By comparison, in dogs the apex closes with blood vessels entering via an apical

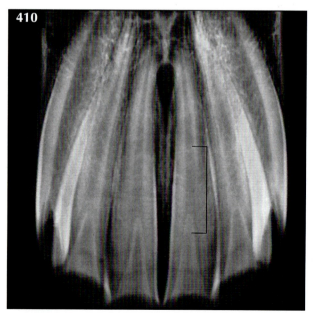

410 Radiograph of a 5-year-old patient demonstrates the parallel sides of the walls of the middle third of the pulp cavity (bracket).

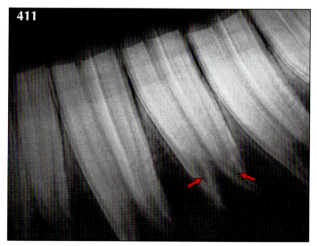

411 The large size of the pulp chamber space of premolars and molars (arrows).

delta, which has numerous openings. The point of entry of blood vessels in the equine tooth may not coincide with the actual apex of the tooth. Geriatric root tips frequently consist only of cementum,[6] laid down by the periodontal tissues. In such cases, vessel and nerve entry is via a lateral orifice. Roots have varying numbers of root canals.[6] Maxillary cheek teeth have one canal in each of two buccal roots, and two canals in the palatal root. Mandibular cheek teeth may have any combination of one or two canals in each of two roots.

The apical opening of the equine cheek tooth root remains until the tooth is 15–20 years of age.[6] The root canal remains open and the pulp remains vascularized in the normal geriatric horse until old age.

ENDODONTIC–PERIODONTIC RELATIONSHIPS

The pulp and periodontium are in intimate contact and communication at points where the neurovascular bundle enters the tooth. Tooth function is best when these tissues are healthy, as nutrition and sensation pass to and from the tooth via both structures. When disease occurs in one of these tissues, it may spread to the other. Understanding of this process and categorizing the types[7] of interrelationships helps with disease diagnosis, treatment, and prognosis.

Class 0 disease is primary endodontic disease with no evidence of periodontal involvement.

Class I lesions are those that begin in the pulp and spread to the periodontium via apical communication. These lesions show radiolucency around the apex and along the PDL. In equines they may also present with cemental lysis in the affected area. An example is seen in figure **412**. Since the primary lesion is endodontic in origin, root canal therapy is helpful and frequently curative if access to the tooth is simple. In incisors, treatment is very effective. In cheek teeth, treatment is effective only if there is no communication of the lesion with the oral cavity. Mandibular cheek teeth are more easily treated than maxillary cheek teeth.

Class II disease begins in the periodontium and extends to the pulp. Communication to the pulp may be at the apex or via open dentinal tubules. Radiographic lesions demonstrate significant periodontal attachment loss. Radiolucency can be tracked from the coronal to apical, as the coronal

attachment is most severe. Clinically, these teeth are easily diagnosed as primary periodontal disease, while radiographs are necessary to evaluate the involvement of the pulp (**413**). These teeth carry a poor prognosis in most cases, as the communication with the oral cavity and the periodontal disease must be resolved before the endodontic problem is addressed. Many of these teeth are so severely diseased when the veterinary dentist encounters them that the severity of attachment loss precludes treatment. Many of these teeth are extracted.

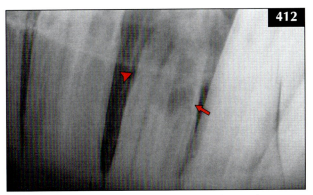

412 Class I endodontic–periodontic relationship exists when a primary endodontic lesion (arrow) extends to the surrounding periodontal structures (arrowhead). Anachoretic (bloodborne) pulpitis resulted in pulp death which extended to periodontal structures causing widened PDL space.

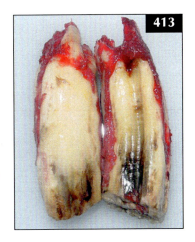

413 Class II endodontic–periodontic relationships exist when primary periodontal disease extends apically to continue as pulp disease. In this case, periodontal disease extended apically to cause sinusitis and pulpitis in both teeth. Both teeth were extracted.

Class III lesions have both primary pulp disease and primary periodontal disease combined. Many of these teeth are so severely diseased as to require extraction.

AGE-RELATED CHANGES OF THE PULP

As pulp tissue ages, many changes occur.[8] Collagen fibers become more numerous and dense, and become organized into bundles. Collagen is denser near the apex in all ages. In the aging and diseased tooth, function and population of all pulp cells are reduced, especially mesenchymal cells. Mineral deposition (pulp stones) may be present. Circulation is reduced.

As a consequence of these changes the pulp is less able to respond to inflammatory stimuli, and is more likely to suffer necrosis when challenged. This is an example of a similarity between aging hypsodont teeth and brachydont teeth.

DENTIN DEPOSITION

Dentin is deposited by odontoblasts that line the pulp cavity. Differences in types of dentin have been identified and characterized.[9] Primary dentin is produced prior to eruption and continues until the tooth is in occlusion. It consists of dentinal tubules filled with intratubular dentin. After the tooth is in occlusion odontoblasts produce secondary dentin. In equine teeth, there is a further classification into secondary regular and secondary irregular dentin. Secondary regular dentin is produced by odontoblasts throughout the normal course of life. It is characterized by dentinal tubules with no intratubular dentin, but surrounded and separated by intertubular dentin. Secondary irregular dentin is produced as a particular portion of pulp is nearly filled. Tertiary dentin is formed in response to noxious stimuli.

Dentin production is stimulated in response to a signal received by the odontoblasts from forces of mastication from the occlusal surface. There is a standard rate of dentin production that can be accelerated or decelerated as odontoblasts sense variation in occlusal forces. This change in rate occurs without a transition from secondary to tertiary dentin. Figures **414** and **415** demonstrate the different rates of dentin production in incisors. If the diagonal malocclusion is reduced to normal, either direct

or indirect pulp exposure of 303 would occur due to its lack of secondary dentin when compared to 302 and 301.

The character of dentin changes in response to stimuli. Moderate to severe inflammatory insults result in production of tertiary dentin. Some severe insults result in pulp necrosis. The transition from secondary dentin to tertiary dentin requires a different or more significant signal than the signal responsible for the change in rate of deposition of secondary dentin. Furthermore, the stimulus received by the odontoblasts results in changes in the pulp that are not equivalent throughout the length of the pulp. A stimulus may result in pulp necrosis, dentin bridge

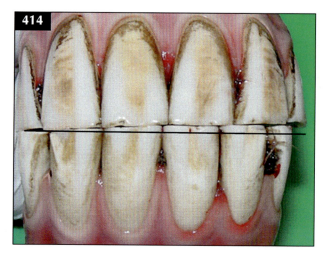

414 Diagonal incisor malocclusion.

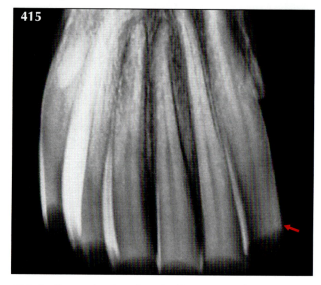

415 Radiograph of patient in figure **414** showing 303 pulp within 3 mm of occlusal surface (arrow).

formation, or pulp canal obliteration, depending on the nature and location of the stimulus and the age and character of the pulp.

Dentin bridge formation as seen in figure **416** is most common in young pulps. The pulp of the young tooth is much more capable responding to and overcoming an insult. It is a larger pulp with more blood supply, has more cells of all types, and is more resilient as cell function is normal. The size of the pulp also helps to diffuse pressure changes that occur with inflammation. Inflammation results in increased circulation and increased pressure within the pulp. As the tooth ages the pulp is less abundant as the pulp canal is narrower. Along with a decreased pulp space, aging changes include reduced numbers of odontoblasts, undifferentiated mesenchymal cells, immune cells, and others. Cell function in the remaining tissue is reduced. Blood supply is reduced as is the volume of pulp tissue. Through these changes, the overall capacity for management of insults is decreased.

Pulp necrosis is more common in incisors of older patient as a result of aging changes, and in cheek teeth of younger horses due to anachoretic (bloodborne) infections. Necrosis may also occur in pulp horns when an apical stimulus has caused either a dentin bridge to form in the pulp chamber or apical portion of the pulp horn. In aged pulps of hypsodont and brachydont teeth, it is the increased pressure that causes most pulp necrosis.[10]

The entire pulp does not respond in the same way to a specific stimulus. The response of the incisor pulp decreases apically from the point of insult. An occlusal insult may result in necrosis of the occlusal portion of the pulp, with either dentin bridge formation or pulp canal obliteration. When a dentin bridge forms, the pulp located apically is vital and normal. In young cheek teeth, necrosis of the coronal portion of the horn may occur and result in dentin bridge formation. Alternatively, anastomosis of circulation in the pulp chamber may be the result of less severe insults.

NVPE of incisor teeth in aged horses presents as a black opening in the occlusal surface (**417**). It is theorized that this is the consequence of reduced mastication forces and pulp aging processes. In some patients, the range of motion of mastication is altered for an extended period of time either by habit or by malocclusion. The altered range of motion reduces the occlusal forces sensed by the odontoblasts. For some of these patients the rate of dentin deposition is slowed in one or more teeth, commonly third incisors. As attrition and eruption occur, the pulp gets closer to the occlusal surface. At some point odontoblasts of the remaining pulp sense an insult. Since the patient has aged, the pulp is limited in its ability to respond to the stimulus. The stimulus, which in earlier years resulted in acceleration of dentin deposition, now becomes sensed as an inflammatory insult to which the pulp is unable to respond. In this circumstance a

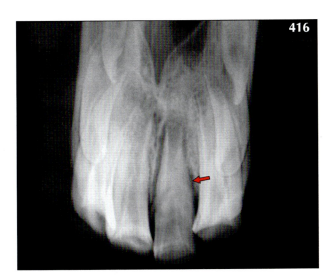

416 Dentin bridge formation in a young incisor subsequent to fracture (arrow).

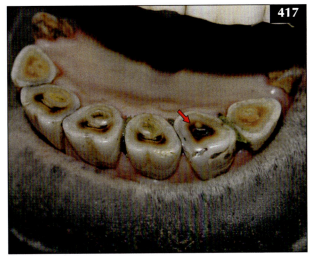

417 NVPE of a 302 (arrow).

portion of the pulp suffers necrosis. Eruption and attrition eventually expose the necrotic pulp to the occlusal surface. In some cases an apical lucency results, as in figure **418**, as a result of necrosis of the entire pulp. However, this is the exception.

The most common condition encountered in incisor NVPE in equine patients is partial necrosis of the pulp. The same age-related changes occur to the pulp, resulting in reduced dentin production, and the same insult occurs as described above. The difference is that either the insult was less severe, or the pulp was more capable of responding to the insult, or both. In this case the pulp produces tertiary dentin resulting in pulp canal obliteration (PCO) (**419**). The same eruptive and attritive processes result in NVPE. Since the pulp has responded in the apical region, no apical lucency is seen on the radiograph. Figures **420** and **421** demonstrate the wide variation in proportions of PCO and NVPE. PCO and dentin bridge formation are radiographic diagnoses. Therefore, it is imperative that radiographs are used to quantify the production of tertiary dentin in the injured tooth.

Premolars and molars can suffer pulp necrosis. The most common pathogenesis is anachoresis.[11] Some equine cheek teeth suffer severe insults resulting in either apical lucency and/or draining tracts in mandibular teeth (**422**), or sinusitis from maxillary teeth pathology. Many of these teeth have complete pulp necrosis. Other teeth that are either more capable of responding, or suffer less severe insults result in clinically diagnosed NVPE (**423**). Many of these have no clinical evidence of apical disease. In these patients the problem develops in a fashion similar to that seen in incisors. Most of these occur in young patients. Since the young pulp retains a capacity for response, it produces a dentin bridge. However, the horns become necrotic as anastomosis of blood vessels near the pulp chamber results in reduced circulation in the coronal pulp horn. Continued eruption and attrition expose the nonvital pulp.

In still other patients a less severe insult or more responsive pulp responds to a stimulus by accelerating the rate of dentin production in pulp horns and pulp chambers. Complete obliteration of pulp horns can result (**424**). Acceleration of separation of pulp chambers can also occur (**425**).

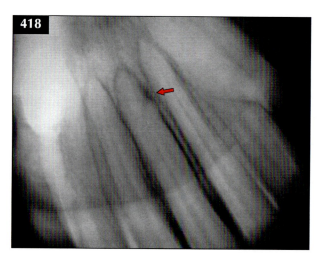

418 Radiograph of NVPE resulting in an apical lucency (arrow).

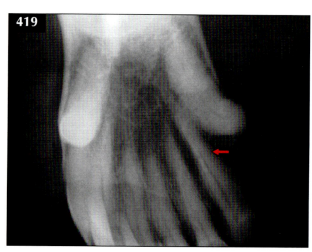

419 Radiograph of a case of NVPE in an incisor showing partial PCO (arrow).

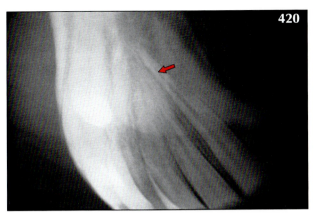

420 Radiograph showing very small proportion of PCO or dentin bridge formation in an incisor with NVPE (arrow).

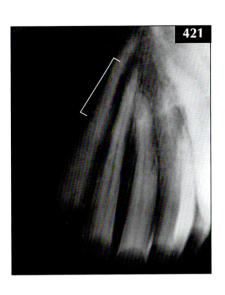

421 Radiograph showing large proportion of PCO in an incisor with NVPE (bracket).

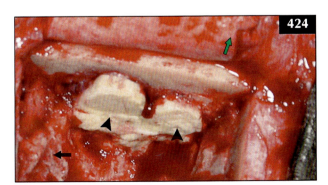

422 Draining tract from an apical abscess of a mandibular cheek tooth (arrow).

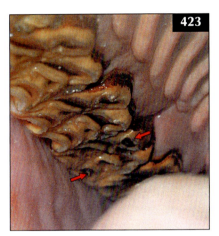

423 NVPE of a maxillary cheek tooth displaying no clinical signs of disease (arrows).

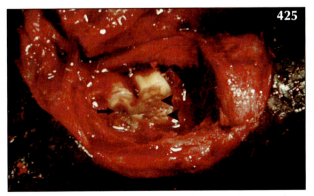

424 Apicectomy at the level of the pulp chamber in a diseased 406 for retrograde endodontic treatment demonstrates obliteration of pulp horns by deposition of tertiary dentin in a young patient (arrowheads). Black arrow: Rostral direction; Green arrow: Occlusal direction

425 A 3-year-old 308 with complete separation of mesial and distal pulp chambers. The arrow points to the mesial chamber and arrowheads indicate distal chambers. Photograph taken after endodontic procedure was performed.

THERMAL DAMAGE

The same pulp pathology is seen as a result of thermal damage to the pulp caused primarily by instrument overheating during occlusal equilibration. The response of the pulp varies with the same characteristics, i.e. age and capacity of the pulp for response to insult.

Thermal damage does not uniformly result in complete pulp necrosis. When resulting in partial pulp necrosis, the remaining tooth and pulp are normal. The response of the tooth can only be determined radiographically. Varying degrees of tertiary dentin formation are seen. Some pulps form dentin bridges while others undergo canal obliteration. In dentin bridge formation the apical portion of the pulp is normal. The tooth undergoes normal eruption and attrition, and wears as a normal tooth.

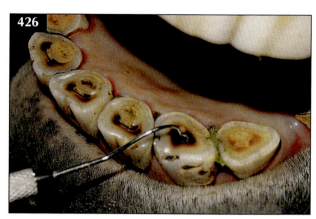

426 A dental explorer is placed in a nonvital pulp canal.

DIAGNOSIS OF PULP DISEASE

The pulp becomes inflamed in response to various types and degrees of stimulus. Continued severe insult causes pulp necrosis. Inflamed pulp swells and suffers increased pressure within the enclosed space of the canal. The increased pressure prevents arterial blood from entering and nourishing pulp tissues, and the pulp dies.

Pulpitis can result from any of the following processes:
- Anachoresis, or bacterial delivery to an inflamed pulp via the bloodstream.
- Extension to the pulp from periodontal disease.
- Bacterial penetration from problems such as caries.
- Direct pulp exposure. Traumatic or iatrogenic exposure of a vital pulp.
- Indirect pulp exposure. Traumatic or iatrogenic exposure of open dentinal tubules near the pulp.

When the patient suffers a pulp exposure, bacteria contaminate the pulp tissue and/or dentinal tubules. Teeth sustaining the first three types of insults usually suffer pulp necrosis before the attending veterinarian or owner is aware of any problem. These teeth may require conventional root canal therapy or extraction.

Severity of trauma and capacity of the pulp's circulatory system to adapt to inflammation are critical factors in determining the outcome of traumatic and iatrogenic pulp exposures. Teeth suffering minimal trauma and those with a large pulp and good circulation have better chance for pulp survival than severely traumatized teeth or those with aging pulps.

Possible outcomes to direct and indirect pulp exposure are:
- Pulp necrosis.
- PCO with tertiary dentin.
- Dentin bridge formation.
- Combination of all the above.

In order to determine which outcome results, radiographic evaluation at 3–6 month intervals is necessary.

Clinical presentation of pulp disease is varied. The following are common presentations in equine patients:
- NVPE.
- Vital pulp exposure (iatrogenic or traumatic).
- Discolored tooth.
- Draining tracts from mandibular teeth.
- Unilateral sinusitis from maxillary teeth.

Clinical examination requires the use of a speculum, head light, mirror, and dental explorer. The dental explorer is drawn along the tooth surface. Necrotic dentin causes the tip of the explorer to 'stick' or 'catch' in the tissue. In these areas, the examiner attempts gently to force the tip of the explorer into the pulp horn (**426**). The use of an endodontic file (**427**) assists in determining the depth of nonvital pulp horn. Systematic examination of the occlusal surfaces results in correct diagnosis of pulp exposures.

Teeth with conditions suspected of pulp disease should always be radiographed for the presence of apical lucencies and to determine the condition of the pulp. PCO and dentin bridge formation can only be diagnosed radiographically.

TREATMENT OF EQUINE PULP DISEASE

Pulp disease is painful. Many apparently nonvital pulps remain painful as the nerve is the last structure to suffer necrosis in the pulp.[12] Fluid-filled dentinal tubules containing viable odontoblastic processes transmit pain. Diseased and necrotic dentinal tubules also contain bacteria which can be transported to other local and systemic locations to cause further disease. When the pulp is compromised, endodontic treatment is indicated. Failure to treat leads to complications that include pulp death, premature tooth loss, local infection, spread of infection to other parts of the body, and other systemic effects.[13] Treatment options include root canal therapy and extraction. The goal is early diagnosis and early intervention in order to relieve pain and maintain tooth function.

THE ENDODONTIC TRIAD
The objectives of treatment[1] of pulp disease are to relieve pain, remove infected tissue and debris, and fill or obturate the canal. These objectives are accomplished by adherence to basic endodontic principles, including the *endodontic triad*:[7]
1. Preparation.
2. Disinfection.
3. Obturation.

Preparation of the canal includes creation of an access and shaping the canal such that placement of obturation material is facilitated. An unrestricted pathway to the apex is necessary. Instrumentation of the canal creates the appropriate shape.

In equine incisors, canal access is either via the necrotic opening on the occlusal surface of a NVPE or by accessing 3–4 mm from the gingival margin. For

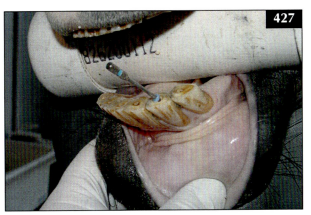

427 An endodontic file with a silicon endo stop is used to measure the depth of necrotic pulp horn.

incisors that require root canal therapy but do not have NVPE, access is gained with a bur and high-speed hand piece by drilling into the canal from the labial surface. Access to c heek tooth canals is routinely gained through the root tip. This is done through by creation of a bone flap and amputating the root tip.

Disinfection of the canal is done by first debriding canal contents with instruments in combination with chemical cleansing agents. An old adage in endodontic therapy is that 'files shape and irrigants clean'.[14] Chemical disinfection is imperative. Many products assist in this process. During instrumentation the disinfecting chemicals diffuse into the dentinal tubules to provide antimicrobial effect.

Obturation is the permanent three-dimensional sealing and filling of the canal. Many materials can be used for this purpose. Sealing the apex and the dentinal tubules of the canal wall is achieved with the use of canal sealing cement. A common sealant is zinc oxide in combination with eugenol, though many canal sealing cements exist. The canal space is filled with inert solid or semi-solid material. Many materials exist for this purpose. Examples include gutta percha and mineral trioxide aggregate (MTA).

ENDODONTIC INSTRUMENTS

Barbed broaches (**428**, **429**) are used for removal or *extirpation*, of residual pulp tissue. These are fragile instruments whose shank is cut and forced open to form barbs. They are inserted to the apex and carefully rotated 180° to engage and remove pulp tissue. The pulp is most fibrous near the apex, therefore it is important to insert the broach all the way to the apex for complete pulp extirpation.

K-files and reamers (**430**) are made of wire machined into a three- or four-sided shaft that is then twisted to create cutting edges. They are inserted into the canal and turned a quarter turn and removed. Reamers are inserted and rotated in a clockwise direction.

Hedstrom files (**431**) are cut from a blank wire to form a spiral groove on a tapered shaft. They are used in a push-pull fashion; twisting these files will frequently result in their fracture.

Many rotary systems exist. They are not yet available for equine use, as their file length is too short for equine pulp canals.

Pluggers and spreaders (**432**) are used to push the filling material against the walls and ends of the canal to create a three-dimensional fill and push the sealer into the dentinal tubules. Pluggers are flat-ended, tapered instruments that compress the filling material toward the apex, or vertically. Spreaders are sharp-pointed, tapered instruments that compress the filling material laterally against the walls.

ENDODONTIC MATERIALS

Irrigants are necessary for flushing debris, necrotic material, and bacteria from the canal. They are essential for debridement and disinfection of the canal and in areas not accessible by instruments. The antibacterial effects of these chemicals extend throughout the canal and dentinal tubules. Lubricants assist in instrument passage and prevention of instrument binding during filing procedures. Sodium

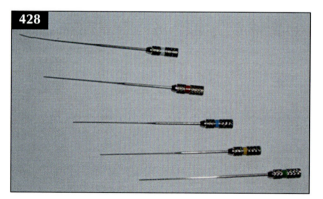

428 Barbed broaches are available in various sizes and lengths. These are 47 mm in length.

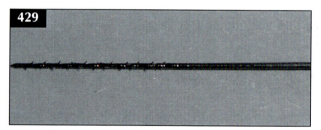

429 Barbs cut into steel shaft of a broach.

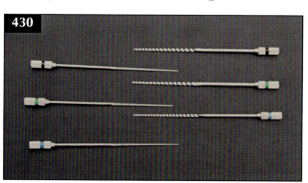

430 Kerr reamers of various sizes are shown in 60 mm length.

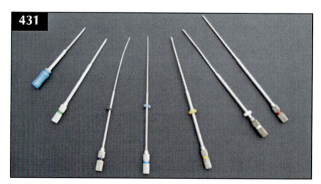

431 Hedstrom files are available in various sizes and lengths.

hypochlorite 3.5–5.25% (bleach) in half-strength solution is an irrigant that dissolves organic material and is antibacterial. Ethylenediaminetetracetic acid (EDTA) and urea peroxidase combined with propylene glycol (RC Prep®) have antibacterial effects in addition to dissolving inorganic debris. Bleach and RC Prep® are commonly used together to debride chemically and lubricate canals. Lubrication aids in instrumentation. Sterile saline is used as a final step to flush chemicals and dentinal shavings created in preparing the canal. A 3 mL syringe with an endodontic irrigation needle works well. Endodontic irrigation needles have a blunt tip and are flexible so as to access any canal opening. Paper points (**433**) are used to dry the canal completely after instrumentation and sterilization. They are available in various sizes that correspond to canal size. The canal must be dry so that sealing cements adhere to the dentin.

Sealing cements are used to seal the apical orifice and the dentinal tubules of the canal wall. They have bacteriostatic effect which prevents infection from recurring or spreading. Many different types of sealing cements are available. A commonly used sealing cement is composed of zinc oxide and eugenol. The mixed cement is introduced into the canal by one of several methods. It can be injected via a polypropylene catheter. However, air pockets are easily created with this method. A file can be dipped in the cement, inserted to the apex and turned to spread cement on to the canal wall. A spiral filler (**434**, **435**) can be used on a slow-speed hand piece to apply the paste to the walls by centrifugal force as the filler is rotated slowly. For equine teeth 60 mm length instruments are needed to reach the apex. The cement can also be applied to the canal as gutta percha points are coated with the paste and inserted.

Gutta percha is an inert rubber material. It is an extract from gummy extract evergreen trees of Southeast Asia, specifically *Pallaquium gutta*.[15]

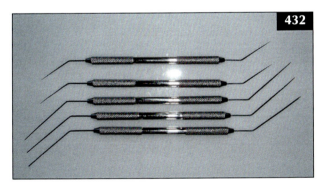

432 Pluggers and spreaders compress the obturation material against the canal apex and walls.

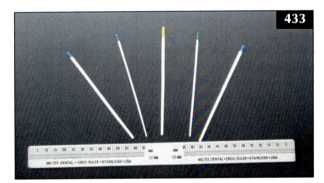

433 Paper points are used to dry the canal.

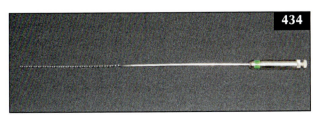

434 A spiral filler is used to spread the cement inside the canal. These instruments are used on a slow-speed hand piece.

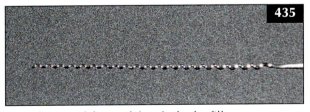

435 The spiral form of the shaft of a filler.

After it is harvested from the trees, it is mixed with other chemicals such as zinc oxide, wax, and resin and formed into cones of various sizes and shapes for insertion into root canals. These cones are called *gutta percha points* and come in two shapes. One is tapered toward the tip, while the other is parallel until it tapers to a point just at the tip. The latter are called *parallax* points (**436**). Gutta percha points are inserted into the canal and pressed both laterally and vertically with pluggers and spreaders.

In the equine patient, if gutta percha is used in young teeth, continual eruption and attrition will eventually expose the gutta percha at the occlusal surface. At that time additional restoration of the tooth is indicated. When this is done, the gutta percha is removed as far apically as possible and a restorative is placed in the cavity. In root canal therapy of late teenage and older patients, eruption will rarely result in exposure of correctly placed endodontic filling material.

MTA is another obturation material that is used primarily in surgical endodontic treatment of equine cheek teeth. It is mixed with water to form a paste that is injected or spiraled in place. This cement material is inert and cures to a very hard surface. It seals tubules and is impervious to bacteria. It does not need additional restoration when exposed and undergoes similar attrition rate as teeth.

After the canal is obturated the access must be closed by placement of restorative material. Incisor root canal filling material should be removed with a bur and high-speed hand piece to the level of the gingiva or slightly below. This will provide the maximum amount of crown eruption prior to exposure of the filling material. In most patients this length is sufficient. In surgical access sites where gutta percha is used, a glass ionomer is used to seal the apex. If MTA is used, additional materials are unnecessary to perfect an apical seal.

ENDODONTIC TECHNIQUE FOR INCISORS: CONVENTIONAL ROOT CANAL THERAPY

Access to the canal depends on the presenting problem. NVPEs are accessed directly at the occlusal surface. Fractured teeth are accessed at the fracture site after debridement of soft tissue and bone and tooth fragments. Discolored teeth are accessed 3–4 mm from the gingival margin with a No. 4, No. 6, or No. 8 round bur as in figure **437**. Access is made on the labial surface at the midline of the tooth. The first 1–2 mm is drilled with the bur perpendicular to the tooth surface. The drill is then angled toward the apex. This prevents the bur from slipping. In some larger incisors a bur in a slow-speed straight hand piece may be necessary. In such cases, water cooling is provided by an assistant.

Residual pulp is extirpated with a barbed broach. The canal is irrigated with half-strength bleach to remove any loose debris. These chemicals are used in a small syringe with a blunt-tipped endodontic needle.

In most cases 60 mm long Hedstrom files are used in equine incisors. These 60 mm files increase in

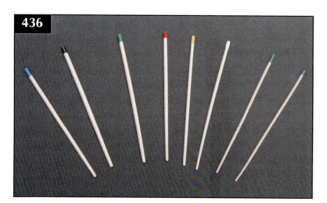

436 Parallax gutta percha points of various sizes fill the prepared canal.

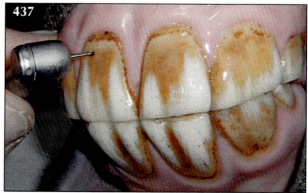

437 Access to the pulp of incisors is made 3–4 mm from the gingival margin on the midline of the tooth. The bur is directed perpendicular to the tooth surface.

diameter. The file that reaches the apical terminus of the canal is called the *master file*. The 60 mm files range in size from 15 to 140. The sizes are numbered by the American National Standards Institute and indicate their relative diameter. All files and gutta percha points are numbered by this system.

After each file is used the canal should be flushed with bleach. The master file is used to clean the canal and assure maintenance of the original canal length. This is called *recapitulation*, and is important to remove filing shavings and other debris so that this material does not become compacted into the apical part of the canal. Urea peroxidase and EDTA combinations are used with half-strength bleach to dissolve and remove organic and inorganic debris and to lubricate the canal. Radiographs are taken initially to determine apical closure, file length compared to canal length (**438**), and to evaluate canal shape. Files are used in the canal until they move freely and reach the apex. The canal is then flushed and the next size larger file is used. This process is continued until clean shavings are removed from the entire canal. This indicates that the canal is clean. The canal is debrided and shaped to the apex with each file. Generally the last file to reach the apex is followed by two additional files and finally recapitulated. Most aged equine incisors require file sizes from 40–90. Younger horses require larger files. The distance to the apex from the access opening is determined with an endodontic stop (**439**) on the file. This distance is confirmed radiographically.

Once the canal is clean, it is flushed with sterile saline. All excess chemicals and debris are removed from the canal. The canal is then dried with paper points.

The goal of obturation is to fill the entire canal completely and accurately. Sealing cement is used in conjunction with gutta percha to fill the apical orifice, dentinal tubules, and canal. Equine teeth require parallax gutta percha cones due to their shape. Their canals are cone-shaped at the apex, while their walls are parallel occlusally to the access.

The initial gutta percha point used in canal obturation is one that is large enough and long enough to fill the canal as completely as possible. It is the same size as the last apical file. Radiographic evaluation assists in determination of quality of fit of this cone. The tip of this point reaches the radiographic apex which is 3–5 mm from the true apex. This point is called the *master cone* or *point*. Its tight fit at the apex can be determined by the presence of 'tug-back' as the cone is fit tightly in the apical canal and tension is felt as the cone is removed. Once appropriate position is determined, the cone is removed and sealing cement is introduced into the canal. The master cone is inserted and condensed and spread into place. Stepwise larger spreaders are used to create space for additional gutta percha points. They are vertically and laterally condensed to perfect a three-dimensional final seal. This process is repeated until the canal is completely obturated.

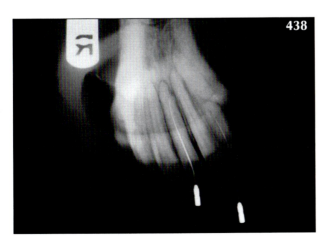

438 A radiograph is taken to determine the position of the file tip within the canal.

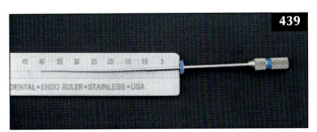

439 Endodontic stops are placed on a file to determine the length of the canal. These stops correspond to the color of the file and slide up and down the shaft.

The gutta percha points are trimmed to the level of the gingival margin. The access opening is undercut with a No. 35 or No. 37 bur. This cavity is lined with a resin-reinforced glass ionomer. Etchant is placed in the cavity and left for 30 s and rinsed thoroughly. A dentin bonding agent and adhesive is placed on to the cavity surface and light cured. Hybrid composite material is placed in 2 mm increments to fill the space. Each layer is light cured. A composite finishing bur is used to smooth the surface. A bonding agent/adhesive is placed and light cured as added insurance against microleakage.

Figures **440** and **441** show results of conventional root canal therapy in equine incisors.

ENDODONTIC TECHNIQUE FOR PREMOLARS AND MOLARS: SURGICAL ENDODONTIC PROCEDURE

Most endodontic procedures for cheek teeth in equines are indicated by the presence of either a draining tract in the mandible or a unilateral sinusitis from infected maxillary teeth. Determination of the affected tooth and affected canal is the first challenge. Radiographs and clinical examination assist in this process. See Chapter 9: Dental radiography, for radiographic details of premolars and molars. In some cases contrast radiography is helpful. Degree of canal filling with secondary dentin is determined both by age of the tooth and by radiography. In most cases, if the tooth is less than 4 years old, the mesial and distal pulp chambers will be in communication.[5] There may be variation in this separation as inflammation may accelerate dentin deposition. Pulp necrosis of long-standing duration may be diagnosed radiographically in patients whose age would indicate separation of the mesial and distal chambers. When in doubt, endodontic treatment of all roots is indicated.

The approach to cheek teeth is retrograde, through the apex of the tooth root. Surgical approach to the roots varies with the location of the affected tooth. Mandibular premolars and molars are approached by creation of a bone flap in the lateral mandible (**442**). Maxillary cheek teeth are accessed either by bone flap for the first two premolars or by sinus flap for other teeth. The teeth most commonly affected are the fourth premolars, third premolars, and the first molars. Success is better in mandibular teeth.[16]

Once adequate exposure to the tooth is achieved, the apical portion of the tooth is amputated with a bur or a diamond cutoff wheel at the level of the pulp chamber. If a diamond wheel is used an assistant cools the wheel and tissue with constant lavage of sterile saline. The pulp chamber in younger teeth is a bulbous shape, and it is not easily instrumented. It must be either chemically debrided and disinfected or it must be amputated. Since it is located near the base of the crown, it can be amputated along with the

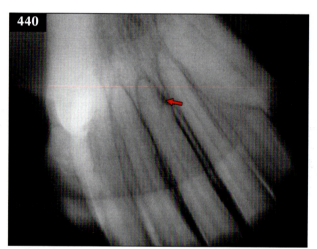

440 Condition of root canal prior to treatment shows open pulp chamber and apical lucency (arrow).

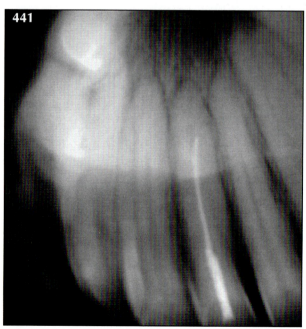

441 Tooth in figure **438** shown 9 months post treatment. Resolution of apical lucency indicates healing.

tooth root(s). This leaves only the pulp horns to be treated. The removal of this extra part of the tooth with the tooth root does not significantly affect the length, life, or function of the remaining tooth. Disinfection and obturation of the remaining pulp horns are facilitated.

Barbed broaches are used to remove remaining pulp from each of the exposed pulp horns. For most cheek teeth there are five pulp horns. For further discussion of numbers of pulp horns see Chapter 3: Anatomical characteristics of equine dentition. Disinfection and preparation of the canal are then done in the same fashion as in conventional root canal therapy. File length of 60 mm is usually sufficient. Radiographs should be taken to confirm various positions and landmarks. In surgical endodontic technique it is particularly important to flush the exposed tissue copiously with sterile saline to prevent tissue irritation from endodontic chemicals such as sodium hypochlorite and urea peroxidase.

Once the canals are prepared, sealing cement is placed and filling material is inserted. As the tooth undergoes attrition, it will wear to the level of the obturation material. If gutta percha is used, restorative should be placed in the same manner as with incisor treatment. The use of MTA alleviates these concerns.

If gutta percha is used, the access is closed with resin-reinforced glass ionomer. If MTA is used, the apex is sealed well with this product. Sharp edges of tooth are removed with a bur and the approach is closed.

FILING TECHNIQUES FOR CONVENTIONAL ENDODONTIC THERAPY

There are two basic canal preparation techniques that apply to equine endodontic treatment: the 'crown-down technique' and the 'step back technique'.

Crown-down technique

The crown-down technique begins at the access point and progresses apically. Initial determination of canal length with the smallest file available is followed by radiography to determine exact length and location of file tip. The file tip should be within 3–5 mm of the radiographic apex. This is the *working length*. If not correctly located or measured, the canal is flushed and debrided and the file advanced; measurement is taken until radiographs determine accurate placement. In canals that have PCO with tertiary dentin at the apex the length is more easily obtained. The importance in determining this length is in maintaining canal cleanliness and prevention of packing of dentinal shavings and debris into the apical canal while the canal is being prepared.

Filing begins at the coronal access with the largest file that fits into the canal opening and continues into the middle third of the canal. This assures that the coronal canal tapers to the diameter of the middle third. Canal preparation is continued with the next two larger files used coronally to create a smooth, tapered access. Recapitulation after each file use is imperative. Next, the middle third of the canal is prepared with the largest file that fits. The next larger file is used and the process repeated until clean shavings are removed. Gradually smaller files are used until the apex is reached. Irrigants, chelators, and disinfecting chemicals are used throughout the process. Once the canal shaping and debriding are completed, a radiograph is taken to determine the canal shape and confirm canal length. Obturation is performed in the conventional manner.

Chelators are used to help lubricate the canal. Sodium hypochlorite is instilled and left in place while filing for its ability to dissolve inorganic material and for its antibacterial effect. Irrigants are used to remove previously used chemicals.

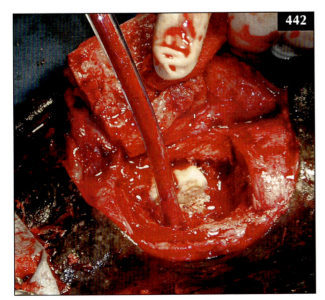

442 A surgical flap is created to allow access to a mandibular cheek tooth (308).

Step back technique

The step back technique begins at the apical terminus of the canal and progresses coronally. After access is created, the canal is flushed with sterile saline to remove debris. The smallest file is inserted into the canal and canal length is measured. Radiographs determine the accuracy of placement of the file and the location of the tip of the file. The next larger file is inserted and its length is measured. This process is continued until the largest file is found that completely enters the canal to its apex. This is the master file size and length. This file is used for recapitulation. The next larger file is used and recapitulated. This file should insert to within 2–3 mm of the length of the previous file. This process is continued until the apical portion of the canal is prepared. The middle third of the canal is prepared in a similar fashion. The difference is that only one or two file sizes are necessary. The coronal canal is prepared using gradually larger file sizes. Again, recapitulation is necessary after each file use. Once prepared, the canal is flushed with sterile saline and dried with paper points. Obturation is conventional.

FOLLOW-UP TO ROOT CANAL THERAPY

Radiographs should be taken at 6 and 12 months postoperatively to determine resolution of apical disease. Thereafter, radiographs at 12 month intervals are used to monitor the condition for recrudescence or new disease. Equine teeth must also be evaluated closely for occlusal exposure of obturation material. Some will require restorative placement.

COMPLICATIONS OF ROOT CANAL THERAPY

Short-term treatment failure is most commonly a result of inadequate debridement or insufficient apical seal. Clinical signs are recrudescence of original presenting problems. Treatment is repetition of conventional root canal therapy on incisors and canines. If this procedure fails, the next option is surgical endodontic treatment. Further failure indicates extraction. Treatment for failed surgical endodontic treatment of premolars and molars is extraction.

Canal perforation during filing is prevented by knowledge of pulp anatomy. Incisor canals have very little dentin on the mesial and distal aspects of the canal. Therefore, canal filing pressure is directed labially and lingually. Canal perforation can be treated with calcium hydroxide placement in the form of a solid cone or a paste. The use of MTA is also

appropriate to fill these areas. In some cases an intermediate restorative material (IRM®, Dentsply Caulk) is used. When this material is placed it is used as a temporary filling material that is replaced in 4–6 weeks. At this time, routine root canal therapy is performed.

Teeth fracture due to either incorrect use of condensers or spreaders or due to mastication forces. Endodontically treated teeth are more fragile than a normal tooth. It is important to maintain correct occlusal forces so that the treated tooth is not stressed by abnormally high occlusal forces. Eruption of these teeth is normal. Treatment of the fractured tooth following endodontic therapy is extraction.

Long-term treatment failure may result from coronal leakage when the restorative undergoes attrition with the remainder of the tooth and the underlying obturation material is exposed. This may also occur if restorative is lost prematurely. This condition is treated with either repeated endodontic therapy or replacement of restorative. Radiographic follow-up is critical.

THERAPY FOR VITAL PULPS

Vital pulp exposures are obvious (**443**). When iatrogenic, as a result of reduction of tooth overgrowth during occlusal equilibration, the duration of exposure is known. When the attending veterinary dentist is presented with a fractured tooth, the duration of exposure is not always known. Radiographs are necessary to determine degree of apical disease and thickness of dentinal deposition on the walls of the pulp canal. Initial radiographs provide data for comparison on follow-up radiographic examination. Vital pulps will continue to

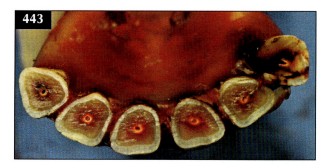

443 A cadaver specimen is prepared to demonstrate vital pulp exposures.

deposit dentin; inflamed vital pulps may deposit dentin at a rate more rapid than normal.

Vital pulps can be protected by various treatment protocols. Once diagnosed, radiographs should be taken initially to evaluate the condition of the apex and the amount of dentin deposition on the walls of the pulp canal. Follow-up radiographs should be taken at 3–6 month intervals to monitor apical health.

TREATMENT FOR DIRECT PULP EXPOSURE

The procedure for treatment of exposed vital pulps is called vital pulpotomy or direct pulp capping. Variations occur from patient to patient in the amount of pulp removed. As the duration of time of pulp exposure increases, such as in a fractured tooth versus an iatrogenic exposure, the amount of inflamed pulp increases. Slight variations in the technique may be found in literature, but the goal is preservation of the vitality of the pulp. Pulp vitality is necessary for further dentin deposition on the walls of the pulp canal and for maturation of the root apex. Both physiological processes contribute to the strength and longevity of the tooth. Stepwise treatment for direct pulp exposure includes:

1. Sedate and perform regional or infiltration anesthesia (see Chapter 11: Regional and local anesthesia).
2. Radiograph to determine degree of dentin deposition and character of root apex.
3. Flush mouth and disinfect local area with 0.12% chlorhexidine solution.
4. Follow sterile technique throughout procedure.
5. Remove 7–10 mm of inflamed or diseased pulp and create sufficient depth in the canal to retain materials used to seal the tooth:
   - Sterile round (No. 4 or No. 6) or diamond bur (No. 879).
   - Copious water or sterile saline to avoid heat necrosis.
6. Hemostasis is achieved with moistened sterile paper points, cotton pellets, or calcium hydroxide. Do not use air to dry the pulp as it may further dessicate the pulp and result in more inflammation. Hemorrhage that is not controlled in 5 minutes indicates inflamed pulp; an additional 1–2 mm of pulp is removed and hemostatic procedures are repeated as needed.
7. There are two options at this point. A temporary filling may be placed if the pulp exposure is diagnosed in the field. If diagnosed in the hospital, a permanent treatment is performed.

When temporary treatment is applied, permanent filling should follow as soon as possible.

- **Temporary procedure:** IRM®, a reinforced zinc oxide/eugenol temporary filling material may be placed on the site. This material self cures. Follow manufacturer's directions. Another useful material is Cavit G® (3M ESPE). This is a resin-based, fiber-reinforced, self-curing composite. The surface is smoothed and sealed with dentin bonding agent. The permanent filling procedure is scheduled.
- **Permanent procedure:**
  (i) The IRM paste is removed to a depth of 3 mm with a high-speed bur.
  (ii) Calcium hydroxide may be chosen to use on a continuously bleeding site and is placed on the remaining pulp. It is a very basic (high pH) substance that accelerates tertiary dentin formation. This forms a dentin bridge. It is not necessary to use this material to stimulate production of tertiary dentin, as the signal for tertiary dentin production is sent to odontoblasts by the process of crown reduction.
  (iii) Access site is undercut to improve mechanical retention with a No. 35 or No. 37 bur.
  (iv) Glass ionomer is placed over the top of the calcium hydroxide. An intermediate layer protects the calcium hydroxide and provides a base for the final restorative. An example of a self-curing resin-reinforced glass ionomer is Ionosit® Microspand® (Zenith/DMG).
  (v) The access site is etched with 37% phosphoric acid.
  (vi) A layer of dentin bonding agent is placed and light cured.
  (vii) Composite resin is used to restore the access site to occlusal level.
  (viii) The access site is sealed with a final layer of dentin bonding agent. This prevents microleakage by enhancing the marginal seal.
  (ix) Antibiotic therapy is instituted as needed.
8. Alternative technique: the use of MTA may be substituted to fill the entire cavity after sufficient pulp is removed and hemostasis is achieved.
9. Follow-up radiographic evaluation is performed at 3–6 month intervals to monitor pulp vitality by dentin deposition in the pulp canal.

Failures occur as a result of any of the following:
- Severe trauma of the initial insult, or irreversible inflammation resulting in pulp death.
- Heat necrosis from insufficient water cooling during the procedure.
- Bacterial contamination at the time of the initial fracture, procedure, or inadequate seal of restorative.

TREATMENT FOR INDIRECT PULP EXPOSURE

When dentinal tubules are opened and the site is within 3 mm of the pulp, bacterial contamination of the pulp can cause pulpitis. The most common cause of indirect pulp exposure is iatrogenic in reduction of overlong teeth. An example is in incisor reductions. In such cases, application of three successive layers of dentin bonding agent and light curing each layer provides adequate protection of the pulp.

SUMMARY

Pulp conditions of equines have many similarities to those of brachydont patients, and many significant differences. Understanding equine endodontics begins with a basic knowledge of endodontics as applied to brachydont species. After gaining basic knowledge, principles are applied to the equine patient and differences observed in pathology and treatment are considered. Further understanding is gained as materials and techniques are adapted to fit the equine patient.

REFERENCES

1. Emily P. Endodontic diagnosis in the dog. *The Veterinary Clinics of North America: Small Animal Practice* 1998: **28**(5); 1189–1202.
2. Torneck CD. Dentin-pulp complex. In: Ten Cate AR (ed) *Oral Histology: Development, Structure and Function*. St. Louis: Mosby, 1998; pp. 150–196.
3. Lyon K. Endodontic anatomy and diagnosis in the veterinary patient. *26th Small Animal Veterinary Association World Congress Proceedings* 2001.
4. Avery JK. Dental pulp. In: Avery JK (ed) *Essentials of Oral Histology and Embryology*. St. Louis: Mosby, 2000; p. 108.
5. Kirkland KD, Baker GJ, Marretta SM, *et al*. Effects of aging on the endodontic system, reserve crown, and roots of equine mandibular cheek teeth. *American Journal of Veterinary Radiology* 1996: **57**(1); 31–38.
6. Gasse H, Westenberger E, Staszyk C. The endodontic system of equine teeth: a re-examination of pulp horns and root canals in view of age-related physiological differences. *Pferdeheilkunde* 2004: **20**; 13–18.
7. Wiggs RB, Lobprise HB. *Veterinary Dentistry: Principles and Practice*. Philadelphia: Lippincott-Raven, 1997; pp. 281–324.
8. Trowbridge H, Kim S, Suda H. Structure and functions of the dentin and pulp complex. In: Cohen S, Burns RC (eds) *Pathways of the Pulp*. St. Louis: Mosby, 2002; pp. 411–455.
9. Dacre IT. Equine dental pathology. In: Baker GJ, Easley J (eds) *Equine Dentistry*. Edinburgh: Elsevier Saunders, 2005; pp. 91–110.
10. Harvey CE, Emily PP. *Small Animal Dentistry*. St. Louis: Mosby, 1993; pp. 156–212.
11. Dacre IT. Fractures and apical abscesses of equine cheek teeth. *Conference Proceedings 18th Annual Veterinary Dental Forum*, 2004.
12. Cohen AS, Brown DC. Orofacial dental pain emergencies: endodontic diagnosis and management. In: Cohen S, Burns RC (eds) *Pathways of the Pulp*. St. Louis: Mosby, 2002; pp. 31–75.
13. DeBowes L. The effects of dental disease on systemic disease. *The Veterinary Clinics of North America: Small Animal Practice* 1998: **28**(5); 1057–1062.
14. Spangberg L. Instruments, materials, and devices. In: Cohen S, Burns RC (eds) *Pathways of the Pulp*. St. Louis: Mosby, 2002; pp. 521–572.
15. Gutta percha. *The Columbia Encyclopedia*, 6th edition. New York: Columbia University Press, 2005, 2001–2004. www.bartleby.com/65/.
16. Baker GJ. Endodontic therapy. In: Baker GJ, Easley J (eds) *Equine Dentistry*. Edinburgh: Elsevier Saunders, 2005; pp. 295–302.

PRINCIPLES OF ORTHODONTICS
David O Klugh and Robert B Wiggs   Chapter 18

Orthodontics is the branch of dentistry addressing alignment and occlusion of teeth. The American Dental Association[1] defines orthodontics as the area of dentistry concerned with the supervision and guidance of the growing dentition and correction of mature dentofacial structures. Included are conditions requiring movement of teeth, correction of abnormal relationships of jaws and teeth and malformations of their related structures. It is clear that orthodontics in all species addresses conditions primarily in young, growing individuals.

Orthodontics in equine dentistry includes several principles and their various effects and conditions seen on a routine basis by the practitioner. Since orthodontics deals with exfoliation of deciduous teeth and eruption of adult teeth in correct order and position, knowledge of the physiological processes of deciduous tooth loss and of the eruption process is important. Since orthodontics addresses conditions of young horses, knowledge of the process of bone growth is also necessary. It is vital to understand how the PDL and alveolar bone respond to forces sensed. The biomechanics of mastication play a central role in orthodontics. The interaction of mastication forces, PDL function, and bone growth is only just beginning to be understood. Further elucidation of how abnormal forces and motions create malocclusions and prevent their correction is necessary. The first step is to classify malocclusions.

CLASSIFICATION OF OCCLUSION AND MALOCCLUSION

Malocclusions can be classified utilizing the same methods as in other species. Wiggs[2] describes the following classifications of normal equine occlusion and malocclusion:

Before attempting to assess an animal's occlusion or malocclusion, a basic understanding of normals for species, as well as the nature of malocclusions is necessary. The horse's normal occlusion is identified by multiple factors:

- The jaws should be of similar length (neutrognathic), but the lower jaw in the cheek tooth area should be slightly narrower than the upper jaws (anisognathic).
- The upper (maxillary) incisors should meet the lower (mandibular) incisors, facial incisal edge to facial incisal edge in a basic 'level bite'.
- If the canine, tush, or cuspid teeth are present, the lower canine teeth should be positioned midway between the upper canine and corner incisor when the mouth is closed.
- With the anisognathic relationship of the jaws, the lingual cusps of the upper premolar and molar arcade should be seated just on top of the buccal or facial cusps of the lower premolar and molar tooth arcade. This means, when the mouth is in occlusion and related in centric relationship, the facial or buccal cusps of the upper cheek teeth and the lingual cusps of the lower cheek teeth are not in occlusal contact.
- The maxillary and mandibular cheek tooth arcades should be almost exactly the same length and fully occlude without teeth or portions of teeth failing to occlude or make contact with their counterparts.

In the equine patient, normal occlusion can also be evaluated from a functional standpoint. With the cheek retracted, the upper and lower cheek teeth arcades can be evaluated for the following characteristics:
- The occlusal surfaces should be even, though not flat, back to the curvature of Spee.
  - The overlong teeth can be identified.
  - The amount of tooth that is too long can be estimated.

- The occlusal surfaces of both arcades should be parallel.
- The occlusal angle should be about 15°.
- When moving the teeth into contact, all teeth should contact at the same time.
- The lateral margin of the lower arcade should contact the occlusal surface of the maxillary arcade at approximately half to two-thirds the distance across the surface. This is referred to as the POC.

Further discussion of these principles is found in Chapter 6: Principles of mastication biomechanics.

After termination of occlusal treatment, the above parameters should be evaluated and should be the same as prior to treatment. This maintains the delivery of forces during mastication. The procedure is referred to as occlusal equilibration.

Classification of malocclusions as defined by Angle[3] and adapted for use in veterinary carnivores by Wiggs and Lobprise[4] can be used for equines. Class 0 is normal occlusion. Class I, or neutroclusion, has both jaws of proper length with teeth in a normal mesiodistal relationship, but with faciolingual alterations. Examples include crowded or rotated teeth. Class II malocclusions are defined as mandibular teeth occluding distally in relationship to the maxillary teeth. Class III malocclusions are defined as mandibular teeth occluding mesially to the maxillary teeth. Class IV includes special malocclusions where one jaw occludes mesially and another occludes distally.

The following is Wiggs' modification[2] of Angle's orthodontic classification system including equines:

BASIC VETERINARY OCCLUSAL CLASSIFICATION

Class 0: Normal (orthoclusion and neutrognathia)

Category or type:
- Normal – brachydont (anterior scissor-type bite) (most omnivores and carnivores).
- Normal – hypsodont (anterior level-type bite) (equine)
- Normal class III occlusion (breed normal prognathia, i.e. the Boxer, Bulldog, and so on).

Class I (neutroclusion or neutrognathia)
- Both jaws in approximately proper length relationship to each other (neutrognathia).

- The neck portion of the tooth is in a normal mesiodistal location (neutroclusion), except in areas where a diastema or tooth void in the arcade exists.
- Teeth may be in any form of version or tilt.
- Teeth may be in any form of intrusion or extrusion.
- In areas of a diastema, teeth may move into the void area and be in a mesial or distal location to their normal expected position in the dental arch.

Class I – division I (neutroclusion and neutrognathia)

Category or type:
- Anterior crossbite (labial or lingual). Minor labial anterior crossbite will appear somewhat similar to a parrot mouth, with the exception that the jaw is neutrognathic rather than distognathic as seen in true parrot mouth.
- Posterior crossbite in a neutrognathic mouth.
- Facial cuspids (base wide canines) in a neutroclusion mouth.
- Lingual cuspids (base narrow canines) in a neutroclusion mouth.
- Crowded or rotated teeth in a neutroclusion mouth.
- Extruded or intruded teeth in a neutroclusion mouth.
- Certain partial level bites in a neutroclusion mouth.
- Waves in a neutroclusion mouth.
- Steps in a neutroclusion mouth.
- Ventral curvature in a neutroclusion mouth.
- Sheared occlusion in a neutroclusion mouth.
- Dorsal curvature in a neutroclusion mouth.
- Diagonal incisors in a neutroclusion mouth.
- Hooks or ramps in a neutroclusion mouth.

Class I – division II (neutrognathia)
In this division of class I, both jaws are approximately proper length (neutrognathia), while individual teeth may be in mesioversion or distoversion, typically associated with a diastema or area void of teeth for some reason. Some cases may have familial or genetic tendencies.

Category or type:
- Mesioversion:
  - Mesioversion (rostroversion) of the crowns of the maxillary cuspids (upper or

maxillary lanced canine) into the maxillary diastema.
- Mesioversion (rostroversion) of the crowns of mandibular cuspids (lower or mandibular lanced canine). Generally causes disruption of the occlusion of the incisors in the area, and may be associated with maxillary lanced canine teeth. When seen with wry mouth, the condition belongs in either class II or III classification.
- Mesioversion (rostroversion) of the upper or lower first cheek tooth resulting in a hook formation on the front of the cheek tooth arcade. Seen in animals with hypsodont teeth.
- Distoversion:
  - Distoclusion of the crowns of the maxillary cuspid (snake teeth) as the roots of the teeth are allowed to move into the tissues below the maxillary diastema.
  - Distoclusion of the crowns of the mandibular cuspid. Typically associated with mesioclusion of the upper cuspid.
  - Distoversion of the upper or lower last cheek tooth (molar) resulting in a hook formed on the last tooth in the arcade. Seen in animals with hypsodont teeth.
- Mesiodistoversion combination: for example, mesioversion (rostroversion) of the upper or lower first cheek tooth and distoversion of the upper or lower last cheek tooth (molar) resulting in a hook or ramp formed at both ends of the arcade. Seen in animals with hypsodont teeth.

Class II (distoclusion and distognathia)

Virtually all of the occlusal conditions seen in class I may also be found in class II, but in association with distoclusion and distognathia. Categories or type (parrot mouth):
- Short mandible – mandibular brachygnathism:
  - Mandibular retrognathism.
  - Mandibular retrusion.
  - Mandibular brachygnathism hooks (anterior, posterior or combined).
  - Unilateral (wry bite).
- Long maxilla – maxillary prognathism:
  - Maxillary protrusion.
  - Maxillary prognathism with hook formation (anterior, posterior, or combined).
  - Unilateral (wry bite).

Class III (mesioclusion and mesiognathia)

Virtually all of the occlusal conditions seen in class I may also be found in class III, but in association with mesioclusion and mesiognathia).
Category or type (sow mouth, monkey mouth, bulldog mouth):
- Long mandible – mandibular prognathism:
  - Mandibular protrusion.
  - Level bite.
  - Mandibular prognathism with hook or ramp formation (anterior, posterior, or combined).
  - Unilateral (wry bite).
- Short maxilla – maxillary brachygnathia and brachycephalics:
  - Maxillary retrusion.
  - Maxillary retraction, maxillary brachygnathia with hook or ramp formation (anterior, posterior, or combined).
  - Level bite.
  - Unilateral (wry bite).

Class IV (mesiodistoclusion)

This is a special classification of wry bite in which one jaw is in mesioclusion and the another in distoclusion.

ETIOLOGY OF MALOCCLUSION

Orthodontic abnormalities can be either developmental or acquired. Developmental problems can be congenital, but are not necessarily genetic. When genetic orthodontic conditions are encountered, counseling of the owner regarding its origins is indicated. Treatment of the affected individual is necessary in all cases where the health of the individual is compromised. Ethical standards of veterinary and breed associations must be followed.

Acquired malocclusions involving uneven occlusal surfaces, such as hooks and waves, are, by definition, malocclusions. Their development and treatment is discussed in depth in Chapter 7: Principles of occlusal equilibration. Periodontal structures respond to forces of mastication. These forces change with hardness of feedstuffs. Correspondingly, the range of motion of the mandible also changes with hardness of feeds. Both concepts are interwoven in their effects on dental eruption and attrition.

DECIDUOUS EXFOLIATION

Exfoliation of deciduous teeth is a complex process. It is not the result of an inflammatory process, but involves resorption of hard tissues and cessation of activity of periodontal and pulpal tissues.

Resorption of dentin in the apices of deciduous teeth occurs by odontoclastic breakdown. Osteoclasts are derived from blood-borne mononuclear cells. Fibroblasts of the PDL appear to either cease the normal collagen secretory mechanism or undergo apoptosis. In either case, the histological appearance is abrupt cessation of activity, with limited inflammatory response present.

Pressure from the erupting permanent tooth plays a role and in cases where the adult tooth is missing, exfoliation is delayed. However, the fact that root resorption occurs in such cases shows that it is a preprogrammed, genetically encoded process.

Occlusal pressure also assists in initiating and promoting resorption. As root structure and PDL attachment are lost, mastication forces delivered to a slightly loose tooth further promote resorption of the support tissues and exfoliation is exacerbated.

The adult incisor tooth bud develops lingually in relation to the deciduous tooth. Eruption involves migration of the adult tooth facially and occlusally. The adult premolar and molar tooth bud develops directly under the deciduous tooth.

PHYSIOLOGY OF BONE GROWTH

The mandible grows in length and thickness by appositional bone growth of the periosteum. It grows in height at the ramus by endochondral growth at the condylar epiphysis. The location and direction of growth are shown in figure **444**. Appositional growth on the posterior surface of the mandible and remodeling of the anterior surface of the ramus of the mandible account for its increase in length. This change in length is so significant that the relative position of the posterior border of the newborn mandibular ramus becomes the relative position of the anterior border in the adult. A smaller amount of growth occurs on the ventral border of the mandible.[5]

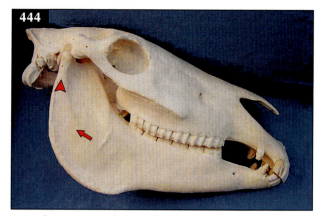

444 The arrow indicates the direction of mandibular growth in length. The arrowhead indicates the location at the condyle of growth in height of the mandible.

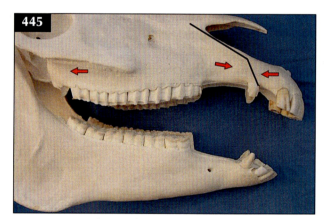

445 Arrows indicate direction and magnitude of growth of the maxillary arcade. Minor growth in length occurs at the suture line between the incisive bone and the maxilla. Major growth in length occurs at the maxillary tuberosity.

The upper dental arcades are positioned in two separate bones. The incisors are in the incisive bone and the cheek teeth and canines are in the maxilla. Both bones grow in length, width, and thickness by appositional growth. The incisive bone and maxilla increase in length by appositional growth at the suture line connecting the two bones. These sites are shown in figure **445**. The maxilla also grows in length at the posterior suture line and by the addition of new bone at the distal tuberosity where the molars develop. The width of the skull increases by appositional growth at suture lines.

PHYSIOLOGY OF TOOTH MOVEMENT

The basic principle of orthodontic therapy is that prolonged pressure applied to a tooth results in its movement. Part of the process involves remodeling of bone. As the tooth moves through the bone it carries with it its attachment apparatus. In short, the socket moves. Cells derived from the PDL mediate the bony response. Movement is primarily a function of the PDL.

Alveolar bone is unique in that it responds to even slight pressure change. It may undergo resorption or deposition, depending on the nature and direction of the forces. Changes occur in both cortical and cancellous bone. Bone remodeling develops that most efficiently withstands the forces acting on it. The result is a structure comprised of the minimal amount of bone needed to support the teeth. The response of bone to forces is described as 'Wolff's law of bone transformation'.[6]

The histological response depends on the degree, direction, and duration of force applied. Light forces not exceeding capillary blood pressure result in frontal resorption through the following effects:

1. Blood flow through the compressed PDL decreases within minutes.
2. In hours the chemical environment changes and a different pattern of cellular activity is produced.
3. Cyclic adenosine monophosphate (AMP) production is increased after about 4 hours. Cyclic AMP is important in cellular differentiation.
4. Osteoclasts develop from monocytes already in the PDL within 36–72 hours.
5. The result is frontal resorption, or resorption of the 'PDL' surface of the alveolar socket.

When the force is heavy, a different series of events occurs:

1. The PDL is compressed, resulting in tissue ischemia and necrosis.
2. In areas of the PDL adjacent to the compressed tissue, cells are transformed and migrate to begin the process of bone remodeling.
3. This results in a delay of the remodeling process for several days.
4. Osteoclasts resorb bone on the borders of the necrotic area and on the medullary side of the alveolar socket. Hence the term 'undermining resorption'.

5. Tooth movement is delayed because:
   i. Chemical stimulus must cross alveolar bone.
   ii. Remodeling of bone must occur from the medullary side, thus the bone is considerably thicker.
   iii. It is painful.

In actual practice, both events occur in orthodontic movement of brachydont teeth. Many factors contribute to variation in rate of movement, including patient growth, type of appliance, and materials used. The scope of this area of orthodontics is beyond this manuscript.

Orthodontic forces can have deleterious effects on teeth. The pulp undergoes varying degrees of inflammation. Heavy forces can cause permanent damage to the apical structures. Cementum and dentin of the root are remodeled as the tooth moves.

In equine dentistry, this may explain in part the development of 'cemental pearls'. A combination of eruptive movement and response to mastication forces may cause remodeling of apical cementum and dentin as the 10s and 11s rotate slightly in their eruptive pattern.

Prolonged heavy forces result in bony adaptation. These forces occur in equine dentistry and result in alveolar sclerosis and ankylosis.

COMMON ORTHODONTIC PROBLEMS OF EQUINES

Several orthodontic problems occur in equines. Most are recognized in young patients, and are best treated in the young, growing patient. Some can be corrected, while others such as genetic dwarfism and related class III malocclusions are not correctable. Many class II malocclusions can be improved to have incisor contact, though cosmetic perfection may not be achieved. Abnormally erupting adult teeth, especially incisors, are addressed as orthodontic problems.

It is also worthwhile to understand the orthodontic effects on teeth of mastication forces. These forces may cause conditions such as tooth shifting and alveolar sclerosis.

CLASS II MALOCCLUSIONS (PARROT MOUTH, OVERBITE)

Class II malocclusions are defined as mandibular teeth occluding distally in relationship to the maxillary teeth and are presented as developmental abnormalities in young foals. A typical presentation is shown in figure **446**. Some cases are presented at birth, while others develop in the first few weeks of life. The malocclusion varies in severity, with some cases having slightly offset incisors and more severe cases having 2–3 cm of space between the lingual margin of the upper incisors and the labial margin of the lowers. Some cases have normal occlusion of the premolars, while others have mandibular premolars in distocclusion. Mandibular brachygnathism is assumed to be the most common presentation, but maxillary prognathism can also occur. Without cephalometric studies in the equine, definitive diagnosis is not possible.

Etiology of class II malocclusions involves expression of multiple genes. Conformation of both parents and their respective proclivity to pass on certain genes play a large role. It is most likely the result of mating parents with differing head conformations. Mating horses with abnormalities is a concern to all in the breeding business. Any defect in the parents can be reproduced in offspring. When presented with a foal with a class II malocclusion, the attending veterinarian is frequently asked about the likelihood of reproduction of this abnormality in a future breeding of the mare or stallion or the affected individual. Breeding horses with any abnormality will ultimately increase the incidence of that condition within the population over time. However, the contribution by a single individual will vary with the frequency of his or her use for breeding. The likelihood of an individual producing additional offspring affected with a condition whose etiology involves multiple genes is reduced by mating to partners that are unrelated to the producer of the animal with the defect. It is wise to avoid repeating a mating that produces a defective offspring.

A clinical feature of many class II malocclusions is the presence of a ventrally deviated incisive bone (**447**). As previously noted, many cases also have malalignment of premolar teeth, with the maxillary teeth positioned mesially to their mandibular counterparts. The result is development of tooth overgrowths in nonoccluding incisors and cheek teeth. Overlong teeth produce dental interlock and restrict the motion and growth of the mandible. One primary goal of treatment is the removal of dental interlock and the re-establishment of normal mastication range of motion.

Failure to address this condition results in permanent ventral deviation of the incisive bone and upper incisors and in the development of dental overgrowths on the first upper cheek tooth and the last lower cheek tooth. These elongated teeth can

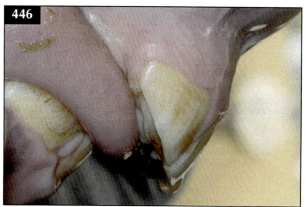

446 A typical presentation of a class II malocclusion in a young foal.

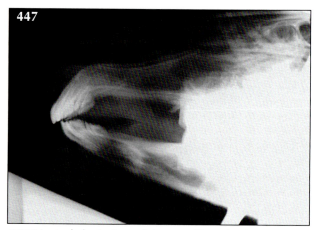

447 Ventral deviation of the maxillary incisors is demonstrated in this radiograph. Slight malalignment of the premolars is also evident.

impact on the range of motion of mastication and can cause trauma to the soft tissue of the opposing arcade. Soft tissue injury can result in significant complications for the patient, including local infection and periodontal disease manifest as chewing or bitting pain.

Objective consideration of therapeutic goals is important. The first consideration in any patient of any age or degree of severity is to maximize the remaining growth potential of the mandible. This may result only in minor improvement in the condition as the patient increases in age. The older the patient is when presented for treatment, the less the condition can be corrected. Reduction of the dental overgrowths allows the mandible to grow normally in patients with reduced but functional incisor occlusion.

The second consideration is the function of the incisors. It is unreasonable to expect normal occlusion of the incisors and cosmetic perfection in all cases. A more reasonable expectation would be to gain some incisor contact, even if it is only one set of teeth. The importance of this distinction is in the maintenance of normal position of the incisive bone and the prevention of the severe dental interlock that results from its ventral deviation.

Treatment in mild cases is regular occlusal equilibration (**448**, **449**). In more severe cases, treatments have included removable bite planes[7], nonremovable bite planes[2] combined with wiring techniques, and wiring techniques alone.[8] These treatments are used in combination with regular occlusal equilibration. All require general anesthesia and some require buccotomy. Risks of complication[7] include wire breakage, soft tissue trauma, mesial displacement of the second premolar, and therapeutic failure.

Nonremovable bite planes can be placed on standing sedated patients.[9] Following the initial treatment, regular occlusal equilibration to maintain optimal occlusion is critical for the long-term health of the animal. Odontoplasty of occlusal abnormalities as the patient matures is performed as needed. Deciduous teeth erupt normally and exfoliate and adult teeth erupt freely.

The bite plane in figure **450** provides a surface for the occlusal forces to be directed such that the incisive bone is maintained in a normal anatomical position. This creates a free range of motion for the mandible so the mandible achieves normal growth potential.

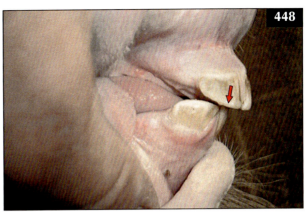

448 A mild class II malocclusion in a young foal. The arrow indicates the rostral limit of occlusion.

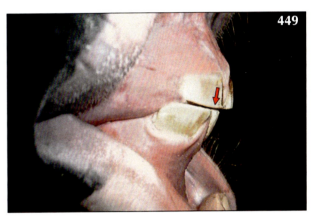

449 After routine occlusal equilibration the rostral limit of occlusion has moved the distance of about half a tooth width (arrow).

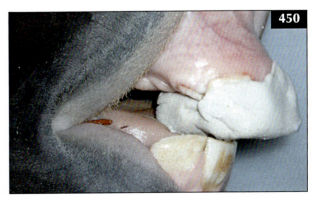

450 The bite plane extends caudally to allow for contact of the lower incisors. It is angled rostrally to encourage active mandibular protrusion. The contact surface is narrowed to allow the third incisors a clear eruptive path.

An additional benefit of the bite plane is that the beveled occlusal surface forces the mandible to slide rostrally during mastication. Rostral movement (protrusion) of the mandible is caused in part by contraction of the lateral pterygoid muscle. Active protrusion of the mandible may be a key to the stimulation of growth.[10]

Wiring techniques that encircle the first or second cheek teeth and the incisors only restrict growth at the anterior suture line. Growth also occurs at the posterior suture line and the distal tuberosity, thus translating the maxilla rostrally in spatial relation to the cranial base. The wiring technique would not be expected to provide sufficient restriction of growth to result in normal incisor alignment. Without restriction of ventral deviation of the premaxilla wiring does not completely address the concept of dental interlock, and may exacerbate it as tension forces pull the incisive bone ventrally.

The following excerpt describes the placement of a bite plane in a standing sedated patient:[9]

Sedation was achieved with intravenous injection of detomidine at 0.02 mg/kg[11] in combination with xylazine at 0.2 mg/kg.[11] After 5 minutes additional xylazine at 0.2 mg/kg together with butorphanol at 0.01 mg/kg[12] was administered.

A full mouth speculum was inserted using gum plates instead of bite plates.

The mouth was rinsed with 0.2% chlorhexidine solution.

After the patient was sedated, routine occlusal equilibration was performed.[13]

Initially the caudal ramps on the mandibular fourth premolars (708 and 808) were removed by the use of a rotary grinder and carbide grit barrel-shaped bur with a water-irrigated extended handpiece attachment. Subsequently the occlusal tables were reduced to an evenly equilibrated level with the use of hand floats, with solid cut carbide steel blades. This step in the procedure also served to reduce the hooks on the maxillary second premolars (506 and 606). The mesial borders of the upper and lower second premolars were rounded. This was done with a carbide grit 'hourglass-shaped' bur. The lingual edges of the lower and the buccal edges of the upper cheek teeth were rounded and their enamel points removed with hand floats and solid cut carbide steel blades. The upper and lower incisors were leveled with a diamond wheel. The occlusion was checked to ensure that all arcades were in full free range of motion and occlusion of the cheek teeth was even and balanced.

The upper incisors were prepared for placement of the acrylic plate. Since the presence of cementum surrounding the tooth precludes adequate bonding, the cementum was removed. A grit bur was used for this purpose.

The enamel surface was acid-etched with 37% phosphoric acid for 30 seconds and rinsed with water for 30 seconds. A bonding agent/adhesive was applied and light-cured for 30 seconds. Dental acrylic was then mixed and applied to the upper incisors, forming a bite plane for occlusion of the lower incisors. The bite plane covered the labial surface and the occlusal surface of the incisors, and extended along the palate far enough so that the lower incisors could contact it during normal mastication. The occlusal surface of the plane was beveled so that the force of mastication of the lower incisors would allow the mandible to slide rostrally during mastication. This procedure assisted in maximizing normal occlusion of the erupting teeth.

CLASS III MALOCCLUSIONS (SOW MOUTH, MONKEY MOUTH, UNDERBITE)

Class III malocclusions, such as the one in figure **451**, are presented as patients of all ages. Many are presented as foals. Some are inherited, as in the achondroplastic dwarf of miniature horses. Individuals of other breeds may also be presented as foals

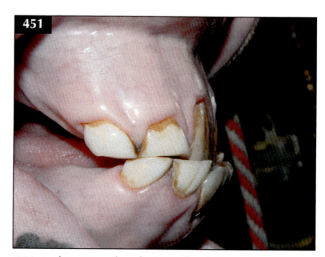

451 A class III malocclusion of mild severity.

with class III malocclusions. The degree of severity of the condition varies with individual and with age. In miniatures displaying the dwarf gene, the condition becomes progressively worse as the foal ages. Once the foal reaches a mature adult age, the occlusal disparity has reached its maximum. It is important to note that not all miniature foals presented with a mild class III malocclusion are genetically affected. As with individuals of other breeds, certain individual miniature horses have the congenital condition, but are not necessarily genetically affected.

Aside from the genetics of achondroplastic dwarfism, the etiology of the class III malocclusions is developmental. If properly addressed, most of these individuals can be dramatically improved and even corrected. Figures **452–454** demonstrate a case of congenital class III maloscclusion that is corrected as an adult. Treatment included regular occlusal equilibration and application of a bite plane as a foal.

A condition of congenital hypothyroidism exists where foals are born with class III malocclusions along with other skeletal abnormalities associated with dysmaturity.[14] These foals were born to mares who had received a diet high in nitrates, causing impairment of thyroid function.

Class III malocclusions develop complications of mastication and bitting as a result of overgrowth of unopposed teeth. As with most malocclusions, failure to address the problem results in progressive worsening of the condition. The dental interlock that develops is similar to that of other conditions. The effects of dental interlock are also the same, in that normal range of motion of the mandible is restricted. Incomplete occlusion can also result in incomplete mastication of feedstuffs. Left uncorrected, individuals that are not genetically affected can suffer impairment of growth of the maxilla from dental interlock.

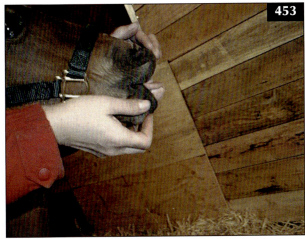

453 The degree of severity of the class III malocclusion in figure **452**. Note the 2 cm disparity in incisor arcade occlusion.

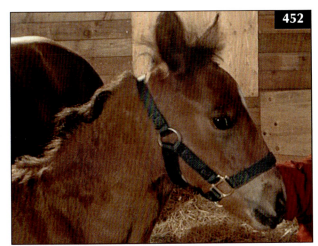

452 A 3-week-old foal with a class III malocclusion. No dished face is evident.

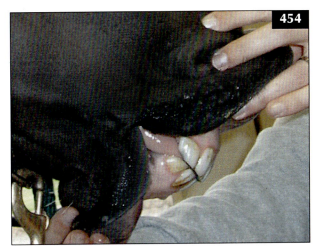

454 The patient with class III malocclusion shown in figures **452**, **453** is shown as an adult with normal occlusion.

In patients with class III malocclusion, whether genetic or developmental, lack of occlusion of the mandibular incisors can result in the appearance of a dorsally curved mandible. This characteristic is evident in the radiograph in figure **455**. This is a result of eruptive migration of incisors carrying the gingiva with them. Migration of gingiva is a result of lack of occlusion. A bite plane in combination with minor dental reduction serves to correct this condition. Placement of the bite plane is demonstrated in figure **456**.

Malocclusions that develop include overlong upper and lower incisors, ramps on lower second premolars, and, in some cases, hooks on upper distal molars. Left unattended, these elongated teeth can directly traumatize the opposing arcade in addition to the previously mentioned impairment of mastication. Secondary conditions include periodontal disease, tooth shifting, and localized infection manifest as pain in chewing or bitting.

Goals of treatment are similar to those of all malocclusions. Removal of obstacles to normal mastication motion is primary. Reduction of overlong teeth also prevents soft tissue damage, local infection, and periodontal disease. Correction of occlusal forces assists in prevention of tooth shifting. An example of the degree of correction of occlusion possible with simple occlusal equilibration is shown in figures **457** and **458**.

Treatment of this condition begins with occlusal equilibration. Overlong teeth are reduced and sharp points and edges are smoothed. In some cases a bite plane may be placed on lower incisors in the same manner as with class II malocclusions.

Radiographs assist in monitoring correction of this condition and diagnosing a potentially genetically affected individual. In dwarfs, the suture line between the maxilla and frontal bone becomes sclerosed and eventually ankylosed. In those not affected by the dwarf gene, this suture line remains normal. Sequential radiographs of young foals provide the necessary information.

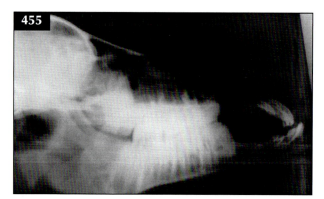

455 The radiograph shows the appearance of dorsal deviation of the incisors and rostral mandible in a class III malocclusion.

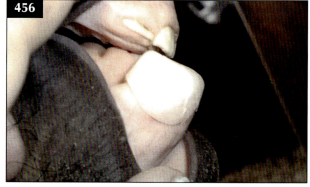

456 Placement of a bite plane on mandibular incisors assists in correcting incisor occlusion in some cases.

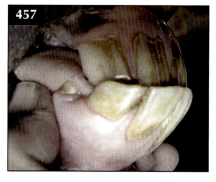

457 A class III malocclusion in an adult miniature horse shows minimal occlusion of the incisors prior to treatment.

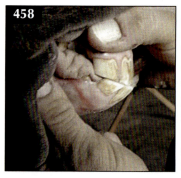

458 The class III malocclusion from figure **457** is improved. Incisor contact is now present after reduction of lower 6 ramps, upper steps, and correction of incisor abnormalities.

CROWDED INCISORS

Individuals of all breeds and especially miniature horses have varying degrees of incisor crowding. The result frequently involves abnormally positioned erupting adult teeth. The etiology is likely one of two pathways: the adult tooth bud may be embryologically positioned inappropriately; or the tooth bud may be positioned within the bone in a correct position; however, due to crowding of multiple teeth in a small space, bone growth results in correct movement of other teeth, while the affected tooth is left in its abnormal position. Support for this theory lies in the fact that most cases in miniature horses involve the third incisor. An example of incisor crowding is shown in figure **459**.

Failure to treat this condition may result in pain in an individual if the deciduous tooth becomes loose. If the deciduous tooth is not removed, it may be delayed in exfoliation for several years. Resulting incorrect occlusion can lead to dental interlock and its associated problems.

Goals of treatment include removal of the deciduous tooth and correction of the malocclusion by correctly repositioning the adult tooth. Many cases require interproximal reduction of nearby teeth to provide a space into which the abnormal tooth can move. Little is required in the way of orthodontic appliance. Abnormally positioned teeth 'want to go home'. Treatment of this condition is shown in figure **460**.

Treatment begins with submucosal infiltration anesthesia of the deciduous tooth. Many of these teeth can be removed by routine elevation and extraction. Others require surgical flap elevation with removal of alveolar bone for extraction. An example of a tooth removed via creation of a gingival flap and alveolar osteotmy is shown in figures **461** and **462**. Interproximal reduction can be done on necessary teeth in order to provide enough room for the malpositioned adult tooth.

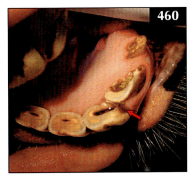

460 After removal of the deciduous tooth and interproximal reduction (arrow) of the 402, the 403 erupts and moves into normal position.

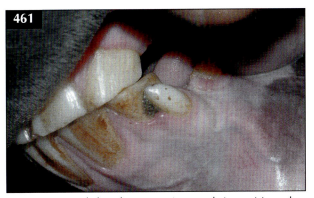

461 A retained deciduous canine tooth is positioned adjacent to the third incisor. The interproximal space retains feed material resulting in periodontal disease. The patient was exhibiting bitting resistance. After extraction, the condition improved.

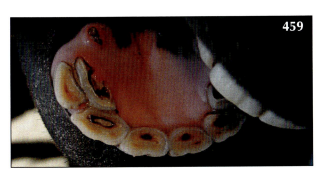

459 Crowded incisors result in malposition of the adult tooth.

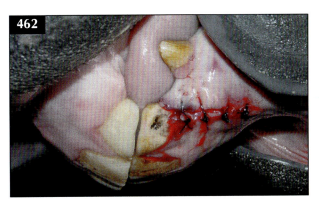

462 The flap necessary for removal of the offending tooth is closed.

EFFECTS ON DENTITION OF ORTHODONTIC FORCES

Orthodontic forces identified and managed in brachydont dentistry have effects in equine dental conditions. Some of these effects are detrimental to the longevity of the arcades and can therefore have unfavorable effects on the health of the patient.

INTERRUPTION OF MESIAL DRIFT

In horses and in man, but not in dogs and cats, it is normal for the distal teeth in the arcades to drift mesially over time. Forces that play roles in mesial drift include the elastic trans-septal fibers of the PDL, the eruptive direction and force of the teeth, and the movement of the tongue to some degree. Trans-septal fibers hold teeth together. Eruption of teeth located distally in the arcade is directed mesially. The second premolar is angled distally and serves as a 'retaining wall' against which the other teeth force themselves (**463**). The tight-fitting battery is thus maintained.

Aging-related changes in these forces dramatically affect mesial drift. As patients age, the trans-septal fibers are reduced in number and size. Aged horses have less eruptive potential in their teeth. Geriatric patients have little if any eruptive potential, thus reducing the ability to correct both the amount and direction of eruption. Tongue and other soft tissue movements are known to affect tooth position in human dentistry and may also affect equine dental position and movement.

Forces can be modified as malocclusions develop. Overlong teeth can either shift or cause other teeth to shift. They can also limit the normal movement of opposing and proximal teeth. One of the primary goals of occlusal equilibration, and a reason for the use of the term, is to maintain normal relationships of occlusal forces. Results of abnormal occlusal forces include enlargement of interproximal spaces, or 'diastema' formation. Additonally, shifting teeth may undergo increased interproximal wear. Both conditions are apparent in figure **464**. Diastema formation may result in damage to the periodontium (periodontal disease). Once diastema and interproximal wear develop in the geriatric horse, their correction is difficult or impossible. Both results of abnormal forces are best prevented.

In some young patients enlarged interproximal spaces develop early in life as a result of arcade and head conformation. Individuals with short heads and crowded teeth may have enlarged interproximal spaces between the lower 10s and 11s or 9s and 10s. This developmental condition results in feed accumulation in these spaces. The space is created when the most distal tooth in the arcade erupts in the part of the mandible where the curvature of Spee is located. This exaggerated angulation results in a triangular space between it and the next mesial tooth. This is referred to as a 'valve diastema'.

Orthodontic principles play a large role in these young patients with developmental enlargement of the interproximal space. The position of the adult tooth at the time of eruption may change over time if occlusal forces are correct. In many cases, the lower distal tooth (either 10 or 11 depending on age) will change its occlusal angulation to be more in line with the rest of the arcade if the ramp on the tooth is corrected and the step or wave on the opposing arcade is reduced. Correct occlusal equilibration will result in normalization of forces keeping the teeth apart, and the space will close over time.

Treatment of enlarged interproximal spaces by space enlargement has been well described.[15] Spaces are enlarged with a diastema bur in order to widen the space and prevent feed accumulation. In some cases, adjunctive perioceutic therapy may be employed.

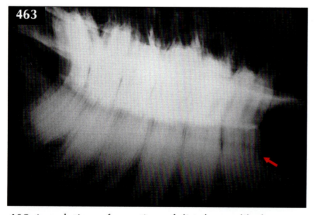

463 Angulation of eruption of distal mandibular teeth is shown as the second premolar (arrow) serves as a 'retaining wall'.

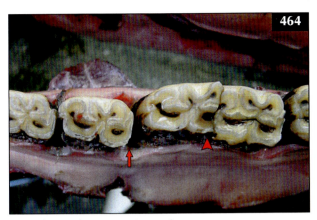

464 This cadaver specimen demonstrates enlargement of an interproximal space (arrow) and excessive wear of proximal tooth margins (arrowhead).

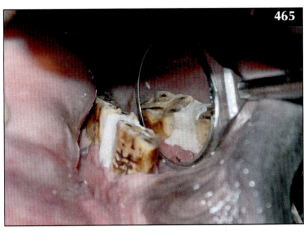

465 Interproximal polymethylmethacrylate prevents feed accumulation and protects the underlying tissue, allowing healing to take place.

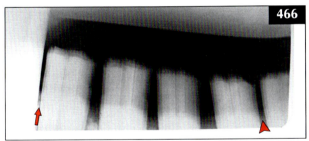

466 Radiograph of case shown in 465 at first presentation shows large interproximal spaces. 306/7 space (arrow) is partially visible at left. 310/11 space is seen at the arrowhead.

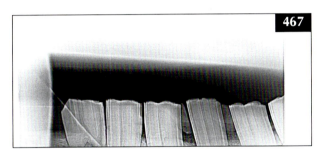

467 Radiograph of the case in figures 465 and 466 taken 3 years later shows significant closure of interproximal spaces. The interproximal spaces at 308/9 and 309/10 have closed to a lesser degree than others and have acrylic patches.

Occlusal equilibration is indicated in all cases. Debridement of necrotic soft tissue is beneficial.

An alternative treatment for enlarged interproximal spaces is the placement of polymethylmethacrylate between teeth (465–467). This is done after debridement of as much necrotic tissue as possible. Filling the interproximal space prevents feed accumulation. The polymethylmethacrylate is left in place for several weeks to months. It is replaced as necessary. In cases where this treatment is used, periodontal damage is improved and even resolved.

In young patients with good eruption potential and normal mesial drift, the spaces frequently close.

TIPPING OF TEETH

Teeth may be tipped by orthodontic forces or may develop in a tipped position. In cases where the cause is developmental, occlusal forces may prevent correction of the condition if the position is extreme. In other cases where the tooth is mildly tipped, occlusal equilibration may assist in correction of the malposition.

Orthodontic forces of mastication and mesial drift cause teeth to move to close spaces where teeth are missing. In other cases, such as in incisors in figure **468**, orthodontic forces work to separate teeth further when an intervening tooth is missing. In all cases, movement can be minimized by occlusal equilibration, as forces and mastication motion are returned to normal.

ALVEOLAR ANKYLOSIS

The tooth erupts and suffers attrition, leaving little reserve crown in aged patients. In such conditions, the PDL may be overwhelmed by the magnitude of occlusal forces, causing it to undergo ankylosis. This is especially common in upper 9s that have undergone premature expiration due to the forces of a wave malocclusion (**469**), particularly in aged patients that have never had prior dental care. Once ankylosed and expired there is little to be done for the tooth. It will not erupt further and will continue to suffer further premature wear, resulting in its loss. This condition is best prevented by early intervention in occlusal equilibration.

ALVEOLAR SCLEROSIS

Sclerosis, or increased radiographic density (**470**) and thickness of the alveolus, is a result of prolonged, heavy compressive occlusal forces. These forces are sensed by the PDL and the bone of the alveolus. They are created by increased mastication forces delivered in a crushing motion and direction to a tooth that is slightly tipped, as in lower molars. The exaggerated crushing forces are a result of consumption of hard feeds. Treatment is by regular occlusal equilibration and by altering the patient's diet to include soft feeds such as grass pasture whenever possible.

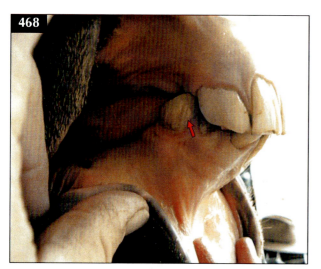

468 Incisor 403 is tipped distally in the arcade (arrow) due to mastication forces from the opposing tooth.

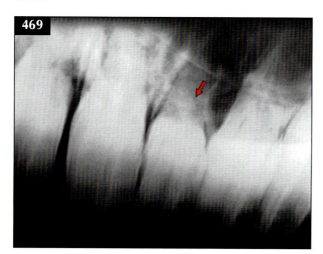

469 The upper 9 (arrow) is near expiration and has undergone ankylosis and alveolar sclerosis.

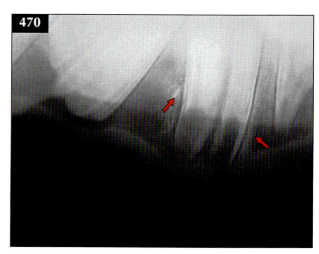

470 Arrows indicate areas of alveolar sclerosis due to increased occlusal forces.

SUMMARY

The orthodontic effects on equine teeth vary in severity and in presentation. Common characteristics include the effects of mastication forces on teeth and the effects of abnormally long teeth on each other. It is helpful to understand the developmental nature of teeth and specific malocclusions in order to address their improvement or correction appropriately.

Equine dentistry has, at its roots, the orthodontic effects of common malocclusions. Understanding the development of malocclusions assists in proper treatment.

REFERENCES

1. *Dentist's Desk Reference*. Chicago: American Dental Association, 1983; p. 182.
2. Wiggs RB. Unpublished manuscript on equine dentistry.
3. Angle EH. *The Angle System of Regulation and Retention of the Teeth and Treatment of Fractures of the Mandible*, 5th edition. Philadelphia: SS White Manufacturing Co, 1899; p. 1.
4. Wiggs RB, Lobprise HB. *Veterinary Dentistry: Principles and Practice*. Philadelphia: Lippincott-Raven, 1997; p. 441.
5. Proffitt WR, Fields HW (eds) *Contemporary Orthodontics*. St. Louis: Mosby, 1986; pp. 16–38.
6. Wolff J. *The Law of Bone Transformation*. Berlin: Hirschwuld, 1892.
7. Easley J. Basic Equine orthodontics. In: Baker GJ, Easley J (eds) *Equine Dentistry*. London: WB Saunders, 1999; pp. 206–219.
8. DeBowes RM, Gaughan EM. Congenital dental disease of the horse. *The Veterinary Clinics of North America: Equine Practice* 1998: **14**(2); 273–289.
9. Klugh DO. Acrylic bite plane for treatment of malocclusion in a young horse. *Journal of Veterinary Dentistry* 2004: **21**(2); 84–87.
10. Proffitt WR. The biologic basis of orthodontic therapy. In: Proffitt WR (ed) *Contemporary Orthodontics*. St. Louis: Mosby 1986; p. 244.
11. Baker GJ, Kirkland KD. Sedation for dental prophylaxis in horses: a comparison between detomidine and xylazine. *Proceedings 41st Annual Convention of the American Association of Equine Practitioners* 1995; pp. 40–41.
12. Orsini JA. Butorphanol tartrate: pharmacology and clinical indications. *Compendium of Continuing Education* 1988: **10**(7); 849–854.
13. Scrutchfield WL, Schumacher J, Martin MT. Correction of abnormalities of the cheek teeth. *Proceedings 42nd Annual Convention of the American Association of Equine Practitioners* 1997; pp. 11–21.
14. Allen AL, Townsend HG, Doige CE, Fretz PB. A case-control study of the congenital hypothyroidism and dysmaturity syndrome of foals. *Canadian Veterinary Journal* 1996: **37**(6); 349–358.
15. Collins NM, Dixon PD. Diagnosis and management of equine diastemata. *Clinical Techniques in Equine Practice* 2005: **4**(2); 148–154.

APPENDIX

MANUFACTURERS

3M Dental Products, St. Paul, MN.

C.E.T. Oral Hygeine Rinse, Virbac Animal Health, Ft. Worth, TX.

D & B Enterprises, Inc., Calgary, Alberta, CAN.

Dentalaire, Fountain Valley, CA.

Dentsply Caulk, Milford, DE.

Dentsply/Tulsa Dental, Johnson City, TN.

Diagnostic Imaging Systems, Rapid City, SD.

Duct Tape, Ace Hardware, Oak Brook, IL.

Equi-Dent Technologies, Sparks, NV.

Float Blades, HL Instrument Co., Inc., Santa Ana, CA.

Foredom Power Tools, Bethel, CT.

Henry Schein, Melville, NY.

Jet Dental Acrylic, Lang Dental Mfg Co., Wheeling, IL.

Lang Dental Mfg Co., Inc., Wheeling, IL.

Medco Instruments, Hickory Hills, IL.

Pfizer Animal Health, Exton, PA.

Premium Stainless Floats, Alberts, Loudonville, NY.

Rena's Equine Dental Instruments, Sparks, NV.

Stubbs Equine Innovations, Johnson City, TX.

Zenith/DMG, Englewood, NJ.

INDEX

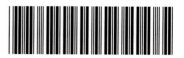